NASOPHARYNGEAL CARCINOMA

NASOPHARYNGEAL CARCINOMA

Second Edition

Editors

C. Andrew van Hasselt

Chief, Division of Otorhinolaryngology,
Professor of Surgery
The Chinese University of Hong Kong

and

Alan G. Gibb

Formerly Visiting Professor, Division of Otorhinolaryngology,
Li Dak Sum Visiting Professor, Department of Surgery
The Chinese University of Hong Kong

Formerly Head of Department of Otolaryngology
University of Dundee, Scotland

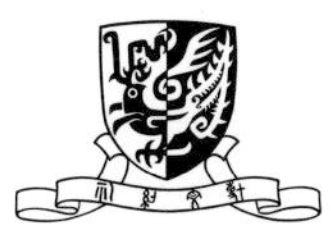

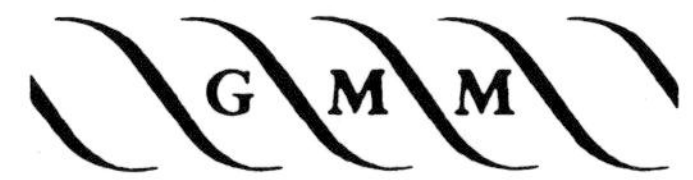

The Chinese University Press

Greenwich Medical Media Limited

First edition 1991
Second edition 1999

THE CHINESE UNIVERSITY PRESS
The Chinese University of Hong Kong
Sha Tin, N.T., Hong Kong
Fax: +852 2603 7355
E-mail: cup@cuhk.edu.hk
www.cuhk.edu.hk/cupress/w1.htm

ISBN 962–201–833–5

GREENWICH MEDICAL MEDIA LTD.
219 The Linen Hall, 162–168 Regent Street
London W1R 5TB, United Kingdom
Fax: +0 171 494 1616
E-mail: gm@greenwich-medical.co.uk
www.greenwich-medical.co.uk

ISBN 1–84110–037–4

A catalogue record for this book is available from the British Library.

Distributed in China Mainland, Hong Kong, Macau, and Taiwan by the Chinese University Press.

Distributed elsewhere worldwide by Oxford University Press.

Printed in Hong Kong

Contents

Foreword

Nasopharyngeal Carcinoma (NPC) represents a major cancer killer in the Cantonese Chinese not only in China but wherever they have settled in South East Asia, North and South America, Australia …

Strangely enough the same tumour is observed among Maghrebin Arabs in North Africa and Greenland Eskimos. Because of such a well defined geographical distribution, it has been a subject of research since 1970 and has become a Rosetta stone for unravelling multi-factorial oncogenesis in humans.

NPC is linked to three factors which play an intermingling role in its pathogenesis. The first is the ubiquitous Epstein-Barr virus (EBV) which is so closely and regularly associated with the epithelial tumour cells in every geographical area that it must play a critical role. The association between the E-B virus and NPC has also led to very useful diagnostic and prognostic applications. The specific IgA responses to the viral structural capsid (VCA) and early (EA) antigens reflects a fundamental process by which the immune system recognizes the viral reactivation associated with pre-cancerous conditions or possibly the first clonal tumour growth in the nasopharyngeal mucosa. Thus the association of EBV with NPC has led to the possibility of early detection of the tumour, permitting early treatment which in turn should lead to a significant decrease in the mortality of this "Cantonese Cancer". One can therefore substantially improve the control of this tumour even without understanding the molecular mechanism by which the E-B virus participates in the pathogenesis of NPC.

The second factor involved in the aetiology of NPC is related to environmental carcinogens and more specifically to certain components present in "Cantonese dried fish". The consumption of such delicacies to the Chinese palate is directly related to an increased risk of developing this tumour in southern China and South East Asia. In Tunisia, it appears that another food item present in the traditional harissa plays a similar role. The chemical carcinogens present in these traditional foods might act in two complementary ways: either by a direct genotoxic effect or through their reactivating potential of E-B viral latency. The future will tell whether this association with food habits can help in preventing NPC either by direct intervention against the consumption or by improved preparation of such food items.

The third factor is of a genetic nature. In fact when multiple cases of NPC among siblings were investigated, there was a 20-fold increase in relative risk of developing NPC in those siblings sharing a similar HLA haplotype with the affected family member.

The question of how this NPC susceptibility gene acts remains unknown. It could either act by controlling the immune response to the virus or as a gene controlling the intermediate metabolism of a pre-chemical carcinogen.

This excellent book covers all the necessary aspects of our knowledge on NPC, from anatomy, histopathology, epidemiology, experimental studies, clinical manifestations, clinical and laboratory diagnostic methods to the latest imaging techniques. It also contains all information necessary for the clinician to reach the proper staging of NPC and to treat the tumour efficiently. In addition, it offers guidance on screening family members in order to better control very early tumours or even precancerous conditions.

Let us hope that before the year 2000 nasopharyngeal carcinoma will be fully controlled by intervention at the pre-cancerous stage made possible by detecting individuals screened for the NPC susceptibility gene.

Pasteur Institute
Paris, France — October 1991

Guy Blaudin de Thé

Preface to the First Edition

The exceptionally high incidence of nasopharyngeal carcinoma in the Cantonese, coupled with excellent facilities available for investigation and research, has given workers in Hong Kong a unique opportunity to advance the study of this poorly understood neoplasm. However, despite expanding knowledge, nasopharyngeal carcinoma remains a dreaded condition and one of the least adequately diagnosed cancers in the world. Delay in reaching a diagnosis is reflected in the unsatisfactory outcome of treatment in a large number of cases. One of the foremost aims of this book is to increase awareness of what can be done to achieve earlier diagnosis and improve treatment.

In the present age of speicalisation and sub-specialisation it is beyond a single author to present this complex disease adequately in all its aspects. We have therefore opted for a team of contributors, each an expert in his own field and with experience of working in Hong Kong. Several authors have also had experience of nasopharyngeal carcinoma in other endemic and non-endemic areas. It is our hope that the experience of our contributors, as imparted in the pages of this book, will assist clinicians, therapists and investigators throughout the world by providing a source of information to which they may refer when dealing with this cancer.

Attention has been given to the need to update existing methods of classification. The section on histopathology includes a new classification which we regard more practical and meaningful than any pre-existing system. A grading system of pre-cancerous changes is also considered of special relevance. The advent of computed tomography and magnetic resonance imaging has added a new dimension to tumour staging. The additional information provided by these techniques forms the basis of the new, up-dated stage-classification presented here.

In any multi-author work duplication of information is an ever-present problem. We have tried to reduce this to a minimum, while taking care that each chapter remains an independent unit, complete and comprehensible without reference to other sections of the book.

We wish to express our gratitude to all those who have supported us in our task, particularly the contributors who have given their services wholeheartedly and shown great patience and tolerance in the face of an extensive amount of editing.

Public concern regarding the lethal effects of nasopharyngeal carcinoma on the young adult population of Hong Kong has stimulated philanthropists in the community to give generous financial support to this cause. In this context, we would express our gratitude to the Shaw Foundation, which has sponsored the costs of publication of this book and thus freed us from any financial obligation in this respect.

It was decided at an early stage that neither the authors nor the editors would derive any financial benefit from sales of this book and that any proceeds accruing would go to research into nasopharyngeal cancer.

CAvH
AGG

Preface to the Second Edition

The main stimulus prompting us to embark on a second edition of this volume was to update the reader on the advances in our knowledge and management of nasopharyngeal carcinoma over the past seven years. Although many questions still remain unanswered, considerable new work has taken place in the fields of genetics, serological testing and management.

The introduction of new authors has brought fresh ideas and the reader will find these reflected in the text. Several chapters have been entirely re-written, while all the others have been subjected to considerable modification from the last edition.

Continuing controversies remain in the classifications on surgical pathology and staging. In the former our author, in common with some renowned pathologists in other countries has reverted to the old term "lymphoepithelioma" believing this best describes the Epstein-Barr virus related undifferentiated tumour arising, in his opinion, deep to the surface epithelium of the nasopharynx. However, we felt justified in retaining the chapters on precancerous changes and cytological examination until there is greater concensus of opinion regarding the origin of the cancer cell.

Other changes worthy of mention are included in the chapters on epidemiology, imaging, stage-classification, chemotherapy, surgical management, recent treatment modalities and the ear in relation to nasopharyngeal carcinoma.

We are again greatly indebted to all authors for their tolerance of our somewhat severe editing regime and for the excellent co-operation from the Chinese University Press. We welcome Greenwich Medical Media Limited as co-publishers as this should ensure an excellent distribution world-wide.

The second edition has provided the stimulus to embark on a Chinese translation which may help those in endemic areas who are unfamiliar with the English language.

Finally, we would thank the secretaries who contributed to the preparation of the scripts and our wives, who patiently tolerated the many long hours we spent in the editing process.

CAvH
AGG

Acknowledgements

In a work of this nature, in which both editors and contributors receive help from a wide range of sources, it is difficult to acknowledge each and every one of these adequately. Valuable contributions were made by Mrs. F. Parkin who created the index and Mr. Y.K. Fung who ensured uniformity in the references. We are greatly indebted to those who checked the proofs and to the secretaries who prepared the scripts, especially Elsie Chu who shouldered the main burden of the work. Finally we wish to thank the Chinese University Press for their close co-operation, guidance and courtesy and our own families for their encouragement, tolerance and loyal support.

Contributors

Ahuja, Anil T., MD, FRCR
Associate Professor
Department of Diagnostic Radiology and Organ Imaging
The Chinese University of Hong Kong

Allen, Philip W., MBBS, FRCPA
Department of Pathology
Flinders Medical Centre
Adelaide, South Australia

Chan, Anthony T.C., MBBS, MD, MRCP, FHKAM(MEDICINE)
Associate Professor
Department of Clinical Oncology
The Chinese University of Hong Kong

Chan, May K.M., MBBS, FHKAM(PATH), MRCPath, FIAC
Adjunct Associate Professor
Department of Anatomical and Cellular Pathology
The Chinese University of Hong Kong
Honorary Consultant, Hong Kong Sanatorium and Hospital

Chang, Alexander R., MBChB, MD(OTAGO), FRCPA, FHKAM(PATH), MIAC, DCP
Professor
Department of Anatomical and Cellular Pathology
The Chinese University of Hong Kong

Choa, George, CBE, KStJ, JP, MBBS, LLD(Hon)HK, FRCS, FHKAM, HonFHKAM(ORL), FRACS, FACS, DLO
Honorary Clinical Associate Professor
Department of Surgery
University of Hong Kong

Gibb, Alan. G., MBChB, FRCS, DLO
Formerly Visiting Professsor, Division of Otorhinolaryngology
Li Dak Sum Visiting Professor, Department of Surgery,
The Chinese University of Hong Kong, and
Head of Department of Otolaryngology
University of Dundee, Scotland

Huang, Dolly P., PhD, FRCPath
Professor
Department of Anatomical and Cellular Pathology
The Chinese University of Hong Kong

King, Ann D., MRCP, FRCR
Associate Professor
Department of Diagnostic Radiology and Organ Imaging
The Chinese University of Hong Kong

Lam, Wynnie W. M., MBBS, FRCR(HK)
Associate Professor
Department of Diagnostic Radiology and Organ Imaging
The Chinese University of Hong Kong

Lee, Anne W.M., FRCR, FHKAM
Consultant and Chief of Service
Department of Clinical Oncology
Pamela Youde Nethersole Eastern Hospital, Hong Kong

Lee, Joseph C.K., MBBS, PhD, Dip Am Board of Patholgy, FRCP(C), FRCPA, FRCPath, FHKAM(PATH)
Professor and Chairman
Department of Anatomical and Cellular Pathology
The Chinese University of Hong Kong

Leung, Sing Fai, FRCR(UK)
Associate Professor
Department of Clinical Oncology
The Chinese University of Hong Kong

Leung, Thomas W. T., MD
Associate Professor
Department of Clinical Oncology
The Chinese University of Hong Kong

Lo, Kwok-wai, PhD
Scientific Officer
Department of Anatomical and Cellular Pathology
The Chinese University of Hong Kong

Metreweli, Constantine, MA, FRCR, FRCP
Professor and Chairman
Department of Diagnostic Radiology & Organ Imaging
The Chinese University of Hong Kong

Soo, Kee Chee, MBBS, MD, FRACS, FACS, FAMS
Head and Clinical Associate Professor
Department of Surgery
Director, Singapore Cancer Centre
Singapore General Hospital

Tam, John S., BSc, PhD
Professor
Department of Microbiology
The Chinese University of Hong Kong

Teo, Peter, MD, FRCR, FHKAM, DMRT
Consultant
Department of Clinical Oncology
The Chinese University of Hong Kong

Tong, Michael C. F., MBBS, FRCS(EDIN), FHKAM(ORL)
Adjunct Associate Professor
Division of Otorhinolaryngology
Department of Surgery
The Chinese University of Hong Kong

van Hasselt, C. Andrew, MBChB, FRCS, FRCS(EDIN), MMED(OTOL), FCS(SA), FHKAM(ORL)
Professor of Surgery
Chief of Otorhinolaryngology
Department of Surgery
The Chinese University of Hong Kong

Woo, John K.S., MBBS, FRCS(EDIN), FHKAM(ORL)
Consultant and Adjunct Associate Professor
Division of Otorhinolaryngology
Department of Surgery
The Chinese University of Hong Kong

The nasopharynx … might well be described as the Cinderella of the nose and throat regions; it has always been and still remains the most difficult area to examine, and consequent upon this the diagnosis of many conditions, frequently serious, has often been incorrect and in most cases delayed …

C.P. Wilson
Ann. Otol. Rhinol. Laryngol. 1957; 66: 5–40

CHAPTER 1

Historical Aspects

Alan G. Gibb and *George Choa*

Ancient Historical Remains

The discoveries of palaeontologists in their examinations of skeletal remains. have led to speculation regarding the possible existence of nasopharyngeal carcinoma (NPC) in ancient times. While the evidence must be treated with due reserve, it must be conceded that the descriptions in certain instances closely resemble the salient features of NPC. In general, evidence of malignant disease, apart from sarcoma, is extremely rare in ancient remains.[1] Careful examination by palaeopathologists of many thousands of skulls and skeletons all over the world, covering the B.C. and early A.D. periods, has furnished positive identification of tumours in only a small number of instances.[2] Yet a surprisingly high proportion of these tumours have been discovered in the region of the nasopharynx.[2]

An ancient Egyptian skull nearly 5,000 years old from the Duckworth Laboratory in England, estimated to belong to the 3rd–5th Dynasty (the Old Kingdom, Pyramid Age), was described in detail by Calvin Wells.[1] The specimen, which was in a perfect state of preservation and thought to be that of a 30–35 year old male subject, showed clear-cut evidence of extensive bone destruction of the skull base together with multiple erosions of the cranial vault. Wells considered that the findings represented a large primary nasopharyngeal cancer with secondary deposits in the skull vault. Ho[3] (1972) however disagreed with Wells' interpretation, favouring a diagnosis of either myeloma or carcinoma arising in the maxillary antrum.

Further possible cases of nasopharyngeal malignancy in ancient times include a specimen from pre-Columbian Chavina, Peru,[4] a skull discovered at the early Iranian site of Tepe Hissar, *circa* 3,500–3,000 B.C.[5] and possibly a skull from the Neolithic period unearthed in Dorset, England.[6]

An extensive search of ancient Egyptian mummies by Elliot Smith[7] revealed no evidence of cancer up to the relatively recent Byzantine era, when two possible specimens of malignant tumour were discovered. One of these, originally described by Derry,[8] belonging to a pre-Christian Nubian, *circa* 4th–6th century A.D., had extensive skull destruction compatible with nasopharyngeal cancer.

Whether the foregoing descriptions in reality represented cases of nasopharyngeal carcinoma is a matter of speculation as several authorities have questioned their interpretation.[9] Furthermore, the apparent rarity of malignant tumours in these researches in ancient times raises doubts as to whether carcinogenic agents indeed existed in that era.

Clinical Recognition

The relatively late recognition of nasopharyngeal carcinoma as a clinical entity is not too surprising when one considers the inaccessibility of the tumour and other problems which confronted the clinician in earlier times.

Difficulties in examining the nasopharynx. Although some very large tumours might have been easily seen, presenting through the nose or mouth, inspection of the nasopharynx to detect smaller growths was not possible until the mid-nineteenth century, the only means of examination being digital palpation. The post-nasal mirror for viewing the nasopharynx was first introduced by Czermak[10] in 1859. However, in the early days, inspection was doubtless compromised by limitations in the brightness of the light source.

Misdiagnosis. There is abundant evidence to suggest that many cases were missed or misdiagnosed in early times due to the lack of knowledge and understanding of cancer spread. It is interesting to note that in 1894, Schmidt[11] did not recognize a single case of NPC in a total of 32,997 ear, nose and throat examinations, although 16 cases of pharyngeal carcinoma and 75 cases of laryngeal carcinoma were diagnosed.[11] At that time, neck swellings or cranial nerve palsies were unlikely to alert the physician to primary disease in the hidden recesses of the nasopharynx. Even as late as 1923, Oscar Thomson,[12] despite living and working in an area in southern China where NPC was extremely common, failed to appreciate that the malignant neck nodes which he constantly encountered, might be related to spread of cancer from the nasopharynx (*vide infra*).

Misinterpretation of histopathology. In the nineteenth and first half of the twentieth centuries, confusion among pathologists over the histogenesis of the tumour resulted in nasopharyngeal tumours masquerading under a variety of different titles. Small, often unrepresentative, biopsy specimens taken by the surgeon contributed to this pathological dilemma. A comprehensive review by Kelsey and Brown[13] of the histopathological appearances of nasopharyngeal neoplasms based on the literature of the early twentieth century, revealed the following tumour types: carcinoma 30%; sarcoma 60% and endothelioma 10%. Comparison of these figures with present day patterns raises the probability that many of the sarcomas, and perhaps all the endotheliomas, would now be classified as carcinomas.

Early Records from Europe and U.S.A.

Although the first clinical description of a case of NPC is attributed to Durand-Fardel[14] more than 150 years ago, histological confirmation was lacking: indeed, writing some years later, Laval[15] maintained that the tumour in question probably arose in the soft palate rather than the nasopharynx.

Laval and Godtfredsen[16] credited the first report to Michaux, who in 1845, described a histologically confirmed tumour in a 45 year old male as "carcinome de base du crane".[17] Towards the end of the last century, Bosworth[18] of New York (1889), outlined details of 5 cases of NPC recorded in the literature, including that of Durand-Fardel, to which he added a further case of his own. Muir, however, having analysed the case records carefully, came to the conclusion that the diagnosis of NPC was suspect in at least half of the cases.[19]

In 1901, Chevalier Jackson,[20] in a comprehensive literature review entitled "Primary Carcinoma of the Nasopharynx" presented at the section of Laryngology and Otology of the American Medical Association, reviewed 7 recorded cases additional to those collected by Bosworth and added a further case of his own. In a detailed analysis of the characteristics of the tumour, he discussed the aetiology, symptomatology and merits of treatment comprehensively.

Meantime, recognition and understanding of the disease was progressing so that by 1904, Laval was able to collect 27 cases of primary NPC.[15]

In Great Britain, all the available evidence points to a general lack of awareness of the disease at the turn of the century, nasopharyngeal carcinoma being considered an extremely rare entity. The first probable case was demonstrated by Waggett[21] to the Laryngological Society of London in 1900. His presentation concerned a lady of 30 years who complained of nasal obstruction, otorrhoea and a painless lump in the neck. The lateral and posterior walls of the nasopharynx were infiltrated with an ulcerating growth spreading towards the soft palate. A neck mass beneath the upper part of the sternomastoid muscle was fixed to the underlying structures. The diagnosis of sarcoma was almost certainly incorrect as the clinical description tallies closely with that of NPC.

By 1906 however, recognition of NPC was obviously on the increase as Parker,[22] already cognisant with Bosworth's report, appeared familiar with all the salient features of the disease. In his textbook published in that year, he pointed out that enlargement of neck glands frequently occurs early, often "out of all proportion to the size and activity of the primary growth" and that "an unobserved epithelioma in the nasopharynx accounts for some of those cases of malignant glands of the neck in which the primary growth has not been discovered".

In 1911, Wilfred Trotter[23] of London proposed a classification of nasopharyngeal tumours: he also gave a detailed and accurate description of their clinical features and discussed their surgical treatment (*vide infra*). Trotter's paper was of special significance in that it underlined the importance of three diagnostic features, namely deafness, neuralgic pain in the distribution of cranial nerve V and asymmetry of the palate. These subsequently became widely known as "Trotter's triad".

By 1920 nasopharyngeal carcinoma had emerged as a widely recognised clinical entity in western countries. In a report of 79 cases of malignant tumours of the nasopharynx at the Mayo clinic, New[24] confirmed that the condition was much more common than had previously been believed. He attributed the paucity of recorded cases to failure on the physician's part to recognise the salient features of the tumour, with the result that many patients received symptomatic treatment without discovery of the primary tumour.

Early Oriental History

In view of the marked geographical prevalence of NPC in southern China and other oriental countries, to which Digby (1930)[25] drew attention, the limited amount of information concerning the early history of the disease in these areas is surprising. The virtual absence of reports emanating from China where nasopharyngeal carcinoma was most common, was considered by Ho[26] to relate to the prevalence of the tumour in the southern part of the country, remote from the main centres of learning and sources of Chinese medical literature, located in northern and central China.

Ancient Chinese writings contain many references to "lo li", meaning neck gland enlargement[27] — a non-specific description covering many different diseases, of which tuberculosis and malignant disease, especially NPC, were the most likely. In the Encyclopaedia of Chinese Medical Terms, Wu[28] and his disciples used the terms "shih ying" and "shih yung", indicating malnutrition in association with a fatal disease with malignant lymph node metastases high up in the neck. Although no supporting clinical information was available, Ho[3] considered that the description might well represent NPC with nodal metastases.

It seems certain however that NPC continued to pass unrecognized for a lengthy period as there is strong evidence to suggest that the condition not only existed but was indeed common. The first clear-cut indication of its probable existence was forthcoming in a series of 121 post-mortems performed on cancer patients in Singapore between 1907 and 1912.[29] The necropsies revealed that over 23% had cancer of the neck glands, most probably secondary to NPC.

Todd of Canton[30] was the first in the Orient to recognize the condition clinically. Reporting a series of 103 cases of enlarged cervical nodes in 1921, he expressed the opinion that "a good many of these followed a malignant focus in the posterior nares". However Todd's observation regarding the metastatic nature of the malignant neck glands appeared to have little impact, as two years later Oscar Thomson, working in the same area, reported a series of 90 cases of malignant cervical nodes which he diagnosed as primary lymphosarcoma.[12] As nearly half of these cases also had nasal problems and over one third had ear symptoms, it is clear that primary carcinoma of the nasopharynx was a far more likely diagnosis

The first histologically confirmed cases in Asia were recorded in the 1924 Annual Report of the Singapore Department of Pathology.[31] This included 40 cancer cases diagnosed at necropsy at Tan Tock Seng Hospital of which 5 were carcinomas of the nasopharynx.

A very comprehensive account of NPC by Digby, Thomas and Hsiu was published in the Hong Kong *Caduceus* in 1930.[25] This was based on the findings of 103 cases and was generously illustrated with drawings giving details of the anatomy, clinical features and histology of the condition (*Figures 1 and 2*).

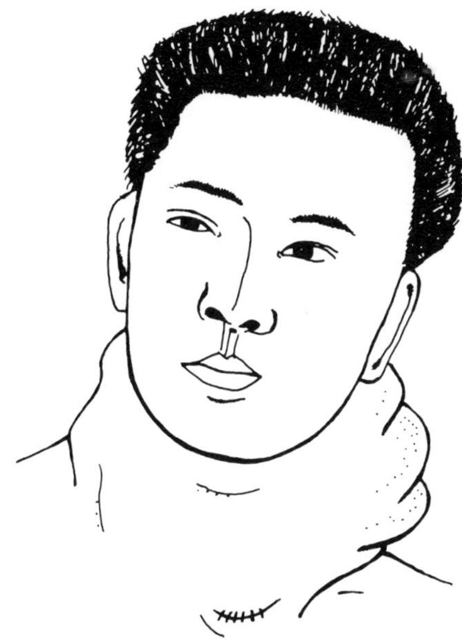

Figure 1

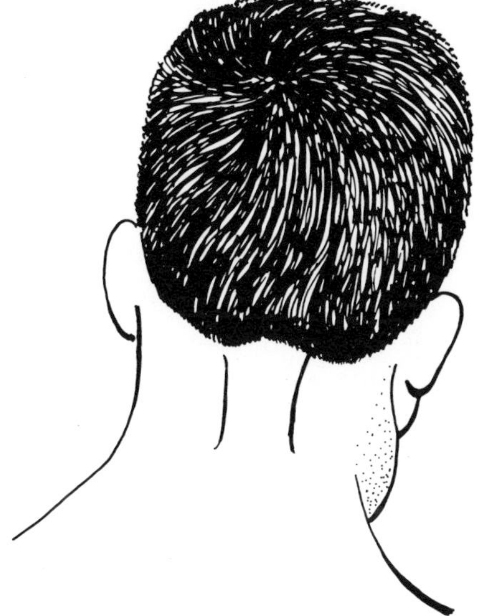

Figure 2

Reproductions of drawings by Digby *et al.* in *Caduceus*, 1930.[25]
Figure 1. Large neck masses after partial excision.
Figure 2. Enlarged glands seen from behind.

The marked prevalence of the tumour in the southern Chinese province of Guangdong (or Kwangtung) and its increasing recognition by the local medical community led to its designation, "Kwangtung tumour" in China and Hong Kong.[26]

Histopathology

Although, as far back as 1901, Jackson[20] considered NPC to be of epithelial origin, it is evident from the early literature that nasopharyngeal carcinomas were frequently mistaken for a wide variety of other tumours. These included endotheliomas (Trotter,[23] Gardham[32]), lymphosarcomas (Thomson[12]), reticulo-endotheliomas (Bonne[33]) and carcino-sarcomas (Von Zalka,[34] Skorpil[35]). Furthermore, the terms "transitional epidermoid carcinoma", and "lymphoepithelioma" were also extensively applied. The former term was proposed by Quick and Cutler[36] who considered the tumour arose from the transitional epithelium lining the junctional area between nose and pharynx. The term "lymphoepithelioma" was initially introduced in 1921 by Regaud[37] and Schmincke[38] independently, as being a tumour of the "lymphoepithelium", a description of the nasopharyngeal mucosa used by Jolly in 1914.[39] The name lymphoepithelioma was, for a period, adopted almost universally to describe the undifferentiated, highly radiosensitive, variety of nasopharyngeal carcinoma. However, considerable confusion ensued, since the term implied an epithelial malignancy, yet Godtfredsen[16] (1944) and Lederman[40] (1961) classified lymphoepitheliomas as sarcomas. Prior to this, Cappell (1934)[41] divided lymphoepithelioma into two sub-types — the Regaud type (carcinomatous) and the Schmincke type (sarcomatous), a classification which many pathologists continue to find useful (Chapter 5). Teoh,[42] New and Kirch[43] regarded both lymphoepitheliomas and transitional cell carcinomas merely as structural variants of squamous cell epitheliomas. However Teoh[42] stressed the difficulties encountered in reaching a clear-cut diagnosis based on small unrepresentative biopsies of the primary tumour or the cervical nodes, both of which contain lymphoid tissue in abundance.

Agreement over an acceptable comprehensive classification proved difficult. Following Cappell's original sub-typing of lymphoepitheliomas,[41] many other classifications were introduced including those of Chen,[44] Shen[45] and Liang,[46] the last named being widely used in China. Although some degree of concensus was eventually restored with the introduction of the World Health Organisation classification in 1978,[47] which underlined the epithelial origin of NPC, this was far from universal and several other classifications have since emerged, some of which are currently in use (Chapter 5).

Exfoliative cytological studies were first applied to nasopharyngeal cancer in 1949 by Morrison *et al.*[48] in San Francisco. This type of investigation had proved of value in the diagnosis of other forms of cancer, such as that of the cervix uteri. However, in NPC, this technique has played a limited role, serving in a few centres to complement, rather than replace, histopathological diagnosis based on biopsy.

Epidemiology

Epidemiological studies related to the aetiology and behaviour of NPC received an important stimulus as a result of the International Union against Cancer (UICC) Symposium on Cancer of the Nasopharynx held in Singapore in 1964.[49] Thereafter this aspect of NPC research was given the attention and support it merited.

The association between NPC and the Epstein-Barr virus was discovered in 1966 thanks to the observations of Old *et al.* (1966),[50] who demonstrated high precipitating antibody levels in undifferentiated or poorly diferentiated types of nasopharyngeal carcinoma, similar to those in Burkitt's lymphoma in African patients. This discovery represented an important milestone in the elucidation of the epidemiology. Old's work was confirmed by De Schryver *et al.* (1969)[51] and Henle *et al.* (1970),[52] while similar studies by Laing in Hong Kong[53] revealed higher titres of antibodies in Asian subjects than those recorded in the other series. All investigators recognized the serological kinship between Burkitt's lymphoma and NPC and were agreed that a viral infection, although not necessarily the cause of NPC, could act as initiator of a malignant process or transformation.

Early theories, initially promoted by Jackson,[20] implicating smoke from various sources. such as fires in poorly ventilated houses,[54] factories, kerosene lamps, joss sticks and opium smoking, as a potential factor in the aetiology of NPC have largely been discounted. In contrast, Ho[55] transferred attention from inhalants to ingestants in the search for causative factors, noting that the highest incidence of NPC in Hong Kong occurs in the "fisher folk" who spend their lives out of doors in boats, fishing and cooking in the open air. He discovered a particularly high intake of salted fish in the this community, which he highlighted as an important factor in the aetiology of this condition if fed to young children over a long period.

Historical Notes on Treatment

The early treatment of NPC, prior to the introduction of radium and X-rays had little to offer the patient. In general, in the 19th and early 20th centuries, tumours were diagnosed at an advanced stage and treatment proved so futile that Bosworth was moved to cynically suggest that the only effective remedies were opium, deception and lying![18]

Chevalier Jackson[20] (1901) discussed the various treatment options in detail, classifying them under two headings, palliative and radical. The objective of the former was to provide comfort "recognizing the hopelessness of thorough removal". The latter aimed at complete extirpation of the tumour. Palliative methods included pain killing drugs such as morphine, absolute alcohol injections, ingested Chian turpentine and local soothing applications, such as aristol in zinc stearate. In addition, the tumour itself was subjected to a variety of measures short of radical removal. These included galvanocautery, electrolysis or removal of obstructing tumour by cold wire snare, curette or cutting forceps and the application of various caustics, such as lactic acid and nitric acid.

Radical procedures with total tumour removal necessitated wide access to the nasopharynx involving resection of variable amounts of the maxilla and/or palate. The exposure however represented only part of the problem, since the subsequent total removal of a massive tumour surrounded by vital structures presented an even more formidable challenge to the surgeon. Having attempted this form of procedure, Jackson[20] concluded that "thoroughness is not attainable at the bottom of a deep artificial pit" and that surgery produces no cures and merely adds "anaemia to cancerous cachexia".

Radical surgery however continued to be employed by other surgeons using a wide variety of techniques. St. Clair Thomson[56] (1911) favoured Moure's approach, while Trotter[23] obtained what he described as excellent and easy access to the nasopharynx by mobilizing a massive "en bloc" osteoplastic flap of the entire maxilla-malar complex. This technique, which he claimed left no deformity, remains a classical precursor of current surgical concepts.

Alternative surgical measures were also tried with limited success. Dawbarn[57] ligated the external carotid arteries and several of their branches to starve the tumour of blood — a method still favoured by Percy[58] as late as 1938. Digby[25] in Hong Kong preferred splitting the soft palate and either cauterizing the tumour or resecting it by diathermy. Wilson[59] of the Middlesex Hospital in London performed palatal fenestration as a routine procedure to facilitate the follow up of NPC cases, regarding this as the only certain way to detect recurrent tumour at an early stage. Block dissections of neck glands with ligation of the common carotid or external carotid arteries were also carried out for cervical metastatic nodes. St. Clair Thomson[56] and Digby[25] considered that tracheostomy and gastrostomy might be required as means of palliation in special cases.

Radiation Treatment

The introduction of radium marked a dramatic change in the management of NPC. This treatment was used in U.S.A. as early as 1918, New[24] reporting that some of the cases remained well for 3–4 years. Many years elapsed however before radium became generally available. Digby[25] reported its early use at the Matilda Hospital in Hong Kong in 1930 in the form of a 25 mg needle introduced along the floor of the nose. He later altered his technique from this simple method to a complicated arrangement involving the use of 27 radium needles.[60] The treatment was of limited success, good initial improvement being invariably followed by tumour recurrence within 6 months, while local radium burns of the skin and palate were common. The 1920s saw the development of deep X-ray therapy machines, followed several years later by their practical application in NPC. In Hong Kong an orthovoltage (400-KV) machine became available at the Queen Mary Hospital around 1938 obviating many of the disadvantages of radium by irradiating the tumour from several fields, thus limiting damage to adjacent structures. The results of this treatment however remained poor, patients seldom surviving for three years.[61] The birth of nuclear medicine following the development of the atomic bomb in the 2nd World War, led to the replacement of radium by radioactive cobalt. The latter was introduced into Hong Kong in 1951 bringing improved treatment results in NPC, while over a decade later, linear accelerators became available, marking the start of the present era of megavoltage radiation for nasopharyngeal cancer.

Tumour Staging

Advances in treatment were immeasurably enhanced by the introduction of tumour staging to which Ho[62] made a major contribution. As a result of this innovation, treatment could be planned more scientifically, and related to the local extent and spread of the tumour. This development proved a major factor in defining and improving the prognosis of NPC.

Concluding Remarks

Those involved in the diagnosis and management of NPC at the present time should be ever aware of the contributions made by the pioneer clinicians, surgeons and scientists of former years. Without the fundamental knowledge resulting from their work and discoveries, the management of nasopharyngeal carcinoma facing the present day oncologist would be even more daunting than it is. To them we pay tribute …

References

1. Wells, C. 1963. Ancient Egyptian pathology. *J. Laryngol. Otol.*; 77:261–265.
2. Wells, C. 1964. Two Mediaeval cases of malignant disease. *BMJ*; 1:1611–1612.
3. Ho, H.C. 1972. *Advances in Cancer Research*, eds. Klein, G., Weinhouse, S., Haddow, A. New York and London: Academic Press, 57–92.
4. Wells, C. 1964. *Bones, Bodies and Disease*. London: Thames and Hudson.
5. Krogman, W.M. 1940. The skeletal and dental pathology of an early Iranian site. *Bull. Hist. Med.*; 8:28–48.
6. Goodman, C.N., Morant, G.M. 1940. The human remains of the Iron Age and other periods from Maiden Castle, Dorset. *Biometrika*; 31:295–312.
7. Smith, G.E., Dawson, W.R. 1924. *In Egyptian Mummies*. London: Allen and Unwin, 157.
8. Derry, D.E. 1909. Archaeological survey of Nubia. Egytian Ministry of Finance. Anatomical Report B. *Cairo Bull.*, No. 3, 4042.
9. Shanmugaratnam, K. — Personal communication.
10. Czermak, J.N. 1860. *Der Kehlkopfspiegel*. Leipzig.
11. Schmidt, M. 1894. *Die Krankheiten der Oberen Luftwege, Wright.*
12. Thomson, J.O. 1923. Cervical lympho-sarcomas, with an analysis of ninety cases. *Chin. Med. J.*; 37:1001–1010.
13. Kelsey, A.L., Brown, J.M. 1913. Malignant tumours of the nasopharynx. *Ann. Otol. Rhinol. Laryngol.*; 22:1147.
14. Durand-Fardel. 1837. Cancer du pharynx — ossification dans la substance musculaire du coeur. *Bull. de la Soc. Anat. (Paris)*; 12:73–80.
15. Laval, F. 1904. *Des Tumeurs Malignes du Naso-pharynx.* (Thèse). Toulouse: Marques.
16. Godtfredsen, E. 1944. Ophthalmologic and neurologic symptoms of malignant nasopharyngeal tumours: a clinical study comprising 454 cases, with special reference to histopathology and possibility of earlier recognition. *Acta Psych. Scand.*; 34 (Suppl.):1–323.

17. Michaux, L. 1845. *Carcinome de base du crane*. (Cited by Godtfredsen, E. 1944.[16]).
18. Bosworth, F.H. 1889. *A Treatise on Diseases of the Nose and Throat*, Vol. 1. New York: William Wood & Coy, 56 & 58.
19. Muir, C.S. 1967. Nasopharyngeal cancer — a historical vignette. In: *Cancer of the Nasopharynx*, eds. Muir, C.S., Shanmugaratnam, K. UICC Monograph No. 1. Copenhagen: Munksgaard.
20. Jackson, C., 1901. Primary carcinoma of the nasopharynx; a table of cases. *J.A.M.A.*; 37:371–377.
21. Waggett, E.B. 1899. Case of sarcoma of the post-nasal space. *Proc. Laryngol. Soc. London*; 7:11.
22. Parker, C.A. 1906. *A Guide to Diseases of the Nose and Throat and Their Treatment*. London: Edward Arnold, 413.
23. Trotter, W. 1911. Certain clinically obscure malignant tumours of the nasopharyngeal walls. *BMJ*; 11:1057–1059.
24. New, G.B. 1922. Syndrome of malignant tumours of the nasopharynx, a report of 79 cases. *J.A.M.A.*; 79(1):10–14.
25. Digby, H.K., Thomas, G.H., Hsiu, S.T. 1930. Notes on carcinoma of nasopharynx. *Caduceus*; 9(2):45–68.
26. Ho, J.H.C. 1976. *Epidemiology of Nasopharyngeal Carcinoma*. Gann Monograph on Cancer Research, Vol. 18, 49–61.
27. Jung, P.F., Yu, C. 1963. Nasopharyngeal cancer in China. *Postgrad. Med.*; A77–A82.
28. Wu, C.H. 1921. In: *The Encyclopaedia of Chinese Medical Terms*, Vol. 1, ed. Wu, C.H. Shanghai: Commercial Press, 756 (in Chinese).
29. Hoffman, F.L. 1915. *The Mortality from Cancer throughout the World*. Newark, New Jersey: Prudential Press.
30. Todd, P.J. 1921. Some practical points in the surgical treatment of cervical tumours. *Chin. Med. J.*; 35:21–25.
31. Shanmugaratnam, K. 1980. Nasopharyngeal carcinoma: epidemiology, histopathology and aetiology. *Ann. Acad. Med. Singapore*; 9:289–295.
32. Gardham A.J. 1929. Endothelioma of the nasopharynx. *Brit. J. Surg.*; 17(66):242–263.
33. Bonne L. 1937. Cancer and human races. *Am. J. Cancer*; 30:435–454.
34. Von Zalka, E. 1934. Über Lymphoepitheliom und Retikulumsarkom. *Krebsforsch*; 41:139–147.
35. Skorpil, F. 1939. Über die lymphoepitheliom (Schmincke) der speicheldrüsen Frankfurt. *Z. Path.*; 53:450–466.
36. Quick, D., Cutler, M. 1927. Transitional cell epidermoid carcinoma. *Surg. Gynecol. Obstet.*; 45:320–331.
37. Regaud, C., Reverchon, L. 1921. Sur un cas d'epithelioma epidermoide developpe dans le massif maxillaire superieur, et endu aux teguments de la face, aux cavities buccale, nasale et orbitaire, ainsi q'aux ganglions du cou, gueri par la curietherapie. *Rev. Laryngol. Otol. Rhinol.*; 42:369.
38. Schmincke, A. 1921. Über Lymphoepitheliale Geschwülste. *Beitr. Path. Anat. Allg. Pathol.*; 58:161–170.
39. Jolly, J. 1914–1915. La Course de Fabricius et les organes lymphoepitheliaux. *Arch. Anat. Microsc. Morphol. Exp.*; 16:363–547.
40. Lederman, M. 1961. *Cancer of the Nasopharynx: Its Natural History and Treatment*. American Lecture Series. Springfield, Illinois: Charles C. Thomas.
41. Cappell, D.F. 1934. On lymphoepithelioma of the nasopharynx and tonsils. *J. Path. Bact.*; 39:49–64.
42. Teoh, T.B. 1957. Epidermoid carcinoma of the nasopharynx among Chinese: a study of 31 necropsies. *J. Path. Bact.*; 73(2):451–465.
43. New, G.B., Kirch, W. 1928. Tumors of nose and throat: a review of literature. *Arch. Otolaryngol.*; 8:600–607.
44. Chen, Q.C., Luo, D.Y. 1959. Nasopharyngeal carcinoma. *Chin. J. Pathol.*; 5:9–11.
45. Shen, Y.Y. 1961. *M. I. Bull. Fujian Med. Coll.*; 1–7, 9–15 (in Chinese).
46. Liang, P.C., Chen, C.C., Chu, C.C., Hu, Y.F., Chu, H.M., Tsung, Y.S. 1962. The histopathologic classification, biologic characteristics and histogenesis of nasopharyngeal carcinoma. *Chin. Med. J.*; 81(10):629–658.
47. Shanmugaratnam, K. 1978. Histological typing of upper respiratory tract tumours. *International Histological Typing of Tumours*, No. 19. WHO, 19–21.

48. Morrison, L.F., Hopp, E.S., Wu, R. 1949. Diagnosis of malignancy of the nasopharynx: cytological studies by the smear technic. *Ann. Otolaryngol.*; 58:18–32.
49. Muir, C.S., Shanmugaratnam, K. (eds.) 1967. *Cancer of the Nasopharynx*. UICC Monograph Series, No. 1. Copenhagen: Munksgaard.
50. Old, L.J., Boyse, E.A., Oettgen, H.F., de Harven, E., Geering, G., Williamson, E., Clifford, P. 1966. Precipitating antibody in human serum to an antigen present in cultured Burkitt's Lymphoma Cells. *Proc. Natl. Acad. Sci. USA*; 56:1699–1704.
51. De Schryver, A., Klein, G., Henle, G., Henle, W., Cameron, H.M., Santesson, L., Clifford, P. 1972. E.B. — Virus associated serology in malignant disease: antibody levels to Viral Capsid Antigens (VCA), Membrane Antigens (MA) and Early Antigens (EA) in patients with various neoplastic conditions. *Int. J. Cancer*; 9:353–364.
52. Henle, W., Henle, G., Ho, H.C., Burtin, P., Cachin, Y., Clifford, P., De Schryver, A., de Thé, G., Diehl, V., Klein, G. 1970. Antibodies to Epstein-Barr virus in nasopharyngeal carcinoma, other head and neck neoplasms, and control groups. *J. Natl. Cancer Inst.*; 44:225–231.
53. Laing, D. 1969. Virus as the cause of rhinopharyngeal carcinoma. *Acta Otolaryngol.*; 67:190–199.
54. Dobson, W.C. 1924. Cervical lymphosarcoma. *Chin. Med. J.*; 38:786.
55. Ho., H.C. 1971. Incidence of nasopharyngeal cancer in Hong Kong. *UICC Bull.*; 9(2):5.
56. Thomson, St., C. 1911. *Diseases of the Nose and Throat*. London, New York, Toronto, Melbourne: Cassell, 328–329.
57. Dawbarn, R.H.M. 1896. Ligation of both external carotids for inoperable nasopharyngeal sarcoma. *Ann. Surg. (Philadelphia)*; 23:189–192.
58. Percy, J.F. 1938. Discussion on paper by Hauser, I.J., Brownell, D.H.: Malignant neoplasms of the nasopharynx. *J.A.M.A.*; 111:2467–2473.
59. Wilson, C.P. 1957. Observation on the surgery of the nasopharynx. *Ann. Otol. Rhinol. Laryngol.*; 66:5–40.
60. Digby, K.H., Fook, W.M.L., Che Y.T. 1941. Nasopharyngeal carcinoma. *Brit. J. Surg.*; 28(112):517–537.
61. Mekie, D.E.C., Lawley, M. 1954. Nasopharyngeal carcinoma. *Arch. Surg.*; 69:841–848.
62. Ho, J.H.C. 1970. The natural history and treatment of nasopharyngeal cancer. In: *Proceedings of the X International Cancer Congress*, eds. Lee-Clark R., Cumley, R.W., McCay, J.E., Copeland, M., Vol. 4. Chicago: Yearbook Medical Publishers, 1–14.

CHAPTER 2

Anatomy and Development

Alan G. Gibb

Definition

The nasopharynx may be defined as that portion of the pharynx which lies behind the nasal fossae and extends inferiorly as far as the level of the soft palate. Its role is solely respiratory, probably functioning as a collecting space where the inspired air is filtered of impurities by the lymphoid tissue.

Since the term "nasopharynx" has an alimentary connotation, the designation has come in for a considerable amount of criticism.[1,2,3] Alternative descriptions such as "posterior nasal passage",[2] "postnasal space"[4] and "epipharynx"[5] have been advocated but have failed to gain universal support and the original title "nasopharynx" has remained in common use. Nevertheless this description is fundamentally appropriate as the nasopharynx in reality comprises two distinct components, an upper anterior segment which developmentally, morphologically and histologically has all the features of the nasal cavity and a lower portion which is developed from the foregut and has similarities to the alimentary tract.

The close proximity to the nose and pharynx, plus its connection with the middle ear via the eustachian tube, identify the nasopharynx as the central hub around which the specialty of otorhinolaryngology revolves.

Development[6]

In early foetal development the expanded cranial extremity of the foregut ends blindly in close proximity to the primitive mouth or stomatodaeum from which it is separated by the delicate buccopharyngeal membrane. This tenuous barrier breaks down and disappears around the 26th–27th day of the foetal life leaving the stomatodeal ectoderm in continuity with the endoderm of the foregut or primitive pharynx.[6] The subsequent evolution of the embryonic nasopharynx, sited at this junctional area, is closely linked on the one hand with the development of the face and nasal cavities and on the other with the disintegration and distribution of the elements of the pharyngeal arches (and their associated clefts and pouches) which lie at either side of the foregut. The upper anterior part of the nasopharynx is derived from ectoderm which extends backwards from the primitive nasal cavities while the lower part develops from endoderm of the foregut. The incongruity of a situation where the gut forms part of the lining of a cavity with an exclusively respiratory role, may be reconciled by an understanding of palatal development. The primordia of the palate, arising from two shelf-like projections of the maxillary processes of the first pharyngeal arch, grow toward the midline and eventually fuse. The plane of this union takes place below the level of the roof of the primitive mouth cavity. Thus areas of stomatodeal ectoderm and foregut endoderm are isolated above the definitive palate and participate in the formation of the nasal and nasopharyngeal cavities. The exact extent of the pharyngeal contribution to the adult nasopharynx remains uncertain but, as the eustachian tube is derived mainly from the first pharyngeal pouch (*vide infra*), it can be inferred that the foregut endoderm reaches at least as high as tubal level. Thus the dual origin of the nasopharynx is reflected in its definitive composition which incorporates both ectodermal and endodermal elements.

Associated vestigial structures

The evolution of the nasopharynx is closely associated with the development of a number of important structures which disappear at a later stage of foetal life. As vestigial remnants of these may assume clinical importance and occasionally appear as swellings which may be confused with nasopharyngeal carcinoma, a knowledge and understanding of their embryology is important to the clinician.

Diverticula

An ectodermal diverticulum, called Rathke's pouch, arises from the deep part of the roof of the stomatodaeum, immediately rostral to the cephalic end of the notochord. It migrates upwards through the mesenchyme, which later forms the body of the sphenoid, and comes to lie in close proximity to a tubular downgrowth from the floor of the diencephalon. The anterior wall of the pouch thickens greatly and gives rise to the anterior pituitary lobe (adenohypophysis). The posterior wall on the other hand remains thin and essentially functionless (pars intermedia) but comes to lie adjacent to a downgrowth from the forebrain (neurohypophysis), forming with it the posterior pituitary lobe. With the continued growth of intervening mesoderm, the connection between the pouch and its point of origin becomes stretched into a slender solid stalk, which subsequently degenerates and disappears. However, a remnant of the stalk is prone to persist on the roof of the nasopharynx at the vomero-sphenoidal articulation, lying in the midline under the mucosa between the posterior border of the nasal septum and the pharyngeal tonsil. This contains active glandular tissue, capable of hormone production and represents the pharyngeal (extra sellar) hypophysis.[7] It has been demonstrated as a constant structure in anatomical dissections and may assume greater importance than is generally acknowledged.[8] Although usually small in size, it may be as large as 10mm and may hypertrophy up to four times its original size in females, but not in males, after the menopause.[8] The stalk of Rathke's pouch disappears but its course through the sphenoid bone from the anterior part of the nasopharyngeal roof to the sella turcica later represents the route of the craniopharyngeal canal.[9] This canal in turn undergoes obliteration but in rare instances a vestigial remnant may persist in the body of the sphenoid as a cyst (cyst of Rathke's pouch) or tumour (craniopharyngioma).

A constant diverticulum, the tubotympanic recess, is derived from the dorsal end of the first branchial pouch, with a similar, albeit smaller, contribution from the second pouch. This is the precursor of the tympanic cavity and eustachian tube and comes into close contact on its lateral aspect with the first branchial cleft, which will eventually form the external auditory meatus.

A median diverticulum termed the pharyngeal bursa, or pouch of Luschka, develops in the caudal portion of the nasopharyngeal tonsil. With the progressive growth of the surrounding tissues, this recess of endoderm is drawn upwards and backwards from its attachment to the point of fusion between notochord and foregut to form a flask-like diverticulum; this may undergo inflammatory change, giving rise to the condition termed Thornwaldt's bursitis.

Notochord

As the notochord ascends in the cervical area, it contributes to the nucleus pulposis of the intervertebral discs, and continues upwards in a longitudinal canal within the odontoid process of C2 before emerging at its tip and traversing the apical ligament.[9] Thereafter it pursues a tortuous course upwards on the superior face of the developing clivus before penetrating downwards and forwards through the basi-occiput to reach its nasopharyngeal aspect deep to the periosteum just behind Rathke's diverticulum. From there it passes dorsally through the sphenoid bone to terminate immediately posterior to the developing sella turcica and the rudiments of the sellar hypophysis.[9] The proximity of the rostral segment of the notochord to the nasopharynx merits attention as, at times, persistence of a vestigial remnant may give rise to a chordoma.

Epithelial changes[10,11]

In the early embryo the lining of the primitive nasopharynx consists of a single layer of cuboidal cells. By the end of the third month the cells have developed cilia and the epithelium has become stratified. By the fifth month the ciliated cells in the anterior part of the nasopharynx have assumed a columnar shape, while in the lower reaches the epithelium is of transitional type interspersed with areas of stratified squamous epithelium. At birth there is little change in this pattern but, during childhood, further metaplastic changes occur in the lower and posterior areas of the nasopharynx. In this transformation of embryonic ciliated epithelium to stratified squamous type, the basal cells serve as a germinal layer to replace the cast-off surface cells.

The metaplastic changes are generally complete by the end of the first decade, by which time 60% of the entire epithelial lining is stratified squamous in type.

The transitional zone where stratified squamous and ciliated epithelia meet is located close to the eustachian orifices. This area may be more liable to metaplastic and neoplastic change in view of the constant shedding and regeneration of the nasopharyngeal epithelium.

The epithelium covering the lymphoid tissue in the nasopharyngeal vault is normally non-ciliated and infiltrated with lymphocytes.

General Description

The nasopharynx is a hollow air-containing passageway featuring an expanded upper portion which tapers downwards like a funnel to the lower limit where it becomes continuous with the oropharynx at the level of the soft palate. It occupies the angle between the base of skull above and the vertebral column behind. The roof and posterior walls merge smoothly into one another and, from above downwards, are supported successively by the posterior part of the basi-sphenoid, the basi-occiput, the atlanto-occipital membrane and the anterior arch of the atlas vertebra. Anteriorly, the nasopharynx communicates with the nasal cavities through the posterior nares (choanae). The lower part of the anterior wall is formed by the soft palate in its resting state. Contraction of the palatal musculature however raises the soft palate to a horizontal plane so that it then forms the floor of the nasopharynx and assists closure of the velo-pharyngeal isthmus. The isthmus, which lies on a plane level with the anterior arch of the atlas represents the lower limit of the nasopharynx: it is bounded by the soft palate, palatopharyngeal arches and the posterior wall of the pharynx, which, when contracted, forms a horizontal fold termed Passavant's ridge. The lateral walls of the nasopharynx are formed by the superior constrictor muscle, apart from a gap between the upper edge of the muscle and the skull base (sinus of Morgagni. — *vide infra*). This defect is sealed off by the pharyngobasilar fascia supported by the levator veli palatini muscle. The medial end of the cartilaginous auditory tube forms a prominent projection (torus tubarius) high up on the lateral wall. From the posterior edge of the eustachian tube orifice, a mucosal fold produced by the underlying salpingopharyngeus muscle, runs downwards and gradually fades out on the lateral pharyngeal wall. A less prominent mucosal fold, due to the levator veli palatini muscle, passes from the anterior margin of the tubal orifice to the upper surface of the soft palate.

Dimensions

The average anterior-posterior dimension of the nasopharynx in adults is 2–3 cm and the transverse and vertical diameters, although subject to considerable variation, measure around 3–4 cm. During muscular contraction the transverse diameter is markedly reduced, even to nearly half the resting dimension.[12]

Motility

The nasopharynx is not, as is commonly supposed, an immobile entity.[12] Such a description is true only of a small area anterior to the eustachian tube orifices which has rigid bony walls. Vigorous contractions, even in the areas of the tubal eminence and the fossa of Rosenmüller, have been demonstrated on contrast radiographic and cinefluorographic studies and on endoscopic observation. Below this level, the nasopharynx is a muscular tube, constantly participating in active contraction during swallowing and speech, especially in the region of the isthmus.

Structure

The walls of the nasopharynx are composed of muscular, fibrous and mucosal layers.

Muscular Layer

The muscular layer comprises outer oblique and inner longitudinal components derived from the superior constrictor muscle. Between the upper edge of this muscle and the base of skull, the muscular layer is absent, the deficiency being strengthened by a thickening of the fibrous layer.

Fibrous Layers

The fibrous coat comprises two layers which provide an outer and inner lining for the constrictor muscles. Both layers are continuous with the general fascia of the neck (*vide infra*). The outer layer, or buccopharyngeal fascia covers the superficial aspect of the superior constrictor muscle. The inner component or pharyngeal aponeurosis, which lies between the mucosal layer and the constrictor muscle is part of the pharyngobasilar fascia. Both fascial layers unite at the upper edge of the superior constrictor muscle and ascend towards the base of skull as a single entity.

Mucosal Layer

The adult nasopharynx is lined mainly by pseudostratified columnar ciliated mucosa near the choanae and adjacent part of the roof, while in the lower and posterior regions of the nasopharynx, the lining assumes a stratified squamous character. Areas of transitional epithelium are encountered at the junctional zone located on the nasopharyngeal roof and lateral walls. The lamina propria is frequently infiltrated by lymphoid tissue, while the submucosal layer contains serous and mucous glands.

Special Features

Pharyngeal Tonsil

A collection of lymphoid tissue, the pharyngeal tonsil, is initially detectable beneath the mucous membrane at the junction of the roof and posterior wall of the nasopharynx around the 4th month of embryonic development. The presence of lymphoid tissue within epithelium during foetal development is unusual. Rapid hypertrophy takes place in early childhood followed by gradual regression after the age of 8–10 years. The lymphoid mass is triangular in shape with the apex pointing towards the posterior free margin of the nasal septum. The surface is irregular with several prominent ridges interrupted by deep furrows lined with epithelium. The lymphoid follicles, embedded beneath the surface epithelium, contain T and B lymphocytes, plasmocytes, reticular cells and fibroblasts.

In childhood, the hypertrophied mass may cause problems and give rise to the clinical condition of "adenoids". Large adenoid masses may extend laterally into the fossa of Rosenmüller, while occasionally, additional lymphoid deposits are encountered in the mucosa surrounding the orifice of the auditory tube, or even in the lining of the tube itself, close to its pharyngeal extremity.

Eustachian Cushion (Torus Tubarius)

The pharyngeal orifice of the eustachian tube lies 1–1.25 cm behind and below the posterior end of the inferior turbinate. The orifice is partially shielded, especially on its posterior and superior aspects, by a prominent comma-shaped elevation termed the eustachian cushion (torus tubarius), which is formed by the medial extremity of the cartilaginous part of the tube.

The eustachian tube, 3 to 4 cm in length, runs laterally and backwards from the nasopharyngeal orifice to the tympanic cavity. The anteromedial two-thirds are composed of cartilage and connective tissue whereas the posterolateral one-third is bony. The cartilaginous segment occupies a groove between the greater wing of the sphenoid and the petrous temporal bone. The cartilage of the tube is elastic in type and has the shape of an inverted "U", the inferior deficiency being closed by connective tissue. The cartilaginous portion of the tube is lined by pseudostratified columnar ciliated epithelium while the bony segment has a non-ciliated cuboidal epithelium.

In recent years it has been shown that opening the eustachian tube is almost totally dependent on the action of the tensor veli palatini muscle which arises from the lateral aspect of the tubal cartilage and is inserted into the aponeurosis of the soft palate. It was previously believed that the levator veli palatini muscle also played a significant role but it has since been shown that its action is limited to dilatation of the pharyngeal orifice of the tube.[13] Interference with the action of the tensor muscle associated with developmental anomalies, such as cleft palate, or tumour infiltration is frequently associated with tubal dysfunction and middle ear problems.

Fossa of Rosenmüller (Pharyngeal Recess) (Figures 1 and 2)

Immediately above and behind the tubal elevation lies the pharyngeal recess or fossa of Rosenmüller. It extends laterally into the sinus of Morgagni immediately above the upper limit of the superior constrictor muscle of the pharynx. The fossa is variable in size and depth and is conical or slit-like in shape. Visualisation of the fossa may be difficult. While the opening is usually wide, in some cases there is a narrow or slit-shaped orifice located superiorly or inferiorly. In children the fossa is usually small and often obliterated with lymphoid tissue, while in adults fibrous trabeculae at the entrance may obscure the view, especially in cases where previous adenoidectomy has caused scarring of the area.

Very large recesses of ovoid-flange shape have been reported, mainly in older age groups.[14] They usually occur bilaterally but unilateral cases have been reported. One such diverticulum measured 2.5–3 cm in vertical height and 2.5 cm in depth. In large diverticula the lining may appear smooth or granular and varying degrees of epithelial metasplasia may be evident on histological examination. The cause of very large fossae is uncertain. Wilson[15] described branchiogenic anomalies in this location which resembled large fossae but Khoo *et al.*[14] firmly rejected the concept of a developmental aetiology. However they postulated that the fossa is frequently deep in southern Chinese, thereby suggesting a possible genetic characteristic.

The fossa of Rosenmüller is of great clinical importance since it represents by far the commonest site of origin of nasopharyngeal carcinoma. Moreover its inaccessable location underlines the problem of the otolaryngologist in performing a thorough examination of the area.

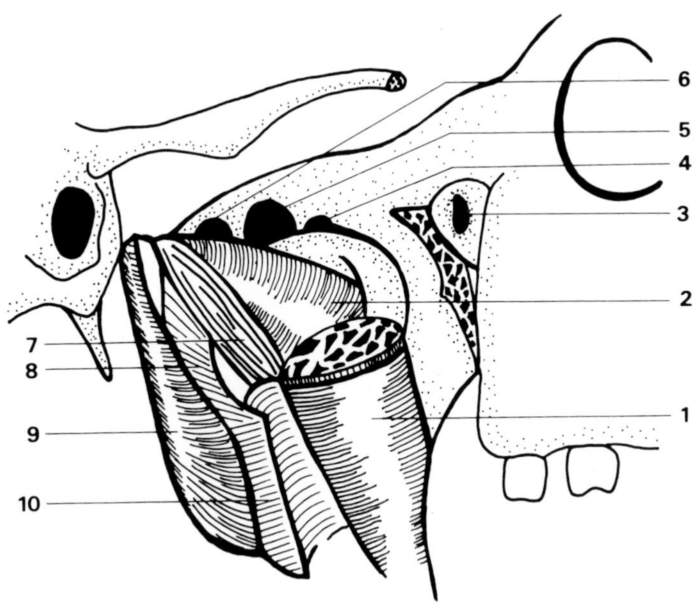

Figure 1. Lateral relations of the fossa of Rosenmüller (*after Cazalas*[6] *and modified from Lederman*[3]).

1. Tensor veli palatini ensheathed by pharygneal fascia
2. Eustachian tube
3. Sphenopalatine foramen
4. Foramen rotundum
5. Foramen ovale
6. Foramen spinosum
7. Levator veli palatini muscle
8. Fascia covering external surface of fossa of Rosenmüller
9. Superior constrictor muscle
10. External lamina of pharyngeal fascia (buccopharyngeal fascia)

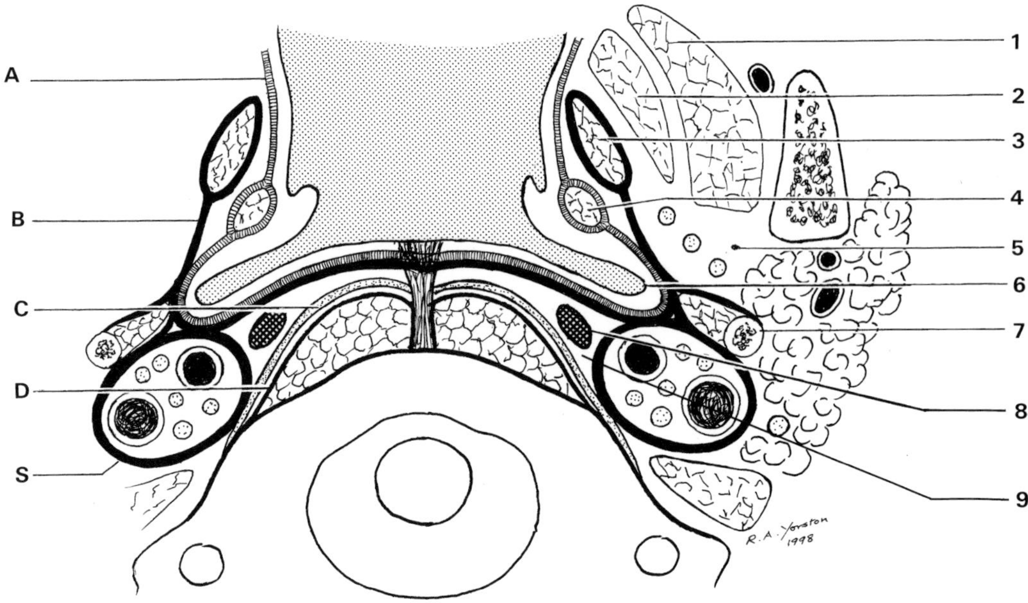

Figure 2. Horizontal section through the nasopharynx at the level of the sinus of Morgagni. Note the fascial layers and spaces and their relationship to the fossa of Rosenmüller. (*Illustration by R.A. Yorston*)

A. Pharyngobasilar fascia
B. Buccopharyngeal fascia
C. Alar fascia
D. Prevertebral fascia
S. Carotid sheath

1. Lateral pterygoid muscle
2. Medial pterygoid muscle
3. Tensor veli palatini muscle
4. Levator veli palatini muscle
5. Parapharyngeal space
6. Fossa of Rosenmüller
7. Styloid process
8. Node of Rouvière
9. Retropharyngeal space

Relations of the Fossa

As tumour spread generally radiates from the fossa of Rosenmüller the anatomical relations are of great clinical significance. They are as follows:

Anterior:	eustachian tube
Antero-lateral:	levator veli palatini muscle
Posterior:	retropharyngeal space
Superior:	foramen lacerum, medially; the petrous apex and carotid canal, posteriorly; the foramina ovale and spinosum (more distant), antero-laterally
Lateral:	tensor veli palatini muscle; pharyngeal space (prestyloid compartment)
Inferior:	superior constrictor muscle (upper edge)

The close proximity of the fossa to the foramen lacerum and other important structures at the skull base readily accounts for the ease and rapidity with which tumour can spread and cause serious neurological complications.

Fascial Layers and Spaces *(Figures 1 and 2)*

The fascial planes of the neck play a central role in determining the direction of spread of infections. Although they constitute a less effective barrier to tumour extension, a knowledge of the anatomy of the fascial planes and spaces is useful to understanding tumour spread and its associated symptomatology in nasopharyngeal malignancy.

Fascial layers

The deep cervical fascia comprises three main layers — investing, visceral and prevertebral — plus a marked condensation around the large vessels, namely the carotid sheath. The investing layer is of little significance in relation to nasopharyngeal carcinoma and will not be considered further. The visceral layer is a continuous sheet enclosing the visceral organs of the neck including the nasopharynx. It is referred to as the buccopharyngeal fascia in the upper part of the neck and the pretracheal fascia lower down. The prevertebral layer envelops the deep neck musculature and vertebral bodies and is thus closely related to the posterior aspect of the nasopharynx.

Visceral Layer

The *buccopharyngeal fascia* is a thin layer covering the outer surface of the constrictor muscles and extending forwards over the pterygomandibular ligament to the surface of the buccinator muscles. Posteriorly it is firmly attached to the prevertebral (and alar) fascia in the midline. Laterally it is attached to the styloid process and its muscles and to the carotid sheath. Superiorly after uniting with the pharyngobasilar fascia to form a single layer in the sinus of Morgagni, it separates and ensheaths the tensor veli palatini muscle as it ascends to gain attachment to the cartilaginous part of the auditory tube medially and the spine of the sphenoid and adjacent base of skull laterally. Inferiorly it is attached to the hyoid bone and laryngeal cartilages, below which it becomes known as the pretracheal fascia.

In the region of the nasopharynx an additional layer of visceral fascia, termed the *pharyngobasilar fascia*, lies deep to the muscular coat forming a connective tissue lining for the lateral and posterior walls of the pharynx. It is thickest above, where it unites with the buccopharyngeal fascia to form a dense layer which compensates for the loss of the muscular coat in the sinus of Morgagni. Superiorly it fuses with the periosteum overlying the pharyngeal tubercle of the basiocciput and the inferior aspect of the petrous temporal bone medial to the carotid canal. Thence the fascia extends anteriorly to gain attachment to the medial pteryoid plate and pterygomandibular ligament. Laterally it splits to embrace the eustachian tube and the levator veli palatini muscle, under which the fascia forms a supporting sling. In the midline posteriorly the fascia is condensed to form a strong band, the median raphe, into which the constrictor muscles are inserted. Below the fascia gradually fades out as a definite structure.

Prevertebral Layer

The *prevertebral fascia* encloses the deep neck musculature, vertebral bodies and the phrenic nerve. In front the fascia lies between the vertebral bodies and the posterior wall of the nasopharynx and extends laterally to the tips of the transverse processes before proceeding backwards to fuse with the spines of the vertebrae.

Although standard anatomical textbooks mention only a single layer of fascia, many modern surgical texts, especially in U.S.A., describe an additional layer, termed the *alar fascia*, between the buccopharyngeal and prevertebral fascial layers. This fascia forms a sheet across the midline between the transverse processes of the cervical vertebrae and extends outwards to fuse with the carotid sheath. In the midline the alar layer is attached to the buccopharyngeal fascia thus dividing the retropharyngeal space (*vide infra*) into two compartments. Above, the alar fascia is attached to the skull base, while inferiorly, usually about the level of C7 vertebra, it fuses with the visceral fascia. The alar and prevertebral layers are separated by a narrow space, the so-called "danger space" (*vide infra*).

Fascial spaces

The complex anatomy of the fascial layers of the neck leads to the formation of a number of compartments which are of great importance to the clinician.

The *retropharyngeal space* lies behind the nasopharynx separating it from the prevertebral (alar) fascia. The firm midline attachment between the buccopharyngeal fascia and the prevertebral (alar) fascia divides the space into two segments. Laterally the space is sealed by the attachments of both these fascial layers to the carotid sheath. The space is of special importance in as much as it contains the median and lateral groups of retropharyngeal lymph nodes, including the node of Rouvière (*vide — lymph drainage*).

The *parapharyngeal space* is triangular on cross-section and lies immediately lateral to the pharynx, extending from the base of skull above, to the superior mediastinum below. In its upper part, it is related laterally to the ascending ramus of the mandible and medial pterygoid muscle in front and to the parotid gland further back. The space is sub-divided into two compartments by the styloid process and attached muscles together with the fascial connections between the carotid sheath and prevertebral (alar) fascia.

The *pre-styloid* compartment is related in its upper part to the lateral wall of the nasopharynx and fossa of Rosenmüller and contains the maxillary artery and inferior dental, lingual and auriculo-temporal nerves. The *retro-styloid* compartment is more deeply placed and contains the carotid sheath and its contents, the upper deep cervical lymph nodes, the cervical sympathetic chain and the last four cranial nerves.

The *"danger space"* is a narrow compartment between the prevertebral and alar fasciae. It lies behind the retropharyngeal space and in front of the vertebral column. It extends from the base of skull above, to a variable level, usually around C7, below. It contains loose areolar tissue which facilitates free movement of the pharynx but also encourages the spread of infection — hence its name.

Blood Vessels

The major *arteries* supplying the nasopharynx — ascending pharyngeal, ascending palatine, descending palatine and pharyngeal branch of the sphenopalatine — all originate from external carotid artery and its various branches.

A *venous* plexus situated beneath the mucous membrane communicates with the pterygoid plexus superiorly and the posterior facial or internal jugular veins below.

Nerves

Sensory

The sensory nerve supply of the nasopharynx, including the posterior part of the soft palate, is derived from cranial nerve IX, excepting an ill-defined area of the nasopharyngeal roof adjacent to the tubal orifices which is supplied by cranial nerve V through its maxillary division.

The glossopharyngeal component is mainly derived through several small branches, including a communicating twig from the tympanic branch of the nerve, which follows the course of the greater superficial petrosal nerve. The supply to the upper surface of the soft palate and adjacent nasopharynx comes directly from the glossopharyngeal nerve as it descends in close proximity to the tonsillar fossa.

The trigeminal component leaves the maxillary division of the nerve in the pterygopalatine fossa and, after traversing the pterygopalatine ganglion (without synapse), it enters the tiny palatinovaginal canal to reach the roof of the nasopharynx.

Motor

The motor innervation is supplied by way of the pharyngeal plexus, comprising cranial nerves IX and X together with branches of the cervical sympathetic. The main innervation to the pharyngeal musculature is derived from the cranial root of the XI nerve passing via cranial nerve X.

Lymphatics *(Figure 3)*

The nasopharynx is the site of a marked aggregation of lymphoid tissue, concentrated mainly in the pharyngeal tonsil, which forms part of the lymphoid ring of Waldeyer.

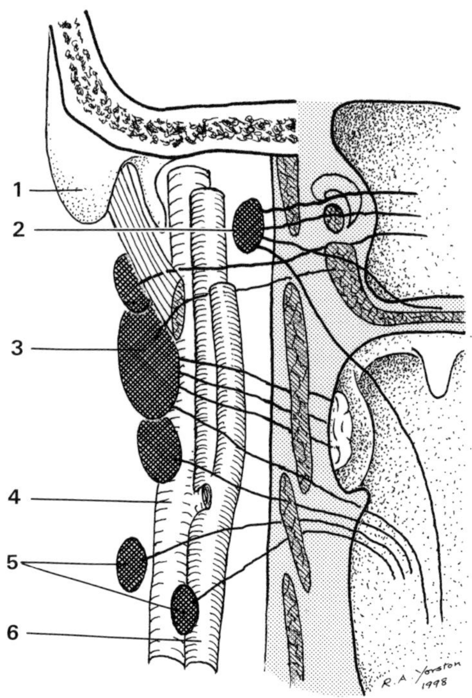

Figure 3. Lymphatic drainage of the nasopharynx (*modified after Rouvière[4] by R.A. Yorston*).

1. Mastoid process
2. Lateral retropharyngeal node of Rouvière
3. Jugulo-digastric node
4. Internal jugular vein
5. Internal jugular chain of lymph nodes
6. Common carotid artery

The lymphatic drainage system is correspondingly extensive.[16] A dense capillary network in the mucosa exists throughout the extent of the pharynx and gives origin to three main groups of submucosal collecting trunks, superior, middle and inferior. The drainage of the nasopharyngeal segment involves the superior, and to a lesser extent the middle, trunks.

The *superior collecting trunks* drain the bulk of the nasopharynx, the posterior part of the nasal fossae, eustachian tube, tympanic cavity, soft palate and oropharynx. They are subdivided into median and lateral groups.

The *median* group of channels, 8 to 12 in number, take origin from the roof and posterior wall of the nasopharynx, especially the area of the pharyngeal tonsil. The majority of channels unite near the midline and perforate the posterior wall of the nasopharynx close to the median raphe but a few pass laterally and traverse the pharyngobasilar fascia. The main destination is the lateral retropharyngeal node but some lymphatic channels by-pass this gland and drain directly to the upper deep cervical nodes situated around the internal jugular vein.

The *lateral* groups, which drain the outer part of the nasopharyngeal network, pass laterally, traversing the superior constrictor muscle and pharyngeal aponeurosis to terminate either in the lateral retropharyngeal node or a node on the lateral aspect of the upper internal jugular chain.

The drainage area of the *middle collecting trunks* includes the soft palate and palatine tonsils but it may extend upwards as far as the eustachian tube orifice. The lymphatic channels run outwards, traversing the lateral wall of pharynx to terminate in the lateral retropharyngeal node.

The *retropharyngeal nodes* are located in the retropharyngeal space between the posterior wall of the nasopharynx and the pre-vertebral fascia. They are prominent in the newborn and in early childhood but tend to atrophy with age and some nodes may disappear by adult life. They comprise two groups, median and lateral.

The *median* retropharyngeal nodes are of limited importance, being inconstant and often absent in adulthood. They consist of one or two small nodes applied directly to the posterior surface of the nasopharynx lying in the course of the median group of collecting trunks as they pass to the lateral retropharyngeal nodes. They are usually located near the midline about the level of the junction of the body and odontoid process of the axis vertebra.

The *lateral* groups of nodes, larger and more constant than the median group, usually consist of a single node on either side, often referred to as the node of Rouvière. The number of nodes, however, is variable and fusion of several nodes into a single one may be evident as surface lobulation. Occasionally the node is absent on one side. Situated in the lateral part of the retropharyngeal space close to the junction of the lateral and posterior walls of the nasopharynx, the node is related to the longus capitis muscle behind and lies medial to the upper pole of the superior cervical sympathetic ganglion (posteriorly) and the internal carotid artery (anteriorly) which it may overlap in front or behind. It is usually found just below the skull base at the level of the arch of atlas but sometimes slightly more inferiorly, at the junction of the body and odontoid process of the axis vertebra. It receives afferent vessels from the median and lateral groups of superior collecting trunks and from the middle collecting trunk. The efferent channels comprise one or two large trunks which proceed laterally, or obliquely outwards and downwards, passing deep to the carotid sheath and contents, to terminate in a lateral node of the internal jugular chain sited at any level between the base of skull and bifurcation of the common carotid artery.

The upper deep *cervical lymph chain* lies mainly along the course of the internal jugular vein between its emergence from the skull and the level of the mylohyoid muscle, some of the nodes lying in front of, and others behind the vein. The uppermost nodes are located in the retro-styloid compartment of the parapharyngeal space, deep to the upper end of the sternomastoid muscle in close relation to the mastoid process and the apex of the posterior triangle of neck. Other nodes in this group follow the course of the accessory and hypoglossal nerves. Lower down, the lymphatic chain lies in the anterior triangle of the neck, where the most important and constant node is the jugulo-digastric gland. The efferent vessels from the upper deep cervical group pass partly to the lower deep cervical nodes, located alongside the internal jugular vein below the level of the omohyoid muscle, and partly into a trunk which joins the efferent vessels from the lower deep cervical nodes to form the jugular trunk. This trunk on the right side ends at the junction of the internal jugular and subclavian veins, while on the left side it joins the thoracic duct.

A thorough understanding of this extensive lymphatic system is of great importance in tumour staging and the detection and management of tumour spread. It should be noted that unlike arteries and veins, lymphatic channels may cross the midline of the body so that contralateral spread of tumour cells may readily occur.

Routes of Tumour Spread

While the spread of disease in general is frequently determined by preformed channels, this is not necessarily the case with malignant tumours which, by their very nature, have the capacity to invade and destroy existing barriers. Nevertheless, nasopharyngeal carcinoma generally follows a number of well established routes. The direction of spread is partly dependent on the site of origin of the neoplasm but in large tumours this may be difficult to determine. Tumours arising near the midline may spread to one or other side but more often spread bilaterally. Tumours of the lateral wall however, also occasionally transgress the midline, so that bilateral, or even contralateral spread *per se*, may occur.

Common Routes

Intralumenary expansion is common and, as the growth enlarges, it may spread from the nasopharynx into the pharynx and nose, causing resorption of adjacent tissues with occasional destruction of the palate, maxillary sinus or orbit. However, spread along the lumen of the auditory tube is extremely rare.

Retropharyngeal Space

This is frequently the first route of spread. Lymphatic spread to the node of Rouvière is commonest but direct invasion also occurs. Further extension of the tumour may result in compression or infiltration of the retro-styloid space and its contents or destruction of the lateral mass of the atlas vertebra.

Parapharyngeal Space

(a) Pre-styloid compartment. This normally takes place by direct extension of the tumour. If this occurs, disturbances of the sensory root of the trigeminal nerve, followed later by the motor root, may become evident. Trismus is also encountered due to invasion of the pterygoid muscles while asymmetry of the palate in the resting position due to infiltration of the levator muscle is frequently encountered. Facial paralysis due to damage to cranial nerve VII is rare. Further spread of the tumour may take place to the palate, sinuses, parotid gland, the pterygo-maxillary fissure and/or the infra-temporal fossa, while very large tumours may invade the maxillary or frontal sinuses.

(b) Retro-styloid compartment. Invasion of the retro-styloid space by direct or, lymphatic spread, may result in paralysis of the last four cranial nerves and the cervical sympathetic chain. The internal carotid artery and internal jugular vein may also be compressed or infiltrated. Upward spread from the parapharyngeal space may lead to erosion of the base of skull, including the sphenoid body and sinus, the foramina ovale, spinosum and rotundum and the greater wing of the sphenoid. In extensive growths, tumour deposits may penetrate the pterygoid muscles and gain access to the infratemporal fossa. Further migration by this route into the orbit and maxillary sinus is possible. Downward extension of the tumour results in invasion of the palate causing associated ear problems, and the parotid and submandibular salivary glands may also be infiltrated.

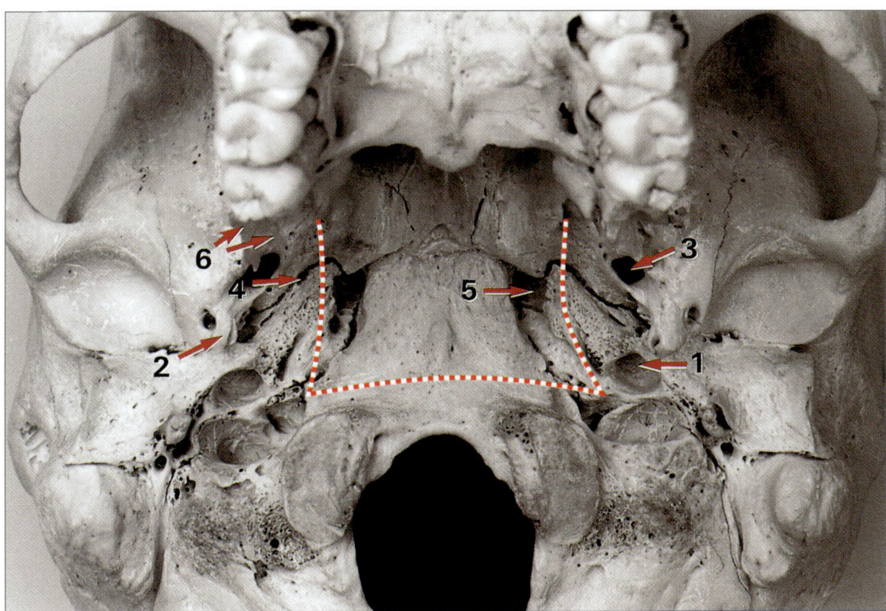

Figure 4. Relationship of the nasopharynx to the skull base. Note the proximity of the carotid canal and foramen lacerum to the fossa of Rosenmüller.

▬▬▬▬ indicates extent of nasopharynx

1. Carotid canal
2. Spine of sphenoid
3. Foramen ovale
4. Petrosphenoidal fissure
5. Foramen lacerum
6. Pterygoid plates

Intracranial

Intracranial spread usually occurs by direct extension of the tumour upwards from the fossa of Rosenmüller and erosion of the skull base. The route may follow the foramen lacerum, but Lederman[17] believes that the fibrocartilage, which partly fills the foramen, is generally resistant to tumour spread and erosion of the floor of the carotid canal is more likely. Thereafter the tumour may follow the course of the internal carotid artery to reach the cavernous sinus *(Figure 4)*. This results in ophthalmoplegia due to functional interference with cranial nerves III, IV and VI. Extradural extension by this route may also cause destruction of the greater wing of sphenoid.

Paranasal Sinuses and Ear

Tumour may also spread directly forwards to the ethmoid and thence occasionally to the frontal and maxillary sinuses and orbit.

Although the cartilage of the auditory tube is relatively resistant to tumour invasion, middle ear involvement may occasionally result from erosion of the petrous bone by upward extension of the tumour. Inner ear involvement is uncommon.

Distant Spread

Distant tumour dissemination may occur via the blood stream or the lymphatic system to liver, bones and lung.

References

1. Negus, V.E. 1929. *The Mechanism of the Larynx*. London: Heinemann.
2. Wood, Jones F. 1940. The nature of the soft palate. *J. Anat.*; 74:147–170.
3. Leela, K., Kanagasuntheram, R., Khoo, F.Y. 1974. Morphology of the primate nasopharynx. *J. Anat.*; 117(2):330–340.
4. Lambert, V. 1960. Malignant disease of the post-nasal space. *J. Laryngol. Otol.*; 74:1–21.
5. Cave, A.J.E. 1960. The epipharynx. *J. Laryngol. Otol.*; 74:713–717.
6. Arey, L.B. 1965. *Developmental Anatomy*, 7th edition. Philadelphia and London: W.B. Saunders.
7. McGrath, P. 1968. Prolactin activity and human growth hormone in pharyngeal hypophyses from embalmed cadavers. *J. Endocrinol.*; 42:205–212.
8. McGrath, P. 1967. Volume and histology of the human pharyngeal hypophysis. *Aust. N.Z. J. Surg.*; 37:16–27.
9. Tobias, P.V. 1981. Review of structure and development with notes on speech, pharyngeal hypophysis, chordoma and the dens. *J. Dent. Assoc. S. Afr.*; 36:765–778.
10. Kanagasuntheram, R., Ramshotham, M. 1968. Development of the human nasopharyngeal epithelium. *Acta Anat.*; 70:1–13.
11. Ali, M.Y. 1965. Histology of the human nasopharyngeal mucosa. *J. Anat.*; 99:655–672.
12. Adams, W.S. 1958. The transverse dimentions of the nasopharynx in child and adult observations on its contractile functions. *J. Laryngol. Otol.*; 72:465–471.
13. Honjo, I. 1988. *Eustachian Tube and Middle Ear Diseases*. Tokyo: Springer-Verlag.
14. Khoo, F.Y., Kanagasuntheram, R., Chia, K.B. 1967. Variations of the lateral recesses of the nasopharynx. *Arch. Otolaryngol.*; 86:456–462.

15. Wilson, C.P. 1955 Lateral cysts and fistulae of the neck of development origin, *Ann. R. Coll. Surg. Engl.*; 17:1–26.
16. Rouvière, H. 1938. *Anatomy of the Human Lymphatic System.* A compendium translated from the original, "Anatomie des lymphatiques de C'homme." Masson, Paris (1932) and rearranged for the use of students and practitioners by M.J. Tobias. Ann Arbor, Michigan: Edwards Bros., Inc.
17. Lederman, M.I. 1961. Anatomy of the nasopharynx in relation to the origin and spread of cancer. In: *Cancer of the Nasopharynx: Its Natural History and Treatment.* Springfield, Illinois: C.C. Thomas.

CHAPTER 3

Aetiological Factors and Pathogenesis

Dolly P. Huang and *Kwok-wai Lo*

Introduction

Nasopharyngeal carcinoma (NPC) is unique among squamous cell carcinomas of the head and neck. In most parts of the world the tumour is rare, the incidence rate for either sex being less than 1 per 100,000 persons per year.[1–5] Notable exceptions however occur in China, Africa, Canada, Alaska and among Greenland Eskimos.[3–8] The highest incidence of all is observed among southern Chinese who reside in central Guangdong province and speak the Cantonese dialect.[3–5,9–13] Male members of this high-risk population exhibit rates of 30–50 per 100,000 persons per year.[3–5,9–11] The incidence is also high in eastern Guangxi province.[14,15] Even in China, however, there are substantial incidence variations. In general, the incidence decreases from south to north so that the rate in Chinese men in the northernmost provinces is no higher than 2–3 per 100,000 persons per year.[3–5,9–11,14] High frequencies of NPC are also observed in emigrant southern Chinese populations in South-east Asia, California and elsewhere.[12,13,16–18] *Table 1* shows the annual incidence rates for nasopharyngeal cancer in China and in Chinese populations elsewhere. The incidence rates for this cancer in emigrant Chinese in southeast Asian countries and in United States (Hawaii and the Bay area) are appreciably higher than those in the respective indigenous populations.[19–21]

Hong Kong is geographically a part of the Cantonese region of Guangdong province. Approximately 98% of the population are Chinese and over 90% are of Guangdong origin and speak the Cantonese dialect.[22] The overall standardised incidence rate for NPC for males is 23.3 per 100,000 per year and 8.9 for females, based on the annual report of Hong Kong Cancer Registry.[23] This cancer ranks 3rd for men and 8th for women in new cancer diagnosis and, 4th and 8th for men and women respectively leading to cancer death (1995). Each year, about 1000 new cases are diagnosed. The age-specific incidence rates for both sexes begin to rise at the early age of 20, reaching a plateau between 35–64 years and declining thereafter. The mean age at diagnosis of this disease is about 50 (*Figure 1*). As illustrated, there is no other cancer that demonstrates this pattern of age distribution. A similar pattern is observed among the Singaporean Chinese.

The marked racial differences and geographical variations in NPC incidence have stimulated much interest in the aetiology of this cancer. Potential aetiological factors

Table 1. Annual incidence rates per 100,000 for nasopharyngeal cancer adjusted to world population distribution.

<table>
<tr><th rowspan="2">Population</th><th colspan="2">Age-standardized (world) incidence</th><th rowspan="2">Key reference</th></tr>
<tr><th>Male</th><th>Female</th></tr>
<tr><td>Southern Chinese (Hong Kong)</td><td>23.2</td><td>8.9</td><td>ref. 23</td></tr>
<tr><td>Chinese (Taipei)</td><td>8.1</td><td>3.2</td><td>ref. 19</td></tr>
<tr><td>Chinese (Shanghai)</td><td>4.4</td><td>2.0</td><td>ref. 19</td></tr>
<tr><td>Northern Chinese (Tianjin)</td><td>1.7</td><td>0.9</td><td>ref. 19</td></tr>
<tr><td>Emigrant Chinese populations in South-east Asia:</td><td></td><td></td><td></td></tr>
<tr><td>Singapore (all Chinese)</td><td>18.7</td><td>7.1</td><td>ref. 20</td></tr>
<tr><td>Singapore (Malays)</td><td>4.8</td><td>0.6</td><td>ref. 20</td></tr>
<tr><td>Malaysia Sabah (Chinese)</td><td>18.6</td><td>8.4</td><td>ref. 20</td></tr>
<tr><td>Malaysia Selengor (Malays)</td><td>2.5</td><td>0.3</td><td>ref. 20</td></tr>
<tr><td>Thailand (Chinese)</td><td colspan="2">10.0</td><td>ref. 21</td></tr>
<tr><td>Thailand (Thasis)</td><td colspan="2">3.0</td><td>ref. 21</td></tr>
<tr><td>U.S.A., Bay area (Chinese)</td><td>19.1</td><td>6.4</td><td>ref. 20</td></tr>
<tr><td>U.S.A., Hawaii (Chinese)</td><td>10.3</td><td>5.1</td><td>ref. 20</td></tr>
<tr><td>U.S.A., Hawaii (Hawaiian)</td><td>4.4</td><td>1.6</td><td>ref. 20</td></tr>
<tr><td>U.S.A., Bay area (Americans)</td><td>0.9–0.5</td><td>—</td><td>ref. 20</td></tr>
<tr><td>Greenland (Eskimo)</td><td>12.3</td><td>8.5</td><td>ref. 20</td></tr>
</table>

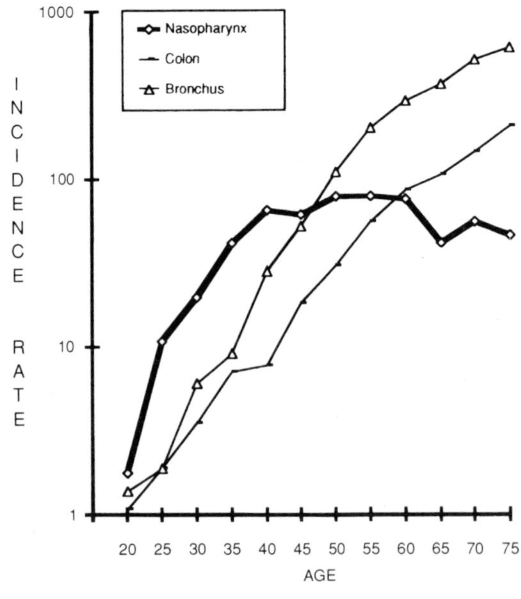

Figure 1. Age specific incidence of cancers of the nasopharynx, bronchus and colon in Chinese males in Hong Kong.[23]

responsible for this 50–100 fold difference in incidence have been the focus of intense investigations over the past two decades. These have revealed strong epidemiological and experimental evidence, linking this cancer with a genetically determined susceptibility associated with specific human leukocyte antigen (HLA) haplotypes,[24–27] early latent infection by the ubiquitous Epstein-Barr virus (EBV) and its reactivation[28–32] and exposure to environmental factors of a chemical nature, in particular, tumour-promoting chemicals in food products, especially early age consumption of salted preserved fish.[19,33–40]

Aetiological Factors

I. Dietary environmental factors

Ho of Hong Kong first proposed that Chinese salted fish, a popular food in southern China, especially favoured by the Cantonese, was a possible aetiological factor in the development of NPC.[19,34,41–43] This theory was based on the fact that the highest incidence of NPC occurs in the fisher folk of Hong Kong,[19,34,41–43] whose diet contains a high proportion of salted fish and a deficient intake of vitamin-rich fresh vegetables and fruit.[19,34,41–45] This salted fish is also a common food item among emigrant Chinese populations,[10,43] the Kadazans in East Malaysia,[46] and other South-east Asian populations.[39] All these groups have intermediate to high susceptibility to NPC.

Case-control studies have suggested that childhood consumption of salted fish is the primary cause of NPC among Cantonese.[45,47–49] In one such study conducted in Hong Kong in 1986, 250 NPC patients below the age of 35 and an equal number of age and sex matched controls were interviewed. It was found that there was a marked increased liability to develop NPC in those who consumed the food during weaning and below the age of 10 years (7.5 and 37.3 fold increased risk respectively). In adults no significant difference in current consumption of salted fish between cases and controls was observed.[49] Association of childhood consumption of salted fish and NPC was confirmed in independent studies in China.[50,51]

It is well known that cancers in the respiratory tract may be induced experimentally by ingested carcinogens. Nitrosamines, being alkylating agents, are known to induce squamous carcinomas, adenocarcinomas and other tumours in the nasal and paranasal cavities or nasopharyngeal tube of experimental animals when administered by the oral, subcutaneous or intravenous routes.[52,53]

Certain traditional southern Chinese foods have been shown to contain mutagenic or carcinogenic components.[54–60] The marine salted fish, referred to above, contain volatile nitrosamines, principally N-nitrosodimethylamine and N-nitrosodiethylamine. In addition, N-nitrosodi-n-propylamine and N-nitroso-n-butylamine have been detected in cooked salted fish samples and in salted fish-head soup.[60] These preserved food items, derived from Cantonese-style salted fish and Muoichoi (salted, preserved vegetable leaves) have shown a dose-dependent effect and produced mutagenic urine when fed to experimental animals.[58] Malignant tumours of the nasal cavity were observed among rats fed on a salted fish diet, a dose-response relationship being demonstrated between level of intake and rate of tumour occurrence. No tumours were observed at any other site and no comparable tumours were found in the control rats.[61,62]

An independent study by Ning *et al.* (1990) in a non-Cantonese rural population of southern Chinese in the city of Tianzin (incidence of 2 per 100,000 persons per year among men) showed that approximately 50% of NPC cases had had exposure to salted fish.[50] In this low incidence region of China the risk of NPC was found to be increased with earlier age at first exposure, frequency and duration of consumption and the method of cooking the salted fish.[50] Early exposure to other salted preserved food items such as shrimp paste and preserved vegetables (chungchoi, a preserved root) have been found to be major independent risk factors for NPC among the people of eastern Guangxi province who exhibit a high incidence of NPC.[15,45,51] Lee *et al.* (1994) have also found an increased risk of NPC in adulthood with the frequent consumption of salted soy beans, salted or pickled vegetables and salted mustard greens among the Chinese in Singapore.[63] Consumption of leafy vegetables was shown to be associated with a decreased risk, and vitamins were found to have a significant protective effect on the development of NPC.[51,63] Moreover, tumour-promoting chemicals such as nitrosamines have been identified in food products in Tunisia, South China and Greenland in high risk areas for NPC.[40]

These findings further strengthen the hypothesis that the risk of developing NPC is diet-related and that Chinese salted fish and other traditional southern Chinese foods are important potential human nasopharyngeal carcinogens. The close correlation between NPC risk and certain traditional southern Chinese dietary factors, in both the low and high incidence regions in China, is more than purely coincidental.

II. Non-dietary environmental factors

A number of non-dietary environmental factors are also thought to be linked to the development of NPC. These include atmospheric agents such as dust, smoke, chemical fumes, domestic smoke from burning wood, grass and incense and active and passive inhalation of tobacco smoke.[15,39,41,43,44,50,64–74] A positive history of nasal disease and the use of Chinese nasal oil and traditional herbal medications have also been suspected.[15,48,64,69,71–73]

Reports from California,[64] Malaysia,[39] Hong Kong[47,48] and Taiwan[66] all incriminate occupational exposure to products of combustion as risk factors for NPC, but no obvious association between the disease and dust or exposure to chemical fumes has been found.[44] Yu *et al.* (1990) reported a significant 3-fold risk in smokers of 30 or more cigarettes per day, while living with a smoker during childhood constitutes a significant and independent risk factor for NPC.[44] Studies of the possible role of previous ear or nose disease suggested by a history of a chronic ear or nose condition (rhinitis, sinusitis, nasal polyp or otitis media) all seem to indicate a positive and significant association with NPC development.[15,44,48,64,69,72] A prior history of nasal disease and its treatment by traditional Chinese medicine, including inhalants,[15,73] has been a relatively constant finding in several studies, although the exact association between these and the development of NPC has not been established.

Hirayama and Ito (1981) demonstrated that the geographical distribution of the plant Croton tiglium, whose seeds are used in Chinese herbs, loosely parallels NPC incidence within China.[70] Moreover, they showed that croton oil induces EBV antigens in human lymphoblastoid cell lines that carry the EBV genome.[75] Because of their extreme potency, croton seeds are reported to be rarely used in herbal mixtures. Epidemiological studies however failed to implicate croton seeds or any of the herbal ingredients, which contain components of the Euphorbiaceae family, as aetiological factors.[44,50,51] Use of certain herbal medicine has also been implicated although not without controversy.[51,63,76]

III. Genetic factors

As stated earlier, the frequency of NPC is nearly 100-fold higher in southern Chinese than in most Caucasian populations. This tremendous disparity in incidence in people of different origin suggests that there may be a genetic factor implicated in the development of NPC.

Several epidemiological features of the disease highlight the possibility of an inherited genetic predisposition to NPC.[36,77] Firstly, markedly higher incidence of NPC occurs in certain well-defined ethnic populations such as the southern Chinese or Cantonese, whereas the disease is rare for other populations in the rest of the world.[5] Secondly, the second generation of the southern Chinese from high incidence areas who emigrated to the low incidence areas in the western countries retains a higher risk than the resident population despite cultural assimilation.[17,18,36] Thirdly, multiple cases of NPC occurring in first degree relatives have been documented in diverse populations.[41,78–80] In fact, the proportion of familial cases is remarkably uniform across southern China — being 7.2% in Hong Kong, 5.9% in Guangzhou and 6.0% in Yulin.[81,82]

Specific haplotypes in the HLA region have been found to be associated with an increased risk of NPC.[24,27,33,83] The HLA loci involved, all of which are situated on the short arm of chromosome 6, include A, B and the DR loci, as shown in *Figure* 2. The association of HLA haplotypes and NPC among Singaporean, Malaysian, Hong Kong and southern Chinese has been well studied by Chan *et al.* (1983, 1990).[25,33] A 3.4-fold increased risk to develop NPC was found for the older age onset in Chinese NPC patients (> 30 years of age) and the specific haplotypes were A2, Cw11, Bw46, together with a missing DR9 locus.[26,33] Patients with this haplotype were reported to be long term survivors.[26,33] On the other hand, a 2.2-fold increased risk was found to be particularly associated with a younger onset (< 30 years) and with a poorer prognosis, involving specific haplotypes Aw33, C3, Bw58 and DR3. A difference in the HLA association between patients with early and late-onset disease was also noted in the northern

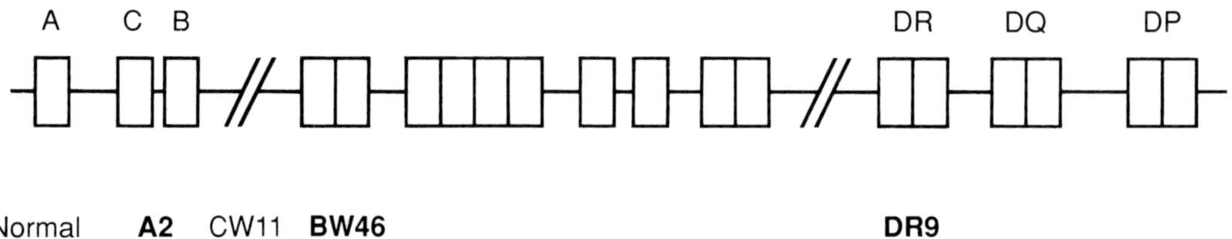

Normal	**A2**	CW11	**BW46**		**DR9**	
	AW33	C3	**B58**		**DR3**	

Two different haplotyes (large portions of chromosome 6) of HLA antigens are found to be associated with nasopharyngeal carcinoma:

						Relative Risk
NPC	**A2**	CW11	**BW46**	(older age onset, > 30 years of age)	**DR9** missing	3.4
NPC	AW33	C3	**B58**	(all ages & especially < 30 years of age — poor prognosis)	**DR3**	2.2

Figure 2. Map showing the Human Major Histocompatibility Complex for normal southern Chinese subjects and NPC patients. A2, Bw46, B58 and DR9 have a proven association with NPC.[3,33] A mutation of DR3 is suggested to have a similar association.[86]

Chinese.[27] On the other hand, a consistent negative association with the alleles A11 and B13 was noted.[33]

Recently, a large scale study on the association between HLA haplotypes and NPC among Caucasians in the United States has been reported.[84] A protective association with HLA-A2 allele specifically in non-Chinese, and with A11 across all races has been found. An increased risk has also been shown to be associated with B5 in the Caucasians. The study further demonstrated that the NPC associated HLA haplotypes were different between the Chinese and the Caucasians.

Other serological evidence indicates that different subtypes of Bw46 exist.[83,85] The gene sequence for Bw46 among Thais and northern Chinese (of low NPC incidence) is reported to be different from that among southern Chinese (of high NPC incidence).[33,83,85] Thus, the gene frequency of Bw46, which seems to correlate with the incidence of NPC, is highest in southern China and decreases with distance from that region. Lower frequencies are also found in other Asian populations and are apparently absent among Caucasians, Indians and Africans.[33] Point mutations, defining positions in HLA-DR3 molecules that affect antigen presentation, have also been observed.[86] It has been suggested that patients with the abnormal DR3 gene haplotype may not be able to mount specific cellular-mediated immunity to viral infection caused by Epstein-Barr virus.[33,86]

NPC susceptibility may also be linked to the different ability of the highly polymorphic HLA molecules in inducing immune responses. HLA molecules perform tasks by presenting antigenic peptides to T cells which are the central component of the immune system. However, it has been shown that HLA molecules vary in their ability to bind and present certain peptides. For the immune response against NPC associated Epstein-Barr virus (EBV) cell-mediated immunity to the product of EBV latent membrane protein-2 gene is only observed when HLA-A2.1 is present.[87] Thus, the degree of susceptibility to NPC may reflect the different ability of HLA haplotypes in controlling Epstein-Barr virus infection.

Other than the association with specific HLA haplotypes, the existence of a recessive NPC susceptibility gene, linked to the HLA region, has been proposed by Lu *et al.* (1990).[88] The pooled data, by linkage analysis on 27 Chinese sib pairs affected with this cancer collected from China, Singapore, Hong Kong and Malaysia, illustrated the existence of a susceptibility gene conferring a highly significant increased risk for NPC. This gene showed a relative increased risk for NPC some 10-fold greater than that associated with Bw46 or B17. This finding provides even stronger evidence to support the hypothesis that HLA-associated genes are related to the high risk group for NPC among southern Chinese. In a recent study, Ooi *et al.* (1997) screened healthy control and NPC samples with HLA haplotypes and highly polymorphic microsatellite markers on MHC regions.[89] Their results showed that the disease susceptibility gene for NPC may be located within the centromeric end of the class-1 and the telomeric end of the class-III regions of the MHC, close to the locus D6S1624.[89]

On the other hand, a large case control study demonstrated an association between the CYP2E1 (cytochrome P420 2E1) genotypes and the risk of developing nasopharyngeal carcinoma in Taiwan.[90] The authors showed that individuals who were homozygous for a specific allele of the CYP2E1 gene had an increased relative risk to develop NPC by 2.6-fold, the effect being restricted to non-smokers. Since the CYP2E1 gene is responsible for the metabolic activation of nitrosamines and the latter have been suspected to be involved in NPC development, this study revealed a possible interaction between genetic factors and environmental factors during disease evolution.

IV. Epstein-Barr virus (EBV)

i. Epidemiology and Natural History of Epstein-Barr Virus Infection

Epstein-Barr virus (EBV) is a herpes virus suspected of being causally related to NPC. EBV is ubiquitous in all human populations and is spread by horizontal infection. Natural primary infection usually takes place in childhood without clinical manifestation. This infection is always accompanied by seroconversion with the development of specific antibodies to virus-determined antigens, and the establishment of permanent immunity to reinfection. The virus is harboured for the rest of the individual's life in one of the following forms:

i. as a silent infection in a small number of circulating B-lymphocytes from a seropositive individual in virus genome form,[91] or
ii. the virus is shed into buccal fluid.[92]

The virus thus released into saliva is responsible for the horizontal transmission which causes natural primary infections such that in developing countries 99.9% of children are already infected by the age of 3 years.[32,93–95] In developed countries, the primary infection is less common in early childhood. However, 80 to 90% of the population ultimately become infected. If natural primary infection is delayed until adolescence or early adult life, there is a 50% chance that it will be accompanied by the clinical manifestation of infectious mononucleosis (IM). The delayed form of infection is more frequent in those enjoying high standards of hygiene than in the lower socio-economic groups.[32,96,97] This explains the characteristic association of IM with the more affluent societies of the Western world.

The annual incidence of heterophile-positive infectious mononucleosis was shown to be 330 times more common in a group of students in California than in a comparable student group in Hong Kong.[98] However, the percentage of EBV excretors was lower (16%) in the Californian based group than in the Hong Kong group (30%). This survey indicates that primary EBV infection among Asian students rarely manifests itself as IM. Independent population surveys carried out in Hong Kong[38,42] have shown that all Chinese children have serological evidence of infection by EBV before the age of 15 years. The early infection is probably related to the higher percentage of EBV excretors and the traditional Chinese eating habit of using chopsticks to pick up food from shared dishes.

ii. Epstein-Barr Virus and NPC

There is no clear-cut evidence showing that viruses cause cancer in man. The close association of the virus with certain human tumours suggests that it may have an oncogenic role in man in specific circumstances and in conjunction with essential co-factors.

EBV is linked to the development of several human cancers and causes lymphoma in immuno-compromised patients. Of particular interest are two human malignancies with which EBV is regularly associated, the endemic (African) Burkitt's lymphoma and NPC.[97,99] Both malignancies have well defined geographical distributions.

The association of EBV with NPC is strong and consistent.[97,99] Higher EBV antibody titres, particularly of the IgA class, occur in NPC patients than in controls.[28–32] These antibody levels rise with the tumour burden regardless of different geographical locations and ethnic groups.[31,32,99] Epstein-Barr virus genome and EBV associated antigens have consistently been found in undifferentiated and in well differentiated NPC tumours.[100–104] EBV contains genes capable of transforming and immortalising B-lymphocytes, monkey kidney and human epithelial cells.[105–107] EBV receptors are reported to be present on normal pharyngeal cell membranes and nasopharyngeal carcinoma cells.[108,109] Even though the virus can enter normal epithelial cells of the pharynx and viral genome is present in the tumour, the causal relationship of the virus and NPC has not yet been proven.

Pathogenesis

I. Epstein-Barr virus

i. Infection and Expression

EBV infection *in vivo* is a complex mixture of latent, reactivated, transforming or replicative types of infection. Sporadic excretions of the replicative virus in the oropharyngeal epithelial cells and persistent latent infection in the bone marrow and peripheral blood lymphocytes have been reported.[110–114] Patients with NPCs have latent EBV infection in their tumours as well as in their circulating blood lymphocytes. The EBV genome and latent gene products are consistently found in the differentiated[104,115,116] and the undifferentiated types of NPC.[101,102,114–124] The latter accounts for the majority of the tumour types in the intermediate and high incidence areas, particularly among the southern Chinese, the Eskimos and some Northern and Eastern African populations. The types of viral gene expressed depend on a specific cellular phenotype. All NPCs express the EBV encoded latent protein, Epstein-Barr nuclear antigen-1 (EBNA-1). This protein binds to the origin of latent viral replication and the binding is essential for the maintenance of the viral episomes. On the other hand, NPCs do not express the immunogenic EBNA2–6 proteins, but 60–90% of them express latent membrane protein 1 (LMP-1).[119,123,124] BZLF (Zebra) protein, which disrupts viral latency, has not been detected confirming that the virus is latent in the NPC tumour cells.[125] The list of EBV encoded latent proteins include EBNA-1, LMP-1 and LMP-2, Bam HI A fragments and the abundantly expressed EBV encoded RNAs, the EBERs. Among all latent antigens expressed by EBV in NPC, LMP-1 has been considered to be the critical factor contributing to the pathogenesis of NPC as it induces cellular growth and affects cellular growth control mechanisms.[114,126,127]

LMP-1 is a viral oncogene of EBV which has been found to transform rat embryo fibroblast cells. The transformed cells have demonstrated tumorigenicity in athymic mice.[128] Expression of this latent protein induced epidermal hyperplasia and altered keratin gene expression.[129] Moreover, its gene expression in epithelial cells has been found to inhibit squamous differentiation and induce down-regulation of cytokeratin expression, accompanied by an up-regulation of the ICAM-1 adhesion molecule and CD40 antigen.[130,131] LMP-1 is also known to activate NF-kB and induce expression of A20 and epidermal growth factor receptor.[132,133] The induction of A20 gene was found to block p53-mediated apoptosis in the epithelial cells.[134] The LMP-1 latent protein has also been thought to bind tumour necrosis receptor associated factor-1, similar to CD30 and CD40 and to function as an active tumour necrosis factor (TNF) receptor.[135] The LMP-1 molecules aggregate in the plasma membrane of the infected epithelial cells, mimicking an active tumour necrosis factor receptor and causing intracellular signal induction.[126,135]

Within the tumour, analysis of the EBV termini showed only one fused terminal fragment, indicating that EBV DNA is homogenous and a clonal cellular proliferation.[136]

Moreover, in the early stages of malignancy such as the dysplastic lesions and carcinoma-in-situ of the nasopharynx, all samples were found to contain monoclonal EBV DNA by the testing of the EBV termini, indicating that these are clonal proliferation from a single EBV-infected cell before expansion of the malignant cell clone.[137] Other latent viral genes expressed in the premalignant lesions included LMP-1 and EBERs. However, EBV has not been detected in normal nasopharyngeal mucosal biopsies from patients at high risk of developing NPC nor in normal mucosa adjacent to EBV-positive NPCs[115,121,122,137,138] (Personal data — Huang). Moreover, from *in vitro* data, it has been demonstrated that stable EBV infection of epithelial cells requires an undifferentiated cellular phenotype, suggesting that EBV infection is not the first step in the carcinogenic process leading to invasive NPC.[139] Taken together, these findings indicate that EBV is an important causal factor in the development of NPC. On the other hand, the ubiquitous nature of the EBV infection in all human populations in contrast to the marked geographical variation in the development of NPC throughout the world, excludes EBV as the sole causative factor of nasopharyngeal carcinoma. It has been suggested that epithelial cells may become susceptible to EBV infection as the result of exposure to mutagenic environmental carcinogens, e.g., in the form of dietary agents implicated in NPC pathogenesis.[127]

It has been previously established that elevated IgA titres to EBV replicative antigens precede the development of NPC and can be used as a marker for tumour progression and remission.[28] Moreover, the secretory IgA has been shown to facilitate EBV entry into epithelial cells suggesting that the IgA antibodies may contribute to the development of NPC by the induction shift of EBV tissue tropism.[140] Infection of epithelial cells by EBV would usually result in viral replication as the epithelial cells matured and differentiated. However, in patients at risk to develop NPC who have IgA to EBV, the increase in viral replication may increase the chance of establishing a latent transforming infection in the nasopharyngeal mucosal epithelium by switching on to another viral expression programme due to tissue tropism.[118] Moreover, the epithelium may also have sustained previous genetic insults that inhibit cellular differentiation or viral replication, and promoted expression of the EBV transforming genes like LMP-1. The expression of the viral latent genes in combination with specific previous cellular genetic changes would result in dysplasia that rapidly progressed to invasive neoplasia, without a long latency period as often indicated by other cancers.

ii. Promoter and Viral Expression Programmes for EBV

The regulation of the membrane antigens expression depends on the phenotype of the host cell. In NPC cells, LMP-1 is expressed in the absence of EBNA2.[118] The latter protein, the EBNA2, is a strong immunogenic antigen as well as a potent transforming protein in most EBV infected cells. In NPCs, viral transcriptions have been found to have switched from the Wp/Cp to the Fp promoter, with down-regulation of the immunogenic EBNA2–6 as a direct, and LMP-1 as an indirect, result. So, only the non-immunogenic EBNA1 protein would be expressed, safeguarding the maintenance of the viral episomes. As for the immunogenic LMP-1, there is evidence showing the presence of some EBV LMP-1 variant strains with specific mutations and deletions which are more oncogenic but less immunogenic favouring virus survival than the prototype (from that of the B95–8 EBV strain).[141–148] One such study even provided evidence that mutations in the Chinese NPC-derived LMP-1 gene have altered the gene into a non-immunogenic protein, being part of the viral strategy to escape the host's cell-mediated immunity in controlling the latent Epstein-Barr virus infection.[146] All together, the latent membrane protein-1 gene in the EBV infected epithelial cells stands out as an important viral factor and may play a significant role in the genesis of NPC.

II. Genetic changes

Cancer is believed to have evolved from the clonal expansion and accumulation of multiple genetic changes in cells. The genetic changes include the inactivation of the tumour suppressor genes and activation of oncogenes.[149] Moreover, the genes related to DNA repair, apoptosis and telomerase activity are also the targets during development of the cancer. Although the correlation of aetiological factors with nasopharyngeal carcinoma have been well documented over the past two decades, the genetic basis for the tumorigensis of this cancer is poorly understood. Like some of the solid tumours, NPC is believed to arise as a consequence of multiple molecular events induced by environmental factors and EBV infection. The neoplastic process may involve alterations of the tumour suppressor genes and oncogenes by genetic damage and interference with the normal cellular functions by the EBV latent gene products. The accumulation of somatic genetic changes in the NPC cells has been investigated by way of cytogenetic and molecular genetic approaches. The studies have led to the identification of many consistent changes affecting chromosomal regions and individual genes.

i. Cytogenetic Observations

Cytogenetic studies of a particular cancer provide the gross and complete investigation of chromosomal aberrations in the cancer cells and indicate the possible target regions involved in the progression of the cancer. Investigation of the chromosome aberrations in tumour cells by cytogenetic analysis has been the first step in identifying genetic lesions which are involved in the development of cancers. Both numerical abnormalities (gains or losses of chromosomes) and structural aberrations (such as deletion, translocation, segmental duplication, inversion etc.) of chromosomes in the cancer cells can be detected by karyotyping analysis. Identification of the region with frequent deletion reveals the inactivation of the tumour suppressor gene in this region while the sites with consistent translocation or amplification indicate the presence of activated oncogenes.

However, classical cytogenetic analysis is limited by difficulties in growing NPC tumours *in vitro* or heterotransplanting them into nude mice. Only a few cytogenetic studies of NPC have been reported previously.[150–159] *Tables 2* and *3* summarize the results of the cytogenetic analysis of NPC cell lines and xenografts. Most of the NPC cell lines are hyper-aneuploid and show multiple chromosomal alterations. Such rearrangements may be induced *in-vitro* and may not represent the primary tumours. NPC xenografts, primary tumours and short-term cultures have a near diploid model number and may show more reliable data, but no consistent chromosome abnormalities common to all NPC have been identified. Abnormal clustering on certain chromosomal regions has been noted. The critical areas of chromosomal loss have been identified in chromosomes 1p, 3p, 9p, 11q, 13q, 14q, 16q and X. Moreover, breakpoints were frequently observed in 1p11–31, 3p12–21, 3q25, 5q31, 11q13, 12q13, 17p13–q25, and Xq24. High frequency of 3p deletion has also been demonstrated in both primary tumours (3/8) and xenografts (2/3).[151] We have recently applied the fluorescence in-situ hybridization (FISH) analysis for the precise location of the deletion regions on chromosome 11q in a NPC cell line cell-666[159] (*Figures 3*). It is suggested that the tumour suppressor gene(s) on these chromosomal regions may be the targets for the development of NPC. On the other hand, consistent chromosomal gains have not been a common finding.

ii. Molecular Genetic Studies

In addition to the cytogenetic studies, the genetic aberrations in nasopharyngeal carcinoma have been identified by molecular genetic approaches. Several chromosomal regions and cancer related genes have been investigated by ourselves and others. Deletions on multiple chromosomal regions have been demonstrated by the loss of

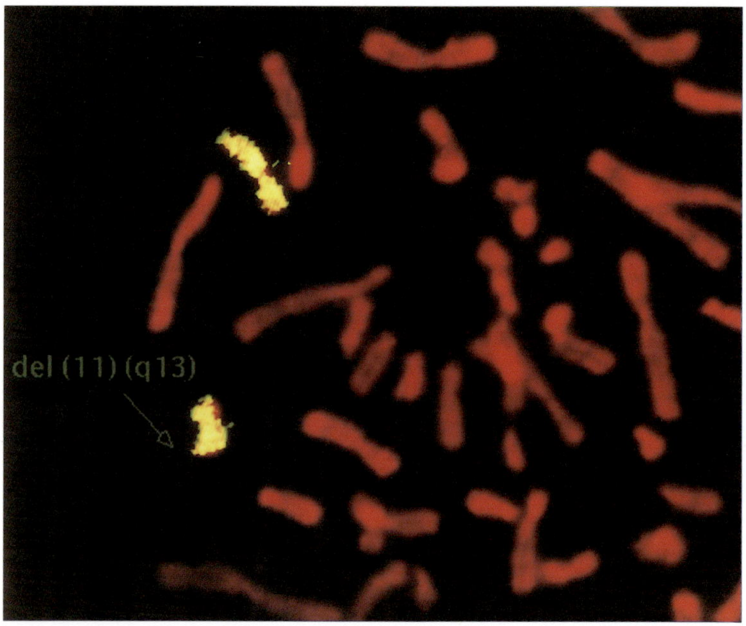

Figure 3. FISH analysis on the deletion of chromosome 11q in a NPC cell line, cell-666.

Table 2 Karyotypes of NPC xenografts.

Xenograft	Karyotypes
Xeno-1 (Huang,1989) [151]	72,XX,+1,+der(1)t(1;12),HSR,+2,+2,+del(3)(p12),+4,+7,+7,+8,+9,+10,12p+?,+14,+15,+16,+16, +18,+18,+19,+19,+20,+20,+21,+22,+22
Xeno-2 (Huang 1989) [151]	61,XX,+1,+2,+6,+7,+8,+9,+10,+11,+15,+der(17)t(11;17)(q13;q23),+18,+19+20,+mar1,+mar2
C15 (Bernheim 1993) [152]	47, X, -X, +i(1q), +2
C17 (Bernheim 1993) [152]	37-40,XY,der(1)t(1;6)(q21;q12),del(1)9q12),der(3)t(3;8)(p22;q11).-4,del(4)9q23), der(5)t(5;8)(q34-35:q1),-6,der(7)t(7:?)(q34-35;?),-8,-9,add(9)(q34),-10,11q-, der(12)t(6;12)(q11:p11),-13,-14,-16,del(17)(p11-12),i(21q),der(21)t(4;21)(p16:q22),+1-4mar
C19 (Bernheim 1993) [152]	49-40,X,-Y,del(1)(p34),der(1)t(1;?)(p31;?)-2,-3,der(4)t(1;4)(p31;p16),14,5p+,der(6)t(6:13(p21;q11), -8,9p-,ins(10;?)(q21;?),-11,-13,-14,-15,-16,der(17)t(2;17)(q13;q25),der (17)t(8;17)(q22;p13),i(21), -22,+mar1,+mar2,+mar3,+mar4
Mbane (Mitelman 1983) [150]	46,XY,ins(3)(q25:?) or dup(3)(q25q27)
Ali bin Ali (Mitelman 1983) [150]	48,XY,der(1)(inv(!)t(1;11)(1pter→p22::q44→cen→p22::11q22→qter),t(1;15)(p11;q21),+del(3)(q12), del(6)(q23),-11,+12,-14,del(16)(q22),+19,+20,-21,+mar1,+mar2

Table 3 Karyotypes of NPC cell lines.

Cell lines	Karyotypes
TW039-N1 (Tien 1990) [156]	95-100,X,del(X)(q24),der(1)t(1;9)(p11;q11),der(3)t(3;9)(p11;q11),der(3)t(3;?;12)(q25;?;q21), der(3)(3pter→3p21::?::3p21→3pter),der(4)t(4;?)(p15;?),del(5)(q13q35),i(5p),der(6)t(6;9)(p22;p23), der(6)t(6;?)(p11;?),del(7)(q22),i(8q),der(8)(8pter→8p22::8p23→8q24::8q23→8qter),der(9)t(6;9)(p22;p23), der(9)t(9;19)(p11q11),del(9)(q22),i(9p)i(10q),del(10)(q22),der(12)t(12;?)(p12;?),i(13q),del(13)9q22q32), der(13)t(13;?)(13;p11.2;?),der(15)t(15;22)(p11;q11),der(15)t(10;15)(p11;p11),der(17)t(17;?)(p13;?), der(19)t(3;19)(p21;p13),der(21)t(21;?)(p11.2;?),der(22)t(22;?)(p11;?),+1-2mar
TW039 (Tien 1990) [156]	95-100,X,del(X)(q24),der(2)t(2;3)(q33;p21),der(3)t(3;9)(p11;q11),der(3)t(3;?;12)(q25;?;q21), der(3)(3pter→3p21::?::3p21→3pter),der(4)t(4;?)(p15;?),del(5)(q13q35),i(5p), der(6)t(6;9)(p22;p23),der(6)t(6;?)(p11;?),del(7)(q22),i(8q),der(8)(8pter→8p22::8p23→8q24::8q23→8qter), der(9)t(6;9)(p22;p23),der(9)t(9;19)(p11;q11),del(9)(q22),i(9p),i(10q),del(10)(q22),der(12)t(12;?)(p12;?), i(13q),del(13)9q22q32),der(13)t(13;?)(13;p11.2;?),der(15)t(15;22)(p11;q11),der(15)t(10;15)(p11;p11), der(17)t(17;?)(p13;?),der(19)t(3;19)(p21;p13),der(21)t(21;?)(p11.2;?),der(22)t(22;?)(p11;?),+1-2mar
CNE (Zhang 1982) [153]	67-68,XX,+1,+2p-,der(3)t(?;3q),+der(5)t(?;5q),+der(7)t(7;?),+der(8)t(8q;8q+),i(8q),+11,+11, +12,der(13)t(?;13q),+der(14)t(14;?),+16,der(18)t(18;?),der(19)t(19;?),-19,+der(20)t(20;?), +20,+22,+22,+mar1 [t(2p;6q),7q-,t(3p+;3q+),+mar2,+mar3]--markers occasionally appeared
CNE-2 (Zhang 1983) [153]	103-104,,XY,+1,+1,+1,+1p-,+2,+3q+,+t(?;3q)+4p+,+5,+6,+7,+7,i(8q),+9,+i(10q)+11,+11, +12,+12p+,+i(13q)+14,+14,+15,+15p+[a],+15p+[b]+16,+16,+17,+17,+t(17;?),+18,+19,+19,+20, +21,+21,+t(22q?;21q)-22,+t(X;?)[a],+t(X;?)[b],+mar1-mar23
Cell-666 (Hui 1997) [159]	45, X, del(X)(q24), -5, der(5)t(5,5,5) (5pter→5q31::5q13→5q31::5p12→5pter) , der(?;6)(p10;q10), add(7)(p22), +9, del(11)(q13),add(12)(p13), -14, -18, -21, +2mar

heterozygosity (LOH) studies and multiplex polymerase chain reaction (PCR) analysis. Alterations of specific genes including tumour suppressor genes and oncogenes have also been reported by different groups.

a. Loss of heterozygosity (LOH) and homozygous deletion

Although cytogenetic analyses provide only limited information on the genetic changes in NPC, frequent abnormalities identified in these studies such as the loss of 3p led us to investigate the involvement of these regions in this cancer by molecular methods. By the LOH study, it was found that the deletion of 3p is the most frequent genetic change in NPC. In our early studies, we confirmed the high frequency (67–100 %) of LOH at chromosome 3 in NPC.[160–161] By detailed deletion mapping using PCR-based microsatellite polymorphic markers, three distinct deletion regions (3p13–14.3, 3p14.3–3p21 and 3p21.3-ter) were identified in the primary NPCs.[161] It is suggested that multiple tumour suppressor genes in this chromosome arm are involved during the development of NPC. The high incidence of LOH at 3p has also been confirmed by other studies.[162,163] Hu *et al.* have identified a homozygous deletion region at 3p26 in which a tumour suppressor may reside.[163] Using microcell fusion to transfer a single normal chromosome 3 into an NPC cell line, Cheng *et al.* (1998) further provided functional evidence of NPC associated tumour suppressor gene(s) activity in chromosome 3p21.3.[164]

In addition to chromosome 3p, we have also demonstrated a high percentage of LOH at chromosome 9p and 11q (61% and 54%, respectively) in NPC. In chromosome 9, homozygous deletions at 9p21 have been found in both NPC xenografts and primary tumours.[165] The region includes the cell cycle regulators, the *p15*, *p16* and *p16β* genes at chromosome 9p21–22 which have been shown to have tumour suppressor properties in human cancers. The involvement of these genes in the NPC tumorigenesis will be discussed in a later section. Our recent study has also defined two distinct deletion regions at 11q13.3–22 and 11q22–24 in primary NPCs.[166] The findings indicate that at least two tumour suppressor genes in 11q may be associated with NPC tumorigenesis. The newly identified MEN 1 gene or ATM gene may be one of the candidate target genes.

Moreover, LOH at chromosome 14q at locus D14S81 (14q31) has also been detected in about 33% of primary NPCs.[167] The deletion of this chromosome region has previously been reported in association with the advanced stages of colorectal and bladder carcinoma. It is suspected that the inactivation of the tumour suppressor in this region may be involved in the progression of NPC. However, no obvious candidate tumour suppppressor genes have been identified in the relevant region.

The status of the loci at chromosomes 1, 2p, 4q, 5, 6q, 13q, 15q, 16, 17q, 22q and X have also been investigated in our recent studies.[167,168] Low frequencies of LOH (0 to 23.3%) at these loci were observed in the NPC samples. Among these regions, a relative higher incidence of deletion was found in 4q (23.3%) and 13q (21.1%). The alterations in these chromosomal regions may be the late events in the progression of this cancer.

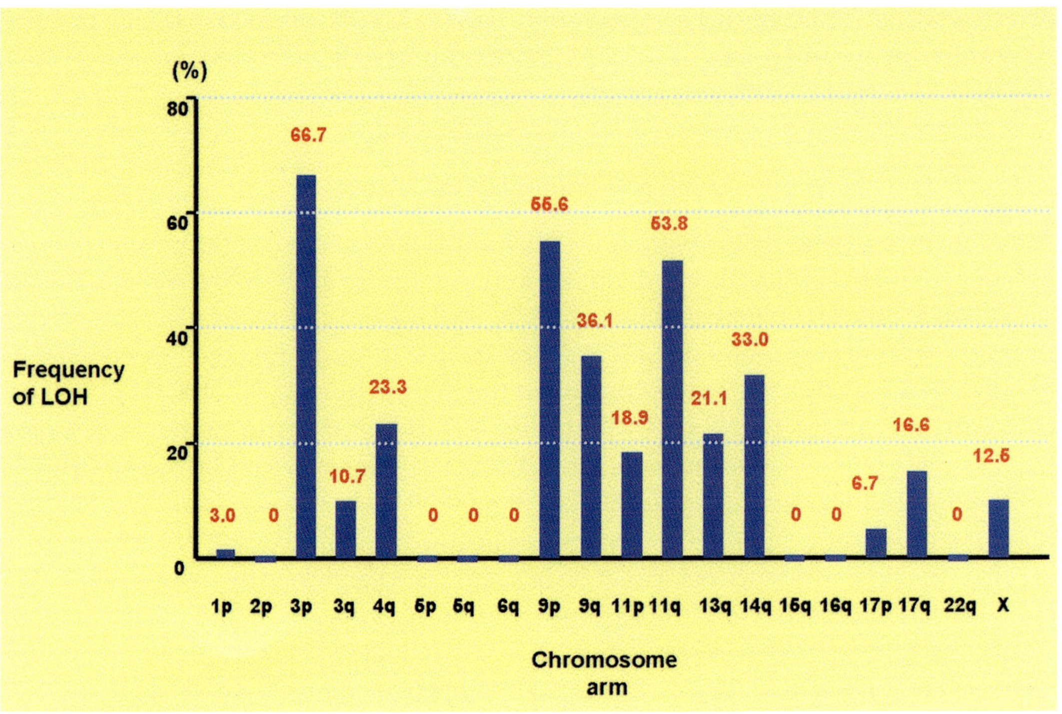

Figure 4. Partial allelotype of NPC.

Figure 4 shows a partial allelotype of NPC and summarizes all of our available data of the LOH studies. The affected chromosome regions are similar to those reported in a recent study by Thailand researchers.[163] However, a comprehensive genome-wide survey of the genetic changes in NPC is not yet available. It would be advantageous to perform comparative genome hybridization (CGH) analysis to identify the other affected regions in NPC.

b. Tumour suppressor genes

The high frequency of the 3p deletion in NPC indicates that the inactivation of the tumour suppressor genes in this chromosome may play an important role in the development of NPC. The tumour suppressor gene at 3p25, the von Hippel-Lindau (*VHL*) gene, may be one of the candidate targets. The *VHL* gene has been demonstrated to have a tumour suppressor function by the inhibition of transcription elongation. However, it was found that no *VHL* gene alterations, either mutation or hypermethylation, occurred in the NPC samples.[168,169] It is not likely that the inactivation of this gene is associated with the development of NPC. Recently, intragenic homozygous deletion and aberration expression of a newly cloned gene at 3p14.2, the *FHIT* (fragile histidine triad) gene, have been shown in 3 NPC cell lines and several primary tumours.[170] However, the role of the *FHIT* gene in human neoplasia is still not clear and is controversial. Further studies are needed to confirm the tumour suppressor function of this gene and its involvement in NPC tumorigenesis.

Based on findings of the homozygous deletions at 9p21, the *p16* gene which resides in this region is likely to be the target for inactivation in NPC. The *p16* gene encodes the negative regulatory protein which prevents the cell cycle progression from G1 to S phase by inhibiting the catalytic activity of the CDK/cyclin D complex and subsequent RB protein phosphorylation.[171,172] By intensive investigation of the status of the *p16* gene in NPC, a high incidence of inactivation of the *p16* gene was found in NPC xenografts (100%), cell lines (100%) and primary tumours (58.3%).[173–175] Major mechanisms for the inactivation of the gene are through homozygous deletion and hypermethylation. Using immunohistochemical analysis, there was no detectable *p16* expression in 64% of primary NPC cases.[176] Sun *et al.* (1995) have also demonstrated the loss or reduced expression of the *p16* gene in 2 NPC xenografts.[177] Thus, the inactivation of the *p16* gene may play an important role in the development of NPC. On the other hand, the *p16* gene alternated transcripts, *p16β* (*p19*) and the *p15* genes were also involved in the 9p21 homozygous deletion regions in NPC samples. Both of these genes are found to have influence on the regulation of the cell cycle progression. We have examined the status of the *p16β* and *p15* genes in NPC and found alterations of both genes were uncommon in samples without homozygous deletion at 9p21.[175] It is suggested that the *p16* gene is the major target on 9p21 for the development of NPC.

Apart from the *p15, p16* and *p16β* genes, the status of several tumour suppressor genes involved in the cell cycle regulation in NPC have been reported previously. No alterations of these genes were identified in this cancer. The study of the *Rb* gene, a gene involved in the restriction point control of progression through G1 to S phase of the cell cycle, demonstrated that the gene is intact in NPC and does not play a role in the development of this disease.[178] The *p53* gene encodes a negative regulation protein which inhibits cell growth and induces apoptosis after DNA damage. The role of *p53* mutations in NPC tumorigenesis appears to be less significant than that in many other tumours. Multiple studies demonstrated that the mutation of *p53* gene is rare (less than 10%) in this cancer.[179–184] On the other hand, overexpression of the *p53* protein is commonly observed in NPC by immunohistochemical analysis.[185–187] The findings indicate accumulation of the wild type *p53* protein in this cancer. This may be due either to inactivation of an enzymatic pathway responsible for the *p53* degradation or some functional interference by the cellular or viral gene products. The alteration of the downstream regulator, *p21*, may be responsible for the loss of the *p53*-mediated G1 arrest function in the NPC cells. Nevertheless, no mutation or gross structural changes of the *p21* gene have been identified in NPC samples.[188,189] It is unlikely that the *p21* gene is the target for inactivation in this cancer. It is suspected that the *p53* function may be inactivated as a result of homozygous deletion of the *p16β* (*p19*) gene in some nasopharyngeal carcinomas. Recent studies have shown that the *p16β* (*p19*) gene product blocks the normal function of inducing MDM2-induced *p53* gene function.[190,191]

c. Oncogenes

The role of oncogenes in the development of NPC appears to be prominent. Overexpression of the bcl-2 protein which inhibits apoptosis has been found in 80% of NPC samples.[192] The consistent overexpression of bcl-2 and the EBV latent gene products (such as LMP-1) in NPC may inhibit apoptosis and contribute to the development of NPC. Immunohistochemical studies also showed that overexpression of the ras and c-myc proteins were common in primary NPC tumours, 76% and 90%, respectively.[193] Over-expression of c-myc has been found to correlate with a poor prognosis in NPC. On the other hand, the genomic alterations such as translocation and mutation have not been identified in these oncogenes. The upregulation of the *bcl-2*, *c-myc* and *ras* gene expression in NPC may be due to the effect of transactivation by other unidentified regulatory factors or alterations in the promotor region of these genes.[155,194,195] Other than the known oncogenes, a unique transformation-associated sequence has also been cloned from the NPC genomic DNA transfectant cell line. The sequence was confined to chromosome 8q23–24.1 and had moderate transforming activity when introduced into JB6 P+ cell. However, the role of this new oncogene in the tumorigenesis of NPC cannot be confirmed as yet.[196,197]

d. Telomerase

A recently described intriguing mechanism of tumorigenesis is the stabilization of chromosome telomeres. The reactivation of telomerase activity has been detected in almost all human cancers and may be a necessary event for their sustained growth. Tsao *et al.* (1996) found evidence of telomerase activity in 100% of stage III and IV, 78.6% of stage II and 80% of stage I NPCs.[198] This pilot study suggests that telomerase plays an important role in the development of NPC. Previous studies have demonstrated that chromosome 3 has an inhibitory role on the telomerase activity in a tumour cell line.[199] The frequent LOH of 3p may be associated with the reactivation of the telomerase activity in this cancer.

e. Comparison between NPC and other head and neck cancers

Figure 5 shows a comparison of the genetic changes, EBV status and telomerase activity between NPC and other head and neck cancers.

Although similar rates of LOH at 3p, 9p, 11q and 14q are demonstrated in both NPC and other head and neck cancers and similar incidence rates are found in their corresponding telomerase activities, NPC stands out as unique by the demonstration of a 100% association with the Epstein-Barr virus. This is in sharp contrast to other head and neck cancers. Other outstanding features include high frequency of bcl-2 over-expression and low incidence of *p53* mutations in NPC. All of the above point to a distinct and different pathway for tumorigenesis of this viral-related nasopharyngeal cancer from other squamous cell head and neck carcinomas, which may also account for the specific undifferentiated phenotype of this cancer.

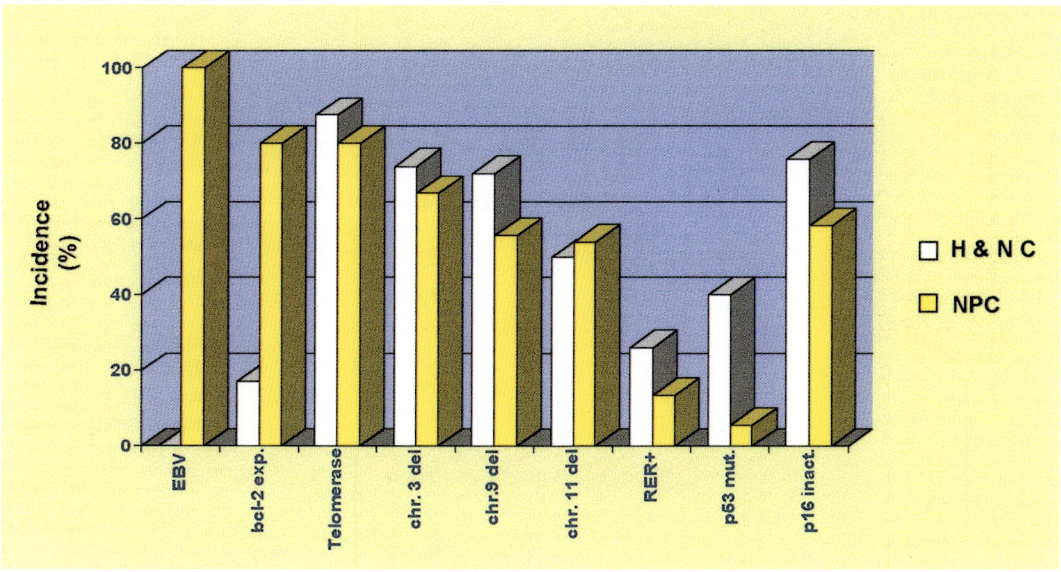

Figure 5. Comparison of genetic changes, EBV status and telomerase activity between NPC and other head and neck cancers.

Insights from Precancerous Lesions of Nasopharynx and a Proposed Tumorigenesis Model

The study of the genetic changes of precancerous lesions of the nasopharynx and correlation of the findings with those of other malignant tumours may provide insights into the genesis of this human cancer.

In NPC, the presence of clonal EBV genome and the expression of the latent EBV gene products EBERs and LMP-1 were previously reported in precancerous lesions which were either high grade or carcinoma-in-situ of the nasopharynx.[200] On the other hand, clonal proliferation of the precancerous lesions has been demonstrated by polymerase chain reaction (PCR)-based X-chromosome restriction fragment length polymorphism (RFLP).[201] Recently, we have further identified clonal alterations of chromosomes 3p and 9p in either low and/or high grade precancerous lesions of the nasopharynx. These findings suggest that genetic alterations at either 3p or 9p are early neoplastic events in the development of NPC. Moreover, evidence of EBV infection and overexpression of bcl-2 were found only in cases of high grade precancerous lesions, nasopharyngeal intraepithetical neoplasia III, but not in those of low grade, indicating that LOH at 3p/9p may occur prior to EBV infection in the NPC tumorigenesis (Personal data — Lo and Huang).

Based on the above findings and those demonstrated previously on malignant tumours, together with the well defined aetiological factors, a conceptual model for multi-stage tumorigenesis of nasopharyngeal carcinoma has been formulated (*Figure 6*). It is

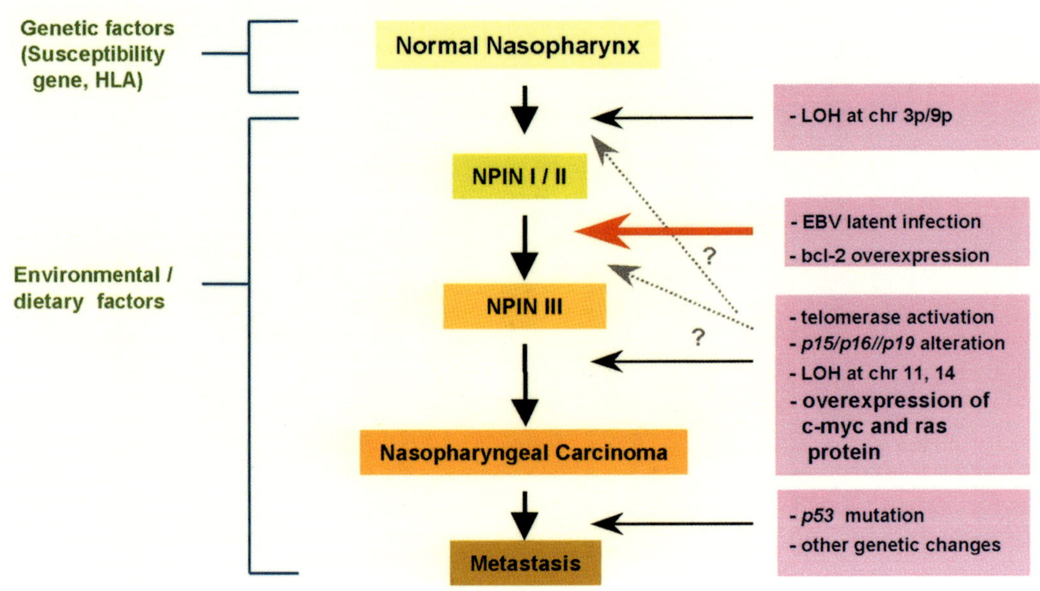

Figure 6. Proposed tumorigenesis model for nasopharyngeal carcinoma.

proposed that NPC may arise as a consequence of multiple genetic changes influenced by environmental factors, both of viral and chemical origin. Involvement of genetic susceptible factor(s) and deletion at chromosome 3p/9p may all play a part in the very early stage of cancer development. It is postulated that the genetic alterations may be induced by chemical carcinogens in the environment which lead to subsequent transformation of normal epithelium to low grade precancerous lesions like NPIN I and II, in which the EBV infection is still absent. Our findings further indicate that latent EBV infection may participate in the progression of low grade to high grade (NPIN III) precancerous lesions of the nasopharynx. Latent EBV infection must be the key event in the clonal selection process in the genesis of NPC and is essential for the further progression to clinically important tumours.

The observation of bcl-2 expression only in the dysplastic cells of the high grade precancerous lesions also suggests that inhibition of the apoptotic pathway may play an important role in the progression of low to high grade precursor lesions. By the continued influence of the environmental factors, some of the genetic changes such as the activation of telomerase, inactivation of the *p16/p15* gene, deletion of chromosome 11q and chromosome 14q may also contribute to the early stage in the development of this cancer. The role of LOH of chromosome 14q and the overexpression of c-myc, ras and p53 protein may participate in further steps in the progression of invasive carcinoma. Moreover, the *p53* gene mutation and perhaps other unknown genetic changes must be associated with the metastatic process of NPC.

References

1. Waterhouse, J., Muir, C., Correa, P., Powell, J. 1976. *Cancer Incidence in Five Continents.* IARC Scientific Publication No. 15. Lyon: IARC.
2. Hirayama, T. 1978. Descriptive and analytical epidemiology of nasopharyngeal carcinoma. In: *Nasopharyngeal Carcinoma: Etiology and Control*, eds. de Thé, G., Ito Y. IARC Scientific Publication No. 20. Lyon: IARC, 167–189.
3. Simons, M.J., Shanmugaratnam, K. (eds.) 1982. *The Biology of Nasopharyngeal Carcinoma. Epidemiology of Nasopharyngeal Carcinoma.* UICC Technical Report Series, Vol. 71. Geneva: International Union Against Cancer, 10–16.
4. Hu, Mengxuan. 1985. Epidemiology of nasopharyngeal carcinoma. In: *Etiology and Pathogenesis of Nasopharyngeal Carcinoma*, eds. Zeng Yi, Ou Baoxiang. Beijing, China: Chinese Academy of Science Press, 1–17.
5. Muir, C., Waterhouse, J., Mack, T., Powell, J., Whelan, S. 1987. *Cancer Incidence in Five Continents.* IARC Scientific Publication No. 88. Lyon: IARC.
6. Mallen, R.W., Shandro, W.G. 1974. Nasopharyngeal carcinoma in Eskimos. *Can. J. Otolaryngol.*; 3:175–179.
7. Lanier, A.P. 1977. Surgery of cancer incidence in Alaskan natives. *Natl. Cancer Inst. Monogr.*; 47:87–88.
8. Nielsen, N.H., Mikkelsen, F., Hansen, J.P. 1977. Nasopharyngeal cancer in Greenland: the incidence in an arctic Eskimo population. *Acta Pathol. Microbiol. Scand. (A)*; 85:850–858.
9. Liang, P.C. 1964. Studies on nasopharyngeal carcinoma in the Chinese: statistical and laboratory investigations. *Chin. Med. J.*; 83:373–390.
10. Ho, J.H.C. 1972. Nasopharyngeal carcinoma (NPC). *Adv. Cancer Res.*; 5:57–92.
11. Ho, H.C. 1975. Epidemiology of nasopharyngeal carcinoma. *J. R. Coll. Surg. Edinb.*; 20:223–235.
12. Shanmugaratnam, K. 1973. Cancer in Singapore — ethnic and dialect group variations in cancer incidence. *Singapore Med. J.*; 14:69–81.
13. Shanmugaratnam, K. 1978. Variations in nasopharyngeal cancer incidence among specific Chinese communities (dialect groups) in Singapore. In: *Nasopharyngeal Carcinoma: Etiology and Control*, eds. de Thé, G., Ito, Y. IARC Scientific Publication No. 20. Lyon: IARC, 191–198.
14. National Cancer Control Office, Nanjing Institute of Geography. 1979. *Atlas of Cancer Mortality in the People's Republic of China.* Shanghai, China: China Map Press.
15. Yu, M.C., Mo, C.C., Chong, W.X., Yeh, F.S., Henderson, B.E. 1988. Preserved foods and nasopharyngeal carcinoma: a case-control study in Guangxi, China. *Cancer Res.*; 48:1954–1959.
16. Shanmugaratnam, K., Lee, H.P., Day, N.E. 1983. *Cancer Incidence in Singapore.* IARC Scientific Publication No. 47. Lyon: IARC, 1968–1977.
17. Buell, P. 1965. Nasopharyngeal cancer in the Chinese of California. *Brit. J. Cancer*; 19:459–470.
18. Buell, P. 1974. The effect of migration on the risk of nasopharyngeal cancer among Chinese. *Cancer Res.*; 34:1189–1191.
19. Yu, Mimi C.C. 1993. Nasopharyngeal carcinoma: epidemiology and dietary factors. *NUH-CME Rev.*; 3:92–96.
20. Simons, M.J., Shanmugaratnam, K. 1982. *The Biology of Nasopharyngeal Carcinoma.* UICC Technical Report Series, Vol. 71. Geneva: UICC, 16.
21. Laing, D. 1967. Nasopharyngeal carcinoma in the Chinese in Hong Kong. *Am. Acad. Ophthalmol. Otolaryngol. Trans.*; 71:934–950.
22. Greenfield, C.C. 1981. *Summary of Results. Commissioner for Census and Statistics, Census and Statistics Dept., Hong Kong.* Hong Kong: Census and Statistics Dept.
23. Hong Kong Hospital Authority. 1995. *Hong Kong Cancer Registry Annual Report 1995.* Hong Kong: Hong Kong Hospital Authority.

24. Simons, M.J., Chan, S.H., Wee, G.B., Shanmugaratnam, K., Day, N.E., de Thé, G. 1975. Probable identification of an HLA second locus antigen associated with a high risk of nasopharyngeal carcinoma. *Lancet*; i:142–143.
25. Chan, S.H., Day, N.E., Kunaratnam, N., Chua, K.B., Simons, M.J. 1983. HLA and nasopharyngeal carcinoma in Chinese — a further study. *Int. J. Cancer*; 32:171–176.
26. Chan, S.H., Chew, C.T., Chandanayingyong, D., Vootiprux, V., Shangruchi, S. 1986. *Proceedings of 3rd Asia-Oceania Histocompatibility Workshop Conference*, ed. M. Aizawa. Japan, 396–400.
27. Zhu, X.N., Chen, R., Kong, F.H., Liu, W. 1990. Human leukocyte antigens -A, -B, -C and -DR and nasopharyngeal carcinoma in northern China. *Ann. Otol. Rhinol. Laryngol.*; 99:286–287.
28. Henle, G., Henle, W. 1976. Epstein-Barr virus specific IgA serum antibodies as an outstanding feature of nasopharyngeal carcinoma. *Int. J. Cancer*; 17:1–17.
29. Ho, H.C., Ng, M.H., Kwan, H.C., Chau, J.C.W. 1976. Epstein-Barr virus specific antibodies in nasopharyngeal carcinoma patients and controls. *Brit. J. Cancer*; 34:655–660.
30. Ho, H.C., Kwan, H.C., Ng, M.H., de Thé, G. 1978. Serum IgA antibody to Epstein-Barr virus capsid antigen preceding symptoms of nasopharyngeal carcinoma. *Lancet*; i:436–437.
31. Huang, D.P., Ho, H.C., Henle, W., Henle, G., Saw, D., Lui, M. 1978. Presence of EBNA in NPC and control patient tissues related to EBV serology. *Int. J. Cancer*; 22:266–274.
32. Henle, W., Henle, G. 1979. Seroepidemiology of the virus. In: *Epstein-Barr Virus*, eds. Epstein, M.A., Achong, B.G. Berlin, Heidelberg, New York: Springer-Verlag.
33. Chan, S.H. 1990 Etiology of nasopharyngeal carcinoma. *Ann. Acad. Med.*; 19:201–207.
34. Ho, J.H.C. 1971. Genetic and environmental factors in nasopharyngeal carcinoma. In: *Recent Advances in Human Tumour Virology and Immunology*, eds. Nakahara, W., Nishioka, K., Hirayama, T. Toyko: University of Tokyo Press, 275–295.
35. Editorial, 1989. Salted fish and nasopharyngeal carcinoma. *Lancet*; i:840–842.
36. Simons, M.J., Shanmugaratnam, K. 1982. *The Biology of Nasopharyngeal Carcinoma*. UICC Technical Report Series. Geneva: UICC, 21–25.
37. Huang, D.P., Ho, J.H.C. 1983. Salted fish and nasopharyngeal carcinoma. In: *Carcinogens and Mutagens in the Environment*, Vol. III, *Naturally Occurring Compounds: Epidemiology and Distribution*, ed. Stich, H.F. U.S.A.: CRC Press, Chap. 3, 21–27.
38. Huang, D.P. 1990. Epidemiology of nasopharyngeal carcinoma. *Ear Nose Throat J.*; 69:222–225.
39. Armstrong, R.W., Armstrong, M.J., Yu, M.C., Henderson, B. 1983. Salted fish and inhalants as risk factors in nasopharyngeal carcinoma in Malaysian Chinese. *Cancer Res.*; 43:2967–2970.
40. Poirier, S., Ohshima, H., de Thé, G., Hubert, A. Bourgade, M.C., Bartsch, H. 1987. Volatile nitroamine levels in common foods from Tunisia, South China, and Greenland, high risk areas for nasopharyngeal carcinoma (NPC). *Int. J. Cancer*; 39:292–296.
41. Ho, H.C. 1972. Current knowledge of the epidemiology of nasopharyngeal carcinoma — a review. In: *Oncogenesis and Herpesviruses*, eds. Bigger, P.M., de Thé, G., Payne, L.N. IARC Scientific Publication No. 2. Lyon: IARC, 357–366.
42. Ho, H.C. 1976. Epidemiology of nasopharyngeal carcinoma. *Gann Monograph on Cancer Research*; 18:49–61.
43. Ho, J.H.C. 1978. An epidemiologic and clinical study of nasopharyngeal carcinoma. *Int. J. Radiat. Oncol. Biol. Phys.*; 4:181–198.
44. Yu, M.C., Garabrant, D.H., Huang, T.B., Henderson, B.E. 1990. Occupational and other non-dietary risk factors for nasopharyngeal carcinoma in Guangzhou, China. *Int. J. Cancer*; 45:1033–1039.
45. Yu, M.C., Huang, T.B., Henderson, B.E. 1989. Diet and nasopharyngeal carcinoma: a case-control study in Guangzhou, China. *Int. J. Cancer*; 43:1077–1082.
46. Rothwell, R.I. 1978. Carcinoma of the nasopharynx in Sabah (Malaysia). *Southeast Asian J. Surg.*; 1:88–91.
47. Anderson, E.N. Jr., Anderson, M.L., Ho, H.C. 1978. Environmental backgrounds of young Chinese nasopharyngeal carcinoma patients. In: *Nasopharyngeal Carcinoma: Etiology and Control*. IARC Scientific Publication No. 20. Lyon: IARC, 231–239.

48. Geser, A., Charnay, N., Day, N.E., Ho, J.H.C., de Thé, G. 1978. Environmental factors in the etiology of nasopharyngeal carcinoma: report on a case-control study in Hong Kong. In: *Nasopharyngeal Carcinoma: Etiology and Control*. IARC Scientific Publication No. 20. Lyon: IARC, 213–229.
49. Yu, M.C., Ho, J.H.C., Lai, S.H., Henderson, B.E. 1986. Cantonese-style salted fish as a cause of nasopharyngeal carcinoma: report of a case-control study in Hong Kong. *Cancer Res.*; 46:956–961.
50. Ning, J.P., Yu, M.C., Wang, Q.S., Henderson, B.E. 1990. Salted fish and other risk factors for nasopharyngeal carcinoma in Tianjin, a low-risk region of China. *J. Natl. Cancer Inst.*; 82:291–296.
51. Zeng, Y.M., Tuppin, P., Hubert, A. Jeannel, D., Pan, Y.J., Pan, Y.J., Xeng, Y, de Thé, G. 1994. Environmental and dietary risk factors for nasopharyngeal carcinoma: a case-control study in Zangwu county, Guangxi, China. *Brit. J. Cancer*; 69:508–514.
52. Pour, P., Stanton, M.F., Kuschner, M., Laskin, S., Shabad, L.M. 1976. Tumours of the respiratory tract. In: *Pathology of Tumours in Laboratory Animals, Vol. 1, Part 2: Tumours of the Rat*. IARC Scientific Publication No. 6. Lyon: IARC, 1–40.
53. IARC, 1978. *Some N-nitroso Compounds*. IARC Monographs on the Evaluation of the Carcinogenic Risk of Chemicals to Humans, Vol. 17. IARC, Lyon.
54. Fong, Y.Y., Chan, W.C. 1973. Dimethylnitrosamine on Chinese marine salted fish. *Fd. Cosmet. Toxicol.*; 11:841–845.
55. Fong, Y.Y., Chan, W.C. 1976. Methods for limiting the content of dimethylnitrosamine in Chinese marine salted fish. *Fd. Cosmet. Toxicol.*; 14:95–98.
56. Huang, D.P., Ho, J.H.C., Gough, T.A. 1978. Analysis for volatile nitrosamines in salted-preserved food stuffs traditionally consumed by southern Chinese. In: *Nasopharyngeal Carcinoma: Etiology & Control*. IARC Scientific Publication No. 20. Lyon: IARC, 309–314.
57. Ho, J.H.C., Huang, D.P., Fong, Y.Y. 1978. Salted fish and nasopharyngeal carcinoma in southern Chinese. *Lancet*; i:626.
58. Fong, L.Y.Y., Ho, J.H.C., Huang, D.P. 1979. Preserved foods as possible cancer hazards: WA rats fed salted fish have mutagenic urine. *Int. J. Cancer*; 23:542–546.
59. Fong, L.Y.Y., Huang, D.P., Lau, S.K.D., Ho, J.H.C. 1980. The Salmonella/Mammalian mutagenicity test to detect chemical mutagens in Chinese preserved foods. In: *Proceedings of the Second Symposium of the Federation of Asian and Oceanian Biochemists*, eds. Khor, H.T., Ong, K.K., Oo, K.C., 157–164.
60. Huang, D.P., Ho, J.H.C., Webb, K.S., Wood, .J., Gough, T.A. 1981. Volatile nitrosamines in salt-preserved fish before and after cooking. *Fd. Cosmet. Toxicol.*; 19:167–171.
61. Huang, D.P., Ho, J.H.C., Saw, D., Teoh, T.B. 1978. Carcinoma of the nasal and paranasal regions in rats fed Cantonese salted marine fish. In: *Nasopharyngeal Carcinoma: Etiology and Control*, eds. de Thé, G., Ito, Y. IARC Scientific Publication No. 20. Lyon: IARC, 315–328.
62. Yu, M.C., Nichols, P.W., Zou, X.N., Estes, J., Henderson, B.E. 1989. Induction of malignant nasal cavity tumours in Wistrar rats fed Chinese salted fish. *Brit. J. Cancer*; 60:198–201.
63. Lee, H.P., Gourley, L. Duffy, S.W., Esteve, J., Lee, J., Day, N.E. 1994. Preserved foods and nasopharyngeal carcinoma: a case-control study among Singapore Chinese. *Int. J. Cancer*; 59:585–590.
64. Henderson, B.E., Louie, E., Jing, J.S., Buell, P., Gardner, M.B. 1976. Risk factors associated with nasopharyngeal carcinoma. *N. Engl. J. Med.*; 295:1101–1106.
65. Yu, M.C., Ho, J.H.C., Ross, K., Henderson, B.E. 1981. Nasopharyngeal carcinoma in Chinese: salted fish or inhaled smoke? *Prev. Med.*; 10:15–24.
66. Chen, C.J., Wang, Y.F., Shieh, T., Chen, J.Y., Liu, M.Y. 1988. Multifactorial etiology of nasopharyngeal carcinoma. Epstein-Barr virus, familial tendency and environmental cofactors. In: *Head and Neck Oncology Research*, eds. Wolf, G.T., Carey, T.E. Amsterdam, Berkeley: Kugler Publication, 469–476.
67. Dobson, W.H. 1924. Cervical lympho-sarcoma. *Chin. Med. J.*; 38:786–787.
68. Djojopranoto, M., Soesilowati, I. 1967. *Nasopharyngeal Cancer in East Java (Indonesia)*. UICC Monograph Series, No. 1, 43–46.

69. Lin, T.M., Chen, K.P., Lin, C.C., Hsu, M.M., Tu, S.M., Chiang, T.C., Jung, P.F., Hirayama, T. 1973. Retrospective study on nasopharyngeal carcinoma. *J. Natl. Cancer Inst.*; 51:1403–1408.
70. Hirayama, T., Ito, Y. 1981. A new view of the etiology of nasopharyngeal carcinoma. *Prev. Med.*; 10:614–622.
71. Shanmugaratnam, K., Higginson, J. 1967. Aetiology of nasopharyngeal carcinoma. In: *Report on a Retrospective Survey in Singapore*. UICC Monograph Series, No. 1, 130–137.
72. Shanmugaratnam, K., Tye, C.Y., Goh, E.H., Chia, K.B. 1978. *Etiological Factors in Nasopharyngeal Carcinoma: A Hospital-based, Retrospective, Case-control, Questionnaire Study*. IARC Scientific Publication No. 20. Lyon: IARC, 19–212.
73. Li, C.C., Yu, M.C., Henderson, B.E. 1985. Some epidemiologic observations of nasopharyngeal carcinoma in Guangdong, People's Republic of China. *Natl. Cancer Inst. Monogr.*; 69:49–52.
74. Mabuchi, K., Bross, D.S., Kessler, I.I. 1985. Cigarette smoking and nasopharyngeal carcinoma. *Cancer*; 55:2874–2876.
75. Ito, K., Kishishita, M., Morigaki, T., *et al.* 1981. Induction and intervention of Epstein-Barr virus expression in human lymphoblastoid cell line: a stimulation model for study of cause and prevention of nasopharyngeal carcinoma and Burkitt's lymphoma. In: *Nasopharyngeal Carcinoma, Cancer Campaign*, eds. Grundman, G., Krueger, G.R.F., Ablashi, D. New York: Gustar Fischer Verlag, 255–263.
76. Hildesheim, A., West, S., DeVeyra, E., Guzman, M.F., Jurado, A., Jones, C., Imai, J., Hinuma, Y. 1992. Herbal medicine use, Epstein-Barr virus and risk of nasopharyngeal carcinoma. *Cancer Res.*; 52:3048–3051.
77. Stinson, W.D. 1940. Epidermoid carcinoma of the nasopharynx occurring in two young brothers. *Ann. Otolaryngol.*; 49:536–539.
78. Brown, T.M., Heath, C.W., Lang, R.M., Lee, S.K., Whalley, B.W. 1976. Nasopharyngeal cancer in Mermuda. *Cancer*; 37:1464–1468.
79. Lanier, A.P., Bender, T.R., Tschopp, C.F., Dohan, P. 1979. Nasopharyngeal carcinoma in an Alaskan Eskimo family: report of three cases. *J. Natl. Cancer Inst.*; 62:1121–1124.
80. Huang, X.L., Wang, Z.J., Luo, F.T., 1980. Familial aggregation and the risk factors of nasopharyngeal carcinoma-a case-control study. *Chung Shan I Hsueh Yuan Hsueh Pao*; 1–50.
81. Yu, M.C. Personal communication.
82. Huang, D.P. 1991. Epidemiology and aetiology. In: *Nasopharyngeal Carcinoma*, eds. van Hasselt, C.A., Gibb, A.G. Hong Kong: The Chinese University Press, 23–35.
83. Chan, S.H., Naito, S. 1984. Report on BW46: histocompatibility testing. In: *Proceedings of 9th International Histocompatibility Workshop Conference, Munich*, ed. Albert, E.D., 153–154.
84. Burt, R.D., Vaughan, T.L., Mcknight, B., Davis, S., Beckmann, A.M., Smith, A.G., Nisperos, B., Swanson, G.M., Berwick, M. 1996. Associations between human leukocyte antigen type and nasopharyngeal carcinoma in caucasians in United States. *Cancer Epidemiol. Biomarkers Prev.*; 5:879–887.
85. Chandanayingyong, D. 1983. BW46. In: *Proceedings of 2nd Asia-Oceania Histopatibility Workshop Conference, Melbourne*, eds. Simons, M.J., Tait, B.D., 127–129.
86. Mellins, E., Arp, B., Singh, D., *et al.* 1990. Point mutations define positions in HLA DR3 molecules that affect antigen presentation. *Proc. Natl. Acad. Sci. USA*; 87:470–471.
87. Murray, R.J., Kurilla, M.G., Brooks, J.M., Thomas, W.A., Rowe, M., Kieff, E., Rickinson, A.B., 1992. Identification of target antigens for the human cytotoxic T-cell response to Epstein-Barr virus (EBV): implication for the immune control of EBV-positive malignancies. *J. Exp. Med.*; 176:157–168.
88. Lu, S.J., Day, N.E., Degos, L., Lepage, V., Wang, P.C., Chan, S.H., Simons, M., McKnight, Easton D., Zeng, Y., de Thé, G. 1990. Lingage of a nasopharyngeal nasopharyngeal carcinoma susceptibility locus to the HLA region. *Nature*; 346:470–47.
89. Ooi, E.E., Ren, E.C., Chen, S.H. 1997. Association between microsatellites within the human MHC and nasopharyngeal carcinoma. *Int. J. Cancer*; 74:229–232.
90. Hildesheim, A., Anderson, L.M., Chen, C.J., Cheng, Y.J., Brinton, L.A., Daly, A.K., Reed, C.D., Chen, I.H., Caporaso, N.E., Hsu, M.M., Chen, J.Y., Idle, J.R., Hoover, R.N., Yang, C.S., Chhabra, S.K. 1997.

CYP2E1 genetic polymorphisms and risk of nasopharyngeal carcinoma in Taiwan. *J. Natl. Cancer. Inst.*; 89:1207–1212.

91. Nilsson, K., Klein, G., Henle, W., Henle, G. 1971. The establishment of lymphoblastoid lines from adult and foetal human lymphoid tissue and its dependence on EBV. *Int. J. Cancer*; 8:443–450.
92. Gerber, P., Nonoyama, M., Lucas, S., Pealin, E., Goldstein, L.I. 1972. Oral excretion of Epstein-Barr virus by healthy subjects and patients with infectious mononucleosis. *Lancet*; ii:988–989.
93. Biggar, R.J., Henle, W., Fleisher, G., Bocker, J., Lennette, E., Henle, G. 1978. Epstein-Barr virus infection in African infants. I. Decline of maternal antibodies and time of infection. *Int. J. Cancer*; 22:239–243.
94. de Thé, G., Geser, A., Day, N.E., Tuker, P.M., Williams, E. H., Beri, D.P., Smith, P.G., Dean, A.G., Bornkamn, G. W., Feorino, P., Henle W. 1978. Epidemiological evidence for a causal relationship between Epstein-Barr virus and Burkitt's lymphoma: results of the Ugandan prospective study. *Nature*; 274:756–761.
95. Epstein, M.A., Achong, B.G. 1979. Introduction and general biology of the virus. In: *The Epstein-Barr Virus*, eds. Epstein, M.A., Achong, B.G. Berlin, Heidelberg, New York: Springer-Verlag.
96. de Thé, G., Day, N.E., Geser, A., Lavoue, M.F., Ho, J.H.C., Simon, M.J., Sohier, R., Tuker, P., Vonka, V., Zavadova, H. 1975. Sero-epidemiology of the Epstein-Barr virus. Preliminary analysis of an international study. In: *Oncogenesis and Herpesviruses II*, Vol. 2, eds. de Thé, G., Epstein, M.A., zur Hausen, H. IARC Scientific Publication No. 11. Lyon: IARC.
97. Henle, W., Henle, G. 1985. Epstein-Barr virus and human malignancies. In: *Advances in Viral Oncology*, ed. Klein, G. New York: Raven Press, 201–238.
98. Chang, R.S., Dan, R., Chan, R. 1988. Epstein-Barr virus infections among university students in a tropical country. *Coll. Health*; 37:115–118.
99. de Thé, G. 1982. Epidemiology of Epstein-Barr virus and associated diseases in man. In: *Herpesviruses*, Vol. 1, ed. Roizman, B. U.S.A.: Plenum Press, 25–87.
100. Desgranges, C., Wolf, H., de Thé, G., Shanmugaratnam, K., Cammoun, N., Ellouz, R., Klein, G., Lennert, K., Munoz, N., Zur Hausen, H. 1975. Nasopharyngeal carcinoma, X. Presence of Epstein-Barr genomes in separate epithelial cells of tumours in patients from Singapore, Tunisia and Kenya. *Int. J. Cancer*; 16:7–11.
101. Zur Hausen, H., Schulte-Holthausen, H., Klein, G., Henle, W., Henle, G., Clifford, P., Santesson, L. 1970. EB virus DNA in biopsies of Burkitt tumors and anaplastic carcinomas of the nasopharynx. *Nature*; 228:1056–1058.
102. Klein, G., Giovanella, B.C., Lindahl, T., Fiakow, P.J., Singh, S., Stehlin, J.S. 1974. Direct evidence for the presence of Epstein-Barr virus DNA and nuclear antigen in malignant epithelial cells from patients with poorly differentiated carcinoma of the nasopharynx. *Proc. Natl. Acad. Sci. USA*; 71:4737–4741.
103. Andersson-Anvret, M., Forsby, N., Klein, G., Henle, W. 1977. Relationship between Epstein-Barr virus and undifferentiated nasopharyngeal carcinoma: correlated nucleic acid hybridization and histopathological examination. *Int. J. Cancer*; 20:486–494.
104. Raab-Traub, N., Flynn, K., Pearson, G. 1987. The differentiated form of nasopharyngeal carcinoma contains Epstein-Barr virus DNA. *Int. J. Cancer*; 39:25–9.
105. Crawford, D.H., Epstein, M.A., Bornkaan, B.W., Achong, B.A., Finerty, F., Thompson, J.A. 1979. Biological and biochemical observations on isolates of EB virus from the malignant epithelial cells of two nasopharyngeal carcinoma. *Int. J. Cancer*; 24:294–302.
106. Huang, D.P., Ho, H.C., Ng, M.H., Lui, M. 1977. Possible transformation of nasopharyngeal epithelial cells in culture with Epstein-Barr virus from B95–8 cells. *Brit. J. Cancer*; 35:630–634.
107. Glaser, R., Lang, C.M., Lee, K. J., Schuller, D.E., Jacobs, D., McQuattie, C. 1980. Attempt to infect non-malignant nasopharyngeal epithelial cells from humans and squirrel monkeys with Epstein-Barr virus. *J. Natl. Cancer Inst.*; 64:1085–1089.
108. Young, L.S., Clark, D., Sixbey, J.W., Rickinson, A.B. 1986. Epstein-Barr virus receptors on human pharyngeal epithelium. *Lancet*; i:240–242.

109. Billaud, M., Busson, P., Huang, D.P., Muller-Lantzch, N., Rousselet, O., Pavlish, H., Wakasugi, J.M., Seigneurin, T., Tursz, T., Lenoir, G.M. 1989. Epstein-Barr virus (EBV) containing nasopharyngeal carcinoma cells express the B-cell activation antigen Blast 2/CD23 and low levels of the EBV receptor/ CR2. *J. Virol.*; 63:4121–4128.
110. Morgan, D.G., Niederman, J.C., Miller, G., Smith, H.W., Dowaliby, J.M. 1979. Site of Epstein-Barr virus replication in the oropharynx. *Lancet*; ii:1154–1157.
111. Sixbey, J.W., Nedrud, J.G., Raab-Traub, N., Hanes, R.A., Pangano, J.S. 1984. Epstein-Barr virus replication in oropharyngeal epithelial cells. *N. Engl. J. Med.*; 310:1225–1230.
112. Gratama, J.W., Oosterveer, M.A.P., Zwaan, F.E., Lepooure, J., Klein, G., Ernberg, I. 1988. Eradication of Epstein-Barr virus by allogeneic bone marrow transplantation: implications for sites of viral latency. *Proc. Natl. Acad. Sci. USA*; 85:8693–8696.
113. Pope, J.H. 1967. Establishment of cell lines from peripheral leukocytes in infectious mononucleosis. *Nature*; 216:810–811.
114. Rickinson, A.B., Kieff, E. 1996. Epstein-Barr Virus. In: *Fields Virology*, 3rd edition, eds. Fields, B.N., Knipe, D.M., Howley, D.M., *et al.* Philadelphia: Lippincott — Raven Publishers, Chap. 75, 2397–2276.
115. Niedobitek, G., Agathanggelou, A., Nicholls, J.M. 1996. Epstein-Barr virus infection and the pathogenesis of nasopharyngeal carcinoma: viral gene expression, tumour cell phenotype, and the role of the lymphoid stroma. *Semin. Cancer Biol.*; 7:165–174.
116. Pathmanathan, R., Prasad, U., Chandrika, G., Sadler, R., Flynn, K., Raab-Traub, N. 1995. Undifferentiated, non-keratizing and squamous cell carcinoma of the nasopharyngeal variant of EBV-infected neoplasia. *Am. J. Pathol.*; 146:1355–1367.
117. Klein, G., Giovanella, B.C., Lindahl, T., Fialkow, P.J., Sing, S., Stehlen, J.S., 1974. Direct evidence fir the presence of Epstein-Barr virus DNA and nuclear antigen in malignant epithelial cells from patients with poorly differentiated carcinoma of the nasopharynx. *Proc. Natl. Acad. Sci. USA*; 7:4737–4741.
118. Klein, G. 1994. The paradoxical coexistence of EBV and the human species. *Epstein-Barr Virus Report*; 1:5–9.
119. Fahraeus, R., Hu, L-F., Ernberg, I., Finke, J. Rowe, M., Klein, G. 1988. Expression of Epstein-Barr virus-encoded proteins in nasopharyngeal carcinoma. *Int. J. Cancer*; 42:329–338.
120. Klein, G. The relationship of the virus to nasopharyngeal carcinoma. In: *The Epstein-Barr Virus*, eds. Epstein, M.A., Achong, B.G. Berlin: Springer-Verlag, 339–350.
121. Niedobitek, G., Hansmann, M.L., Herbst, H., *et al.*, 1991. Epstein-Barr virus and carcinoma: undifferentiated carcinomas but not squamous cell carcinomas of the nasopharynx are regularly associated with the virus. *J. Pathol.*; 165:17–24.
122. Weiss, L.M., Movahed, L.A., Butler, A.E., Swanson, S.A., Friesson, H.F., Cooper, P.H., Colby, T.V. 1989. Analysis of lymphoepithelioma and lymphoepithelioma-like carcinomas for Epstein-Barr virus by in situ hybridization. *Am. J. Surg. Pathol.*; 13:625–631.
123. Young, L.S., Dawson, C.N., Clark, D. Rupain, H., Busson, P., Tursz, T., Johnson, A., Rickinson, A.B. 1988. Epstein-Barr virus gene expression in nasopharyngeal carcinoma. *J. Gen. Virol.*; 69:1051–1065.
124. Brooks, L. Yao, Q.Y., Rickinson, A.B., Young, L.S. 1992. Epstein-Barr virus latent gene transcription in nasopharyngeal carcinoma cells: coexpression of EBNA1, LMP1 and LMP2 transcripts. *J. Virol.*; 66:2689–2697.
125. Niedobitek, G., Young, L.S., Sam, C.K., Brooks, L., Prasad, U., Rickinson, A.B. 1992. Expression of Epstein-Barr virus genes and of lymphocyte activation molecules in undifferentiated nasopharyngeal carcinoma. *Am. J. Pathol.*; 140:879–887.
126. Kieff, E. 1995. Epstein-Barr virus — increasing evidence of a link to carcinoma. Editorial. *N. Engl. J. Med.*; 333:724–726.
127. Raab-Traub, N. 1996. Pathogenesis of Epstein-Barr virus and its associated malignancies. *Seminar in Virol*; 7:315–323.

128. Wang, D., Liebowitz, D., Wang, F., Gregory, C., Rickinson, A., Larson, R., Springer, T., Kieff, E. 1988. Epstein-Barr virus latent membrane protein alters the human B-lymphocyte phenotype: deletion of the amino terminus abolishs activity. *J. Virol.*; 62:41173–84.
129. Wilson, J., Weinberg, W., Hohnson, R., Yuspa, S., Levine, A. 1990. Expression of the BNLF-1 oncogene of Epstein-Barr virus in the skin of transgenic mice induces hyperplasia and aberrant expression of keratin 6. *Cell*; 61:1315–1327.
130. Dawson, C.W., Rickinson, A.B., Young, L.S. 1990. Epstein-Barr virus latent membrane protein inhibits human epithelial cell differentiation. *Nature*; 344:777–780.
131. Fahraeus, R., Rymo, L., Rhim, J.S., Klein, G. 1990. Morphological transformation of human keratinocytes expressing the LMP gene of the Epstein-Barr virus. *Nature*; 345:447–449.
132. Miller, W.E., Earp, H.S., Raab-Traub, N. The Epstein-Barr virus latent membrane protein 1 induces expression of the epidermal growth factor receptor. *J. Virol.*; 69:4390–4398.
133. Paine, R., Scheinman, R.I., Baldwin, A.S., Raab-Traub, N. 1995. Expression of LMP1 in epithelial cells leads to the activation of a select subset of NF-kB/Rel family proteins. *J. Virol.*; 69:4572–4576.
134. Fries, K.L., Miller, W.E., Raab-Traub, N. 1996. Epstein-Barr virus latent membrane protein 1 blocks p53-mediated apoptosis through the induction of the A20 gene. *J. Virol.*; 70:653–8659.
135. Mosialos, G., Birkenbach, M., Yalamanchili, R., VanArsdale, T., Ware, C., Kieff, E. 1995. The Epstein-Barr virus transforming protein LMP1 engages signaling proteins for the tumor necrosis factor receptor family. *Cell*; 80:389–399.
136. Raab-Traub, N., Flynn, K. 1986. The structure of the terminal of the Epstein-Barr virus as a marker of clonal cellular proliferation. *Cell*; 47:883–889.
137. Pathmanathan, R., Prasad, U., Sadler, R., Glynn, K., Raab-Traub, N. 1995. Clonal proliferations of cells infected with Epstein-Barr virus in preinvasive lesions related to nasopharyngeal carcinoma. *N. Engl. J. Med.*; 333:693–698.
138. Sam, C.K., Brooks, L.A., Niedobitek, G., Young, L.S., Prasad, U., Rickinson, A.B. 1993. Analysis of Epstein-Barr virus infection in nasopharyngeal biopsies from a group at high risk of nasopharyngeal carcinoma. *Int. J. Cancer*; 53:957–962.
139. Knox, P.G., Li, Q.X., Rickinson, A.B., Young, L.S. 1996. In vitro production of stable Epstein-Barr-positive epithelial cell clones which resemble the virus:cell interaction observed in nasopharyngeal carcinoma. *Virology*; 215:40–50.
140. Sixbey, J.W., Yao, Q.Y. 1992. Immunoglobulin A-induced shift of Epstein-Barr virus tissue tropism. *Science*; 255:1578–1580.
141. Hu, L-F., Zabarovskv, E.R., Chen, F., Cao, S.L., Ernberg, I., Klein, G., Winberg, G. 1991. Isolation and sequencing of the Epstein-Barr virus BNLF-1 (LMP-1) from Chinese nasopharyngeal carcinoma. *J. Gen. Virol.*; 72:2399–2409.
142. Chen, M.L., Tsai, C.N., Liang, C.L., Shu, C.H., Huang, C.R., Sulitzeanu, D., Liu S.T., Chang, Y.S. 1992. Cloning and characterization of the latent membrane protein (LMP) of a specific Epstein-Barr virus variant derived from nasopharyngeal carinoma in the Taiwanese population. *Oncogene*; 7: 2131–2140.
143. Hu, L.F., Chen, F., Zheng, X., Ernberg, I., Cao, S.L., Christensson, B., Klein G., Winberg, G. 1993. Clonability and tumorigenicity of human epithelial cells expressing the EBV encoded membrane protein LMP1. *Oncogene*; 8:1575–1583.
144. Zheng, X., Yuan, F., Hu, L.-F., Chen, F., Klein, G., Christensson, B. 1994. Effect of B-lymphocytes and NPC-derived EBV-LMP1 gene expression on in vitro growth and differentiation of human epithelial cells. *Int. J. Cancer*; 57:747–753.
145. Li, S.N., Chang, Y.S., Liu, S.T. 1996. Effect of a 10-amino acid deletion on the oncogenic activity of latent membrane protein 1 of Epstein-Barr virus. *Oncogene*; 12:2129–2135.
146. Trivedi, P., Hu, L.F., Christensson, B., Masucci, M.G., Klein, G., Winberg, G. 1994. Epstein-Barrr virus (EBV)-encoded membrane protein LMP1 froma nasopharyngeal carcinoma is non-immunogenic in a murine model system, in contrast to a B cell derived homologue. *Eur. J. Cancer*; 30A:84–88.

147. Cheung, S.T., Lo, K.W., Leung, S.F., Chan, W.Y., Choi, P.H.K., Johnson, P.J., Lee, J.C.K., Huang, D.P. 1996. Prevalence of LMP1 deletion variant of Epstein-Barr virus in nasopharyngeal carcinoma and gastric tumors in Hong Kong. *Int. J. Cancer*; 66:711–712.
148. Miller, W.R., Edwards, R.H., Walling, D.M., Raab-Traub, N. 1994. Sequence variation in the Epstein-Barr virus latent membrane protein 1. *J. Gen. Virol.*; 75:2729–2740.
149. Vogelstein, B., Kinzler, K.W. 1993. The multistep nature of cancer. *Trends Genet.*; 9:138–141.
150. Mitelman, F., Mark-Vendel, E., Mineur, A., Giovanella, B., Klein, G. 1983. A 3q+ marker chromosome in EBV-carrying nasopharyngeal carcinomas. *Int. J. Cancer*; 32:651–655.
151. Huang, D.P., Ho, J.H.C., Chan, W.K., Lau, W.H., Lui, M. 1989. Cytogenetics of undifferentiated nasopharyngeal carcinoma xenografts from southern Chinese. *Int. J. Cancer*; 43:963–969.
152. Bernheim, A., Rousselet, G., Massaad, L., Busson, P., Tursz, T. 1993 Cytogenetic studies in three xenografted nasopharyngeal carcinomas. *Cancer Genet. Cytogenet.*; 66:11–15.
153. Zhang, S., Gao, X., Zeng, Y. 1983. Cytogenetic studies on an epithelial cell line derived from poorly differentiated nasopharyngeal carcinoma. *Int. J. Cancer*; 31:587–590.
154. Chang, Y.S., Lin, S.Y., Lee, P.F., Durff, T., Chung, H.C., Tsai, M.S. 1989. Establishment and characterization of a tumor cell line from human nasopharyngeal carcinoma tissue. *Cancer Res.*; 49:6752–6757.
155. Lin, C.T., Chan, W.Y., Chen, W., Huang, H.M., Wu, H.C., Hsu, M.M., Chuang, S.M., Wang, C.C. 1993. Characterization of seven newly established nasopharyngeal carcinoma cell lines. *Lab. Invest.*; 68:716–727.
156. Tien, H.F., Lee, F.Y., Chuang, S.M., Lin, C.T. 1990. Cytogenetic characterization of a nasopharyngeal carcinoma cell line and its subline. *Cancer Genet. Cytogenet.*; 49:31–36.
157. Mitelman, F., Mark-Vendel, E., Mineur, A., Giovanella, B., Klein, G. 1983. A 3q+ marker chromosome in EBV-carrying nasopharyngeal carcinomas. *Int. J. Cancer*; 32:651–655.
158. Kristensen, M., Quek, H.H., Chew, C.T., Chan, S.H. 1991. A cytogenetic study of 74 nasopharyngeal carcinoma biopsies. *Ann. Acad. Med. Singapore*; 20:597–600.
159. Hui, A.B.Y., Cheung, S.T., Fong, Y, Lo, K.W., Huang, D.P. 1998. Characterization of a new EBV-associated nasopharyngeal carcinoma cell line. *Cancer Genet. Cytogenet.*; 101:83–88.
160. Huang, D.P., Lo, K.W., Choi, P.H.K., Ng, A.Y.T., Tsao S.Y., Yiu, G.K.C., Lee, J.C.K. 1991. Loss of heterozygosity on the short arm of chromosome 3 in nasopharyngeal carcinoma. *Cancer Genet. Cytogenet.*; 54:91–99.
161. Lo, K.W., Tsao, S.W., Leung, S.F., Choi, P.H.K., Lee, J.C.K., Huang, D.P. 1994. Detailed deletion mapping on the short arm of chromosome 3 in nasopharyngeal carcinoma. *Int. J. Oncol.*; 4: 1359–1364.
162. Hu, L.F., Eiriksdottir, G., Lebedeva, T., Kholodniouk, I., Alimor, A., Chen, F., Luo, Y., Zabarovsky, E.R., Ingvarson, S., Klein, G., Ernberg, I. 1996 Loss of heterozygosity on chromosome 3p in nasopharyngeal carcinoma. Genes Chrom. *Cancer*; 17:118–126.
163. Mutlrangura, A., Tanunyutthawongese, C., Pornthanakasem, W., Kerehanjanarong, V., Sriuranpong, V., Yenrudi, S., Suplyaphun, P., Voravud, N. 1997. Genomic alterations in nasopharyngeal carcinoma: loss of heterozygosity and Epstein-Barr virus infection. *Brit. J. Cancer*; 76:770–776.
164. Cheng, Y., Poulos, N.E., Lung, M.L., Hampton, G., Ou, B., Lerman, M.I., Stanbridge, E.J. 1998. Functional evidence for a nasopharyngeal carcinoma tumor suppressor gene that maps at chromosome 3p21.3. *Proc. Natl. Acad. Sci. USA*; 95:3042–3047.
165. Huang, D.P., Lo, K.W., van Hasselt, A., Woo, J.K.S., Choi, P.H.K., Leung, S.F., Cheung, S.T., Cairns, P., Sidransky, D., Lee, J.C.K. A region of homozygous deletion on chromosome 9p21–22 in primary nasopharyngeal carcinoma. *Cancer Res.*; 55:2039–2043, 1995.
166. Hui, A.B.Y., Lo, K.W., Leung, S.F., Choi, P.H.K., Fong, Y., Lee, J.C.K., Huang, D.P. 1996. Loss of heterozygosity on the long arm of chromosome 11 in nasopharyngeal carcinoma. *Cancer Res.*; 56:3225–3229.
167. Cheng, R.Y.S., Lo, K.W., Huang, D.P., Tsao, S.W. 1997. Loss of heterozygosity on chromosome 14 in primary nasopharyngeal carcinoma. *Int. J. Oncol.*; 10:1047–1050.

168. Lo, K.W., Huang, D.P. Unpublished data.
169. Sun, Y., Hildesheim, A., Li, H., Lanier, A.P., Cao, Y., Yao, K.T., Yang, C.S., Colburn, N.H. 1995 The von Hippel-Lindau (VHL) disease tumor-suppressor gene is not mutated in nasopharyngeal carcinoma. *Int. J. Cancer*; 60:437–438.
170. Ohta, M., Inoue, M., Cotticelli, M.G., Kastury, K., Baffa, R., Palazzo, J., Siprashvili, Z., Mori, M., McCue, P., Druck, T., Croce, C.M., Huebner, K. 1996. The FHIT gene, spanning the chromosome 3p14.2 fragile site and renal carcinoma-associated t(3;8) breakpoint, is abnormal in digestive tract cancers. *Cell*; 84:587–597.
171. Serrano, M., Hannon, G.J., Beach, D. 1993 A new regulatory motif in cell-cycle control causing specific inhibition of cyclin D/CDK4. *Nature*; 366:704–707.
172. Kamb, A., Gruis, N., Feldhaus, J., Liu, Q., Harshnman, K., Tavtigian, S., Stockert, E., Day, R., Johnson, B., Skolnick, M. 1994. A cell cycle regulator potentially involved in genesis of many tumor types. *Science*; 264:436–439.
173. Lo, K.W., Huang, D.P., Lau, K.M. 1995. p16 gene alterations in nasopharyngeal carcinoma. *Cancer Res.*; 55:2039–2043.
174. Lo, K.W., Cheung, S.T., Leung, S.F., van Hasselt, A., Tsang, Y.S., Mak, K.F., Chung, Y.F., Woo, J.K.S., Lee, J.C.K., Huang, D.P. 1996. Hypermethylation of the p16 gene in nasopharyngeal carcinoma. *Cancer Res.*; 56:2721–2725.
175. Lo, K.W., Huang, D.P. Unpublished data.
176. Gulley, M.L., Nicholls, J.M., Schneider, B.G., Amin, M.B., Ro, J.Y., Geradts, J. 1998. Nasopharyngeal carcinomas frequently lack the p16/MTS1 tumor suppressor protein but consistently express the retinoblastoma gene product. *Am. J. Pathol.*; 152:865–869.
177. Sun, Y., Hildesheim, A., Li, H., Lanier, A.E.P., Cao, Y., Yao, K.T., Raab-Traub, N., Yang, C.S. 1995. No point mutation but decreased expression of the p16/MTS1 tumor suppressor gene in nasopharyngeal carcinomas. *Oncogene*; 10:785–788.
178. Sun, Y., Hegamyer, G., Colburn, N.H. 1993. Nasopharyngeal carcinoma shows no detectable retinoblastoma susceptibility gene alterations. *Oncogene*; 8:791–795.
179. Lo, K.W., Mok, C.H., Huang, D.P., Liu, Y.X., Choi, P.H.K., Lee, J.C.K., Tsao, S.W. 1992. p53 mutation in human nasopharyngeal carcinomas. *Anticancer Res.*; 12:1957–1964.
180. Effert, P., McCoy, R., Abdel-Hamid, M., Flynn, K., Zhang, Q., Busson, P., Tursz, T., Liu, E., Raab-Traub, N. 1992. Alterations of the p53 gene in nasopharyngeal carcinoma. *J. Virol.*; 66:3768–3775.
181. Chakrani, F., Armand, J., Lenoir, G., Ju, L.Y., Liang, J.P., May, E., May, P. 1995. Mutations clustered in exon 5 of the p53 gene in primary nasopharyngeal carcinomas from southeastern Asia. *Int. J. Cancer*; 61:316–320.
182. Spruck III, C.H., Tsai, Y.C., Huang, D.P., Yang, A.S., Rideout III, W.M., Gonzalez-Zulueta, M., Choi, P., Lo, K.W., Yu, M.C., Jones, P.C. 1992. Absence of p53 gene mutations in primary nasopharyngeal carcinomas. *Cancer Res.* ; 52:4787–4790.
183. Sun, Y., Hegamyer, G., Cheng, Y.J., Hildesheim, A., Chen, J.Y., Chen, I.H., Cao, Y., Yao, K.T., Colburn, N.H. 1992. An infrequent point mutation of the p53 gene in human nasopharyngeal carcinoma. *Proc. Natl. Acad. Sci. USA*; 89:6516–6520.
184. Sun, Y., Dong, A., Nakamura, K., Colburn, N.H. 1993. Dosage-dependent dominance over wild-type p53 of a mutant p53 isolated from nasopharyngeal carcinoma. *F.A.S.B.*; 7:944–949.
185. Niedobitek, G., Agathanggelou, A., Barber, P., Smallman, L.A., Jones, E.L., Young, L.S. 1993. p53 expression and Epstein-Barr virus infection in undifferentiated and squamous cell nasopharyngeal carcinomas. *J. Pathol.*; 170:457–461.
186. Porter, M.J., Field, J.K., Lee, J.C.K., Leung, S.F., Lo, D., van Hasselt, C.A. 1994. Detection of the tumour suppressor gene p53 in nasopharyngeal carcinoma in Hong Kong Chinese. *Anticancer Res.*; 14: 1357–1360.
187. Sheu, L.F., Chen, A., Tseng, H.H., Leu, F.J., Lin, J.K., Ho, K.C., Meng, C.L. 1995. Assessment of p53 expression in nasopharyngeal carcinoma. *Human Path.*; 26:380–386.

188. Sun, Y., Hildesheim, A., Li, H., Li, Y., Chen, J.Y., Hayes, R.B., Pothman, N., Bi, W.F., Cao, Y., Yao, K.T., Lanier, A.P., Hegamyer, G., El-Deiry, W.S., Xiong, Y., Colburn, N.H. 1995. No point mutation but a codon 31 ser > arg polymorphism of the WAF-1/CIP-1/p21 tumor suppressor gene in nasopharyngeal carcinoma (NPC): the polymorphism distingushes Caucasians from Chinese. *Cancer Epidemiol. Biomarkers Prev.*; 4:261–267.
189. Qian, W., Hu, L.F., Chen, F., Wang, Y., Magnusson, K.P., Kashuba, E., Klein, G., Wiman, K.G. 1995. Infrequent MDM2 gene amplification and absence of gross WAF1 Gene alterations in nasopharyngeal carcinoma. *Eur. J. Cancer B Oral Oncol.*; 31B:328–332.
190. Pomerantz, J., Schreiber-Agus, N., Liegeois, N.J., Silverman, A., Alland, L., Chin, L., Potes, J. Chen, K., Orlow, I., Lee, H.W., Cordon-Cardo, C., Depinho, R.A. 1998. The Ink4a tumor suppressor gene product, p19Arf, interacts with MDM2 and neutralizes MDM2's inhibition of p53. *Cell*; 92:713–723.
191. Zhang, Y., Xiong, Y., Yarbrough, W.G. 1998. ARF promotes MDM2 degradation and stabilizes p53: ARF-INK4a locus deletion impairs both the Rb and p53 tumor suppression pathways. *Cell*; 725–734.
192. Lu, O.L., Elia, G., Lucas, S., Thomas, J.A. 1993. Bcl-2 proto-oncogene expression in Epstein-Barr-virus-associated nasopharyngeal carcinoma. *Int. J. Cancer*; 53:29–35.
193. Porter, M.J., Field, J.K., Leung, S.F., Lo, D., Lee, J.C., Spandidos, D.A., van Hasselt, C.A. 1994. The detection of the c-myc and ras oncogenes in nasopharyngeal carcinoma by immunohistochemistry. *Acta Otolaryngol.*; 114:105–109.
194. Harn, H.J., Ho, L.I., Liu, C.A., Liu, G.C., Lin, F.G., Lin, J.J., Chang, J.Y., Lee, W.H. 1996. Down regulation of bcl-2 by p53 in nasopharyngeal carcinoma and lack of detection of its specific t(14; 18) chromosomal translocation in fixed tissues. *Histopathology*; 28:317–323.
195. Yung, W.C.W., Sham, J.S.T., Choy, D.T.K., Ng, M.H. 1995. ras mutations are uncommon in nasopharyngeal carcinoma. *Eur. J. Cancer B Oral Oncol.*; 31B:399–400.
196. Cao, Y., Sun, Y., Poirier, S., Winterstein, D., Hegamyer, G., Seed, J., Malin, S., Colburn, N.H. 1991. Isolation and partial characterization of a transformation-associated sequence from human nasopharyngeal carcinoma. *Mol. Carcinog.*; 4:297–307.
197. Sun, Y. 1995. Molecular oncology of human nasopharyngeal carcinoma. *Cancer J.*; 8:325–330.
198. Cheng, R.Y.S., Yuen, P.W., Nicholls, J.M., Zheng, Z., Wei, W., Sham, J.S.T., Yang, X.H., Cao, L., Huang, D.P., Tsao, S.W. 1998. Telomerase activation in nasopharyngeal carcinomas. *Brit. J. Cancer*; 77:456–460.
199. Ohmura, H., Tahara, H., Suzuki, M., Ide, T., Shimizu, M., Yoshida, M.A., Tahara, E., Shay, J.W., Barrett, J.C., Oshimura, M. 1995. Restoration of the cellular senescence program and repression of telomerase by human chromosome 3. *Jpn. J. Cancer Res.*; 86:899–904.
200. Pathmanathan, R., Prasad, U., Chandrika, G., Sadler, R., Flynn, K., Raab-Traub, N. 1995. Clonal proliferations of cell infected with Epstein-Barr virus in preinvasive lesions related to nasopharyngeal carcinoma. *N. Engl. J. Med.*; 333:693–698.
201. Xin, J., Yao, K.T. 1996. The clonal progression in the neoplastic process of nasopharyngeal carcinoma. *Biochem. Biophys. Res. Commun.*; 221:122–128.

CHAPTER 4

Precancerous Changes

Joseph C.K. Lee

Historical Review

Precancerous changes, defined as "conditions of organs and tissues which sometimes, often or regularly lead to the genesis of cancer", have been described in humans[1] and in experimental animals.[2] Much is known about the histopathological changes in the oesophagus, upper aerodigestive tract, skin and in particular the uterine cervix, where extensive cytological and histological studies have been reported.[3,4,5,6] These observations have emphasized the nature and characteristics of precancerous lesions, their biological behaviour and application in early diagnosis and management of patients.

The earliest reference to pre-invasive cancerous change in the nasopharynx was in a 1957 report, in which Teoh[7] carried out a detailed study of 31 autopsies on Chinese patients with nasopharyngeal carcinoma (NPC). He documented carcinoma *in situ* (CIS) in the posterior wall of the nasopharynx of a patient adjacent to the primary growth and suggested "multiplicity of origin" of NPC. Liang *et al.* 1962[8] studied 500 biopsies and 300 complete autopsies in Canton and discovered 16 cases of precancerous changes and 17 cases of CIS. They found "squamous metaplasia to be of great significance in the histogenesis of nasopharyngeal carcinoma". Shen,[9] after reviewing 300 biopsies of the nasopharynx and 10 nasopharynges from autopsies, defined atypical hyperplasia and CIS. Shanmugaratnam and Muir[10] and Yeh[11] also reported CIS in tissue adjacent to NPC. Zong and his group in China[12] reported two sub-types of nasopharyngeal carcinoma *in situ* (NPCIS) and demonstrated an increase in DNA content in NPCIS over that in non-cancerous nasopharyngeal tissue. They postulated that "reserve cells or indifferent cells having undergone dysplasia may transform into malignant CIS cells". All these studies are reported from southern China, Taiwan, and Singapore.

In our studies on biopsies of human nasopharynges (NP) and autopsy specimens,[13] we have observed a spectrum of pathological changes in the mucosa ranging from acute inflammation to early invasive cancer.

Table 1 gives a chronological summary of reports on this subject.

Table 1. Review of literature on precancerous changes in NP.

Author	Year	Description	Reference
Teoh	1957	CIS in posterior wall	(7)
Liang *et al.*	1962	NPCIS, Metaplasia	(8)
Shen	1964	Atypical hyperplasia, CIS	(9)
Shanmugaratnam	1967	CIS	(10)
Yeh	1967	CIS	(11)
Zong and Li	1986	NPCIS — Columnar & Squamous	(12)
Lee	1986	NPIN	(13)

CIS: Carcinoma in situ
NP: Nasopharynx
IN: Intraepithelial neoplasia

Pathological Changes in the Nasopharyngeal Mucosa

Inflammation

Acute and chronic inflammation are commonly present in the nasopharynx. The former is usually associated with mucosal ulceration containing varying amounts of polymorphonuclear leukocytes, plasma cells and some eosinophils. Where chronic inflammation exists, lymphocytes and fibrosis are present. These are usually aggregated below the mucosa.

The role of regeneration and repair, if any, in predisposing the mucosa to cancerous changes is unknown at present. The association of regeneration of ulcerated pseudo-stratified columnar epithelium with resultant metaplastic and dysplastic changes, as observed in the bronchial mucosa,[14] is distinctly possible, but this sequence of events would require substantiation in experimental animal models.

Hyperplasia

Hyperplasia has been observed in the epithelial lining cells of the nasopharyngeal mucosa, in the glands and ducts, as well as in the lymphoid tissue. Glandular hyperplasia is often associated with inflammation, while lymphoid hyperplasia may be present with or without acute inflammation. Germinal centres are frequently seen. Recent work on the lymphocytic infiltration in NPC tissue has demonstrated the presence of a variety of lymphokines and the sharing of some lymphoid receptors with nasopharyngeal epithelial cells.[15] Billaud *et al.* detected the presence of the receptor Blast2/CD23, which normally activates B-cells, in medium taken from short-term cultures of NPC cell lines.[16] This finding suggests expression of the lymphoid receptor in epithelial cells and "a possible role for this molecule in the pathogenesis of NPC".[16]

Hyperplasia of the stratified squamous epithelium results in an orderly increase in the thickness of the mucosa from the normal 4 to 5 cells to a thickened mucosa 12 cells in depth. In the columnar epithelial areas, simple hyperplasia and basal cell hyperplasia are seen. This is analogous to the changes seen in the cervix of the uterus.

Zong[17] classified the epithelial changes into simple hyperplasia, reserve cell hyperplasia, goblet cell hyperplasia and endophytic simple hyperplasia. He observed, as we did, that hyperplasia of the columnar epithelium was more common than simple hyperplasia of the stratified squamous epithelium.

Metaplasia

This is commonly seen in the columnar epithelial areas of the nasopharynx (NP) where there is focal replacement by stratified squamous epithelium. Li[18] subclassified metaplasia into: (a) transitional metaplasia, (b) superficial squamous metaplasia, (c) deep squamous metaplasia, (d) thin full-thickness squamous metaplasia, (e) thick full-thickness squamous metaplasia, (f) thick full-thickness squamous metaplasia forming regular stratified squamous epithelium and (g) squamous metaplasia with atypical hyperplasia. These changes are probably a reflection of varying degrees of severity. The significance of such a subclassification remains to be demonstrated. We prefer to combine together all groups, except those with atypical changes, under "squamous metaplasia" as has been accepted practice for the uterine cervix. According to Liang, 50% of biopsies, positive for NPC, contain additional foci of squamous metaplasia.[8] In our own experience the incidence of squamous metaplasia varies between 16.8% and 45.3% (*Table* 2).

Intraepithelial Neoplasia (NPIN)

In 1957 Teoh, in his classic report of autopsy findings on 31 NPC patients, was the first to observe intraepithelial neoplastic changes in the nasophyarnx.[7] In case number 6 of his report, he observed, "besides primary growth in the left tubal elevation, multiple sections reveal the epithelial changes of carcinoma *in situ* in the posterior wall". Liang *et al*., of Guangzhou, China, reported in 1962 "Among the biopsy specimens in which a portion of the nasopharynx mucosa was included, there were found to be 54 cases with

Table 2. Nasopharyngeal Intraepithelial Neoplasia (NPIN).

Type of specimen	Number	Hyperplasia (%)	Squamous metaplasia (%)	Koilocytic changes (%)	NPIN (%)
Autopsies	137	58 (42.3)	23 (16.8)	1 (0.7)	2 (1.5)
Surgical biopsies	266				
Positive for NPC	86	42 (48.8)	39 (45.3)	10 (11.6)	63 (73.3)
Negative for NPC	180	45 (25.0)	64 (35.6)	7 (3.9)	23 (12.8)

NPC: Nasopharyngeal carcinoma

carcinomatous change.[8] Among the 54 cases with malignant change, 17 showed carcinoma *in situ*, and 34 showed early invasive carcinoma. The malignant change was multicentric in 33 cases (61%)". Based on the study of 300 biopsies and 10 autopsies, Shen made a distinction between atypical hyperplasia and carcinoma *in situ* and defined the two types of change. In carcinoma *in situ* there were features of malignant changes in cells, such as nuclear pleomorphism, hyperchromatism and clumping of chromatin, whereas in atypical hyperplasia such changes were observed to a lesser extent. Carcinoma *in situ* displayed malignant cells through the full-thickness of the mucosa, while atypical hyperplasia usually contained abnormal cells in the basal part of the epithelium.[9] More recently, Zong and Li[12] further characterized carcinoma *in situ* after reviewing 2,742 biopsies. In these they found 64 specimens with "paracancerous CIS", which they further divided into "Columnar type" and "Squamous type", both of which showed an increase in nuclear DNA content over that in normal epithelium and metaplastic squamous epithelium.

We have studied 266 consecutive biopsies of the nasopharynx and 137 nasopharynges removed at autopsy.[19] The results are shown in *Table 2*. The NP mucosa showed varying degrees of intraepithelial neoplasia (NPIN) ranging from mild to severe changes or CIS (*Figure 1*).

With the current concepts on intraepithelial neoplastic changes in other sites of the body in mind, we have defined NPIN as follows:

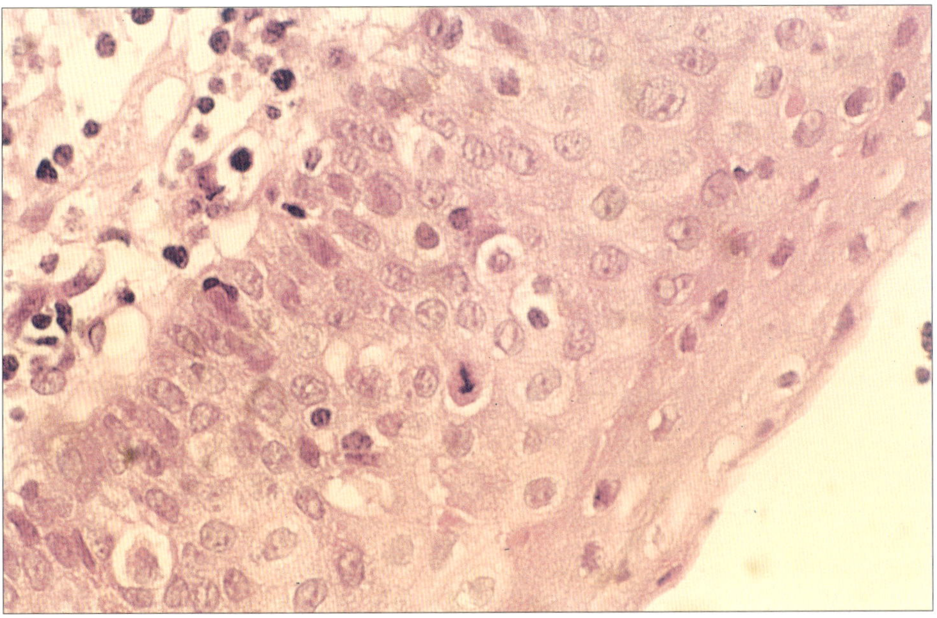

Figure 1. Photomicrograph of a histological section of an intraepithelial lesion of the nasopharynx showing involvement of the lower two-thirds of the epithelium by abnormal cells, NPIN-II changes. Haematoxylin and eosin stain. Mag. ×1250.

NPIN 1: Isolated atypical cells in the lower 2/3rd of the epithelium or numerous undifferentiated cells in the lower 1/3rd.
NPIN II: Undifferentiated cells in the lower 2/3rd of the epithelium.
NPIN III: Undifferentiated cells in the full thickness of the epithelium.

In further work Wai and McGuire[20] conducted a morphometrical analysis of histological sections of nasopharyngeal biopsies utilizing an interactive semi-automatic image analyzer. The results supported the above 3-tiered grading system of NPIN which is identical to that used in the cervix uteri.

Yuen, Chew and Lee[21] have studied the cell surface carbohydrate profiles using a variety of lectins. These studies showed marked differences in the binding ability of these reagents to normal, NPIN or invasive cancerous tissue. These findings may be used as a basic guide in the evaluation of pre-invasive and invasive lesions of the nasopharynx.

Pathmanathan *et al.*[22] presented evidence of Epstein-Barr Virus (EBV) in "pre-invasive lesions" and the clonal proliferation of such cells which might lead to carcinoma. Our studies[23] showed loss of heterozygocity (LOH) at 3p and 9p and the absence of EBV in the early precancerous lesions suggesting that LOH at 3p or 9p may occur prior to EBV infection.

While it is clear that pre-invasive carcinoma can exist in the nasopharynx, the extent of this condition, its biological behaviour and clinical significance require further exploration. However, it is hoped that, as is the case with CIN in the uterine cervix, early diagnosis of pre-invasive carcinoma in the nasopharynx as NPIN may be possible.

Experimental studies

Early attempts failed to induce cancer in the nasopharynx of mice, rabbits, rats or dogs.[24] Wang in 1964[25] instilled benzo(a)pyrene, dimethylbenantracene and methylcholanthrene into the posterior nasal orifice through bent needles and was successful in inducing "*in situ* nasopharyngeal cancer of squamous and columnar cell types". The tumours were mainly located on the hard palate and within the nasal cavity. It should be noted however that the cancers produced were of squamous cell type and not the typical undifferentiated carcinoma seen in the human nasopharynx. Huang[26] induced cancers in the nasal and paranasal regions of rats fed with preserved salted marine fish. These tumours were presumably induced by chemical carcinogens in the preserved fish.

Concluding remarks

While much progress has taken place on clinical staging and treatment of NPC, studies on precancerous changes and early invasive carcinoma of the nasopharynx have not been keeping pace with these advances. A thorough documentation of NPIN, both histologically and cytologically, would be most beneficial in designing strategic methods for early diagnosis and screening of populations at risk. At the same time a better understanding of the histogenetic origin of NPC would contribute towards the identification of carcinogenetic vents and provide further clues to the aetiology.

Reference

1. Henson, D.E., Albores-Saavedra, J. (eds.) 1986. *The Pathology of Incipient Neoplasia*. Philadelphia: W.B. Saunders Company.
2. Suss, R., Kinzel, V., Scriber, J.D. (eds.) 1973. *Cancer, Experiments and Concepts*. New York: Springer-Verlag.
3. Rubio, C.A., Liu F-S, Zhao, H-Z. 1989. Histological classification of intraepithelial neoplasias and microinvasive squamous carcinoma of the esophagus. *Am. J. Surg. Pathol.*; 13:685–690.
4. Crissman, J.D., Zarbo, R.J. 1989. Dysplasia, *in situ* carcinoma, and progression to invasive squamous cell carcinoma of the upper aerodigestive tract. *Am. J. Surg. Pathol.*; 13 (Suppl. 1):5–16.
5. Reagan, J.W., Seidemann, I.L., Saracusa, Y. 1953. The cellular morphology of carcinoma *in situ* and dysplasia or atypical hyperplasia of the uterine cervix. *Cancer*; 6:224–235.
6. Richart, R.M. 1966. Colpomicroscopic studies of cervical intraepithelial neoplasia. *Cancer*; 19:395–405.
7. Teoh, T.B. 1957. Epidermoid carcinoma of the nasopharynx among Chinese: a study of 31 necropsies. *J. Path. Bact.*; 73:451–465.
8. Liang, P.C., Chén, C.C., Chu, C.C., Hu, Y.F., Chu, H.M., Tsung, Y.S. 1962. The histologic classification, biological characteristics and histogenesis of nasopharyngeal carcinomas. *Chin. Med. J.*; 81:629–658.
9. Shen, Y.Y. 1964. General pathological changes in the mucosal epithelium, atypical hyperplasia and carcinoma *in situ*. *Chin. J. Pathol.*; 388–391 (in Chinese).
10. Shanmugaratnam, K., Muir, C.S. 1967. *Nasopharyngeal Carcinoma Origin and Structure in Cancer of the Nasopharynx*, Vol. 1, eds. Muir, C.S., Shanmugaratnam, K. UICC Monograph Series. Copenhagen: Munksgaard, 152–162.
11. Yeh, S. 1967. *Histology of Nasopharyngeal Cancer in Cancer of the Nasopharynx*, Vol. 1, eds. Muir, C.S., Shanmugaratnam, K. UICC Monograph Series. Copenhagen: Munksgaard, 147–152.
12. Zong, Y.S., Li, Q.X. 1986. Histopathology of paracancerous nasopharyngeal carcinoma *in situ*. *Chin. Med. J.*; 99:763–771.
13. Lee, J.C.K., Suen, M.W.M. 1986. Intraepithelial neoplasia in mucosa of human nasopharyngeal carcinoma. In: *Abstracts of the XVI International Congress of the International Academy of Pathology, Vienna.*
14. McDowell, E.M., Hess, F.G., Trump, B.F. 1980 Epidermoid metaplasia, carcinoma in situ and carcinomas of the lung. In: *Diagnostic Electron Microscopy*, Vol. 3, eds. Trump, B.F., Jones, R. New York: John Wiley and Sons, 37–96.
15. Lin, H. 1990. *Lymphoinfiltration and Nasopharyngeal Carcinoma*. Thesis, The University of Hong Kong, Hong Kong.
16. Billaud, M., Busson, P., Huang, D., Mueller-Lantzch, N., Rousselet, G., Pavlish, O., Wakasugi, H., Seigneurin, J.M., Tursz, T., Lenoir, G.M. 1989. Epstein-Barr Virus (EBV) — containing nasopharyngeal carcinoma cells express the B-Cell activation antigen Blast2/CD23 and low levels of the EBV receptor CR2. *J. Virol.*; 63:4121–4128.
17. Zong, Y.S. 1987. Histopathology of nasopharyngeal carcinoma. In: *Etiology and Pathogenesis of Nasopharyngeal Carcinoma*, eds. Zeng, Y., Ou, B. Beijing: The People's Medical Publishing House, 122–153.
18. Li, C.C., Pan, Q.C., Chen, C.C. 1983. Hyperplasia and metaplasia in the nasopharynx. In: *Nasopharyngeal Carcinoma, Clinical and Laboratory Researches*, eds. Li, C.C., Pan, Q.C., Chen, C.C., 143–153 (in Chinese).
19. Szanto, P.B. 1944. A modified technique for the removal of the nasopharynx and accompanying organs of the throat. *Arch. Path.*; 38:313–320.
20. Wai, C.W.G. 1990. *Morphometric Studies of Intraepithelial Neoplasia and Associated Lesions in the Cervix Uteri and the Nasopharynx*. Thesis. The Chinese University of Hong Kong, Hong Kong.

21. Yuen, K.W., Chew, E.C., Lee, J.C.K. 1990. Studies of lectin binding to the normal and neoplastic nasopharyngeal epithelium. In: *Abstracts of the XVIII International Congress of the International Academy of Pathology, Buenos Aires.*
22. Pathmanathan, R., Prascad, U., Sadler, R., Flynn, K., Raab-Traub, N. 1995. Clonal proliferation of cells infected with Epstein-Barr virus in preinvasive lesions related to nasopharyngeal carcinoma. *N. Engl. J. Med.*; 333:693–698.
23. Lo, K.W., Huang, P.W.S.D., Lee, J.C.K. 1997. Genetic changes in nasopharyngeal carcinoma. *Chin. Med. J.*; 110:548–559.
24. Pan, S-C, Yao, K-T. 1987. Chemical etiology of nasopharyngeal carcinoma. In: *Etiology and Pathogenesis of Nasopharyngeal Carcinoma*, Beijing: The People's Medical Publishing House, 48–89.
25. Wang, H.W., Jiang, F.L. 1965. Study on the *in situ* induced experimental nasopharyngeal carcinoma of mice. *Acta Biol. Exper. Sinica*; 10:190–199 (in Chinese).
26. Huang, D.P., Ho, J.H.C., Saw, D., *et al.* 1978. Carcinoma of the nasal and paranasal regions in rats fed Cantonese salted marine fish. In: *Nasopharyngeal Carcinoma, Etiology and Control*, eds. de Thé, G., Ito, Y. IRAC Science Publication No. 20, 315–318.

CHAPTER 5

Surgical Pathology

Philip W. Allen

Nomenclature

In the broadest sense, the term "nasopharyngeal cancer" could encompass many different nasopharyngeal tumours, from carcinomas of minor salivary glands to primary mucosal malignant melanoma, malignant lymphomas and even various sarcomas. However, in South East Asia, nasopharyngeal carcinoma generally means the common tumour now known either as lymphoepithelial carcinoma of the nasopharynx[1] or undifferentiated nasopharyngeal carcinoma. The word "lymphoepithelial" does not imply or indicate a peculiar kind of lymphoma. It is purely descriptive of the benign, reactive lymphocytes that infiltrate the tumour tissue.

This tumour, which is so common in Southern China, is hardly ever seen in non endemic areas such as Australia. Thus, I saw no cases over a period of 32 years of pathology practice in large and small Australian hospitals and regional pathology services nor during my three years in the Soft Tissue Branch at the Armed Forces Institute of Pathology in the United States. I saw my first case in 1989, when I first worked in Hong Kong and I expect that many other pathologists from non endemic areas would be equally unfamiliar with the tumour.

According to Choa and Gibb,[2] the histology was delineated in 1921 by Schmincke in the German literature and by Regaud and Reverchon in the French. After these publications, two histological patterns of lymphoepithelial nasopharyngeal carcinoma were recognized. The more common "Schmincke" pattern consisted of diffuse sheets of undifferentiated tumour cells with poorly demarcated cytoplasmic borders. The sheets of tumour cells were infiltrated by numerous lymphocytes which prompted the name "lymphoepithelial carcinoma." The second and less common "Regaud" pattern was characterized by trabeculae, columns and nests of undifferentiated tumour cells with well defined cytoplasmic borders surrounded by a supporting loose fibrous stroma infiltrated with lymphocytes. The inflammatory infiltrate was restricted to the supporting stroma surrounding the trabeculae of tumour cells.

This histological classification was generally accepted for over 40 years. Thus, in the 1964 first series tumour fascicle,[3] lymphoepithelial carcinoma of the nasopharynx was still subclassified into the Schmincke and Regaud types. The term "lymphoepithelial carcinoma" was preferred, to distinguish it from squamous cell carcinoma and

Schneiderian papilloma. Those authors also noted that "pathologic material collected in the (American) Registry, especially during the Korean conflict, contains many such tumours from men in their second and third decades. Incidence is particularly high in the Chinese and other Oriental groups."

This simple and straightforward classification was thrown into confusion with the publication in 1978 of the World Health Organization classification of upper respiratory tract tumours,[4] the scientific influence of which seems to have been magnified by its association with the Organization. The short monograph had minimal text and no references. The Schmincke and Regaud histological variants were not mentioned and the interpretation of the classification depended mainly on eight color photomicrographs with no clinical details in the captions. Two illustrations were captioned "nasopharyngeal carcinoma — squamous cell carcinoma". Three illustrations, which seem to be of the Regaud pattern, were captioned "nasopharyngeal carcinoma — non-keratinizing carcinoma" while the other three, which seem to be of the Schmincke pattern, were captioned "nasopharyngeal carcinoma — undifferentiated carcinoma." The explanatory notes indicate that lymphoepithelial carcinoma "is used to describe nonkeratinizing and undifferentiated nasopharyngeal carcinomas in which numerous lymphocytes are found amongst the tumour cells," but the classification table (page 19) lists squamous cell carcinoma, non-keratinizing carcinoma and undifferentiated carcinoma as variants of the one and the same nasopharyngeal carcinoma. While this classification might satisfy a pure pathologist, it does not take into account the extraordinarily specific clinical and radiological features of lymphoepithelial carcinoma.

The authors of the 1988 second series tumour fascicle[5] disregarded the classification in the first series fascicle and supported the World Health Organization views, classifying lymphoepithelial carcinoma as a variant of squamous cell carcinoma because the tumour cells produce desmosomes and poorly defined tonofilaments.

In 1987, Hsu *et al.* from Taipei[6] proposed a slightly different classification, adding a spindle cell variant and grading each group on the basis of histological atypia and pleomorphism. They confirmed that squamous cell carcinoma had a worse prognosis than the other types while the differences between the non squamous cell types were not great. However, on the basis of their pictures, I do not believe that I personally could reliably and consistently subclassify lymphoepithelial nasopharyngeal carcinomas according to their criteria.

The World Health Organization classification has now been questioned by French[7] and German[8] experts.

The most recent edition of Ackerman's Pathology supports the Europeans' views[1] and stresses the difference between the rare squamous cell carcinoma arising in the nasopharynx, which is not associated with geographical clustering nor with a high percentage of cases with raised Epstein-Barr virus serology, and lymphoepithelial carcinoma, which is.

The controversies over the nomenclature have been largely due to the undifferentiated histological appearance of the tumour. Hematoxylin and eosin (H and E) stained sections of undifferentiated or dedifferentiated carcinomas from many different primary sites can, when they are associated with a lympho-plasmacytic infiltrate, exactly simulate a nasopharyngeal lymphoepithelial carcinoma. Thus, poorly differentiated squamous carcinomas of the oropharynx or vallecula may spread locally and extensively to involve the region of the fossa of Rosenmüller. If they are associated with a pronounced local lymphoid reaction, the appearances may be indistinguishable from a primary lymphoepithelial carcinoma of the nasopharynx, even in a fairly large biopsy. However, these patients are likely to be smokers, the Epstein-Barr (EB) virus serology is usually normal, the EB virus-encoded RNAs(EBER) stain is negative and squamous pearls, intercellular bridges or individual cell keratinization are usually found somewhere in larger samples.

Carcinomas histologically similar to lymphoepithelial nasopharyngeal carcinoma may occur in many different sites (see below). A few are associated with raised EB virus serological titers and EB virus genomes in the tumour cells and are probably the same type of lymphoepithelial carcinoma occurring in ectopic locations. However, most such ectopic lymphocyte-rich carcinomas are negative for the EB virus (see below).

Accordingly, I do not believe that the generally characteristic histological picture of nasopharyngeal lymphoepithelial carcinoma is, by itself, diagnostic. The diagnostic criteria for both nasopharyngeal and ectopic lymphoepithelial carcinomas of the nasopharyngeal type should include combined clinicopathological and serological factors as well as studies for EB viral elements in the tumour cells rather than histological features alone.

The Diagnostic Criteria for Lymphoepithelial Carcinoma of the Nasopharyngeal Type

Based on a review of archived sections of over 600 nasopharyngeal tumours, most of which were lymphoepithelial nasopharyngeal carcinomas, and my five year's experience at the weekly head and neck conferences at the Prince of Wales Hospital, where the clinical, radiological and histological sections of head and neck malignancies are reviewed, I believe the location of the tumour, the status of the EB virus serological titres and the presence of Epstein Bar Virus-encoded RNAs (EBER) in the sections should be included in the diagnostic criteria for lymphoepithelial carcinoma of the nasopharyngeal type. I propose the following three diagnostic criteria.

1. *Histology*. The primary, untreated tumour should be a poorly differentiated, carcinoma without keratin pearls, intercellular bridges or individual cell keratinization, must exhibit either the Shmincke (syncytial) (*Figures 1, 2, 3*) or the Regaud (trabecular) (*Figures 4, 5, 6*) pattern and should be keratin positive by immunohistochemistry (*Figure 3*). Pearls, bridges and individual cell keratinization must be definite and unequivocal before a tumour can be rejected as a lymphoepithelial carcinoma and classified as a squamous cell carcinoma. The "squamoid" features characteristic of the Regaud type of lymphoepithelial

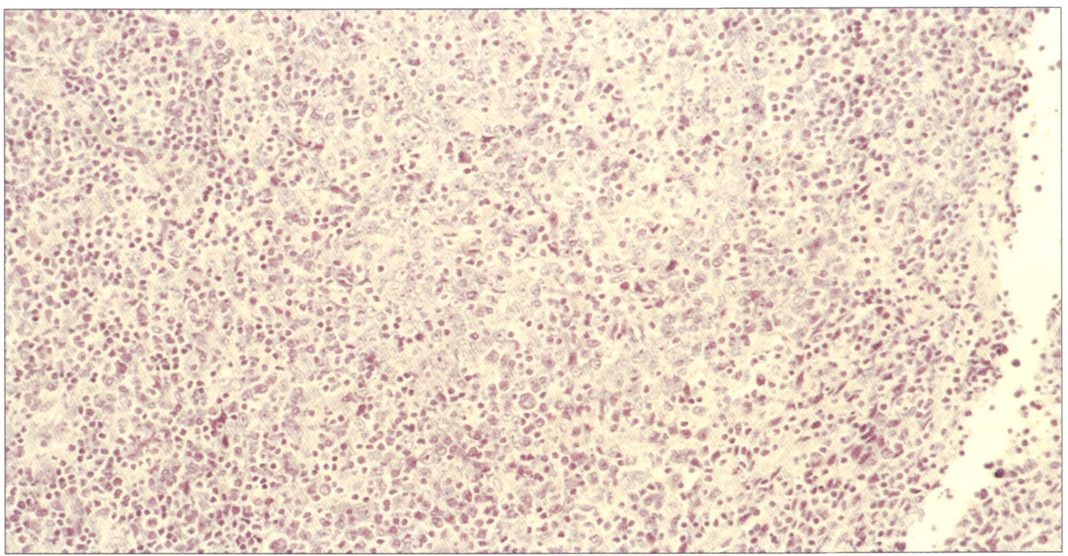

Figure 1. Schmincke pattern of undifferentiated (lymphoepithelial) nasopharyngeal carcinoma. Syncytial sheets of tumour cells are diffusely infiltrated by lymphocytes.

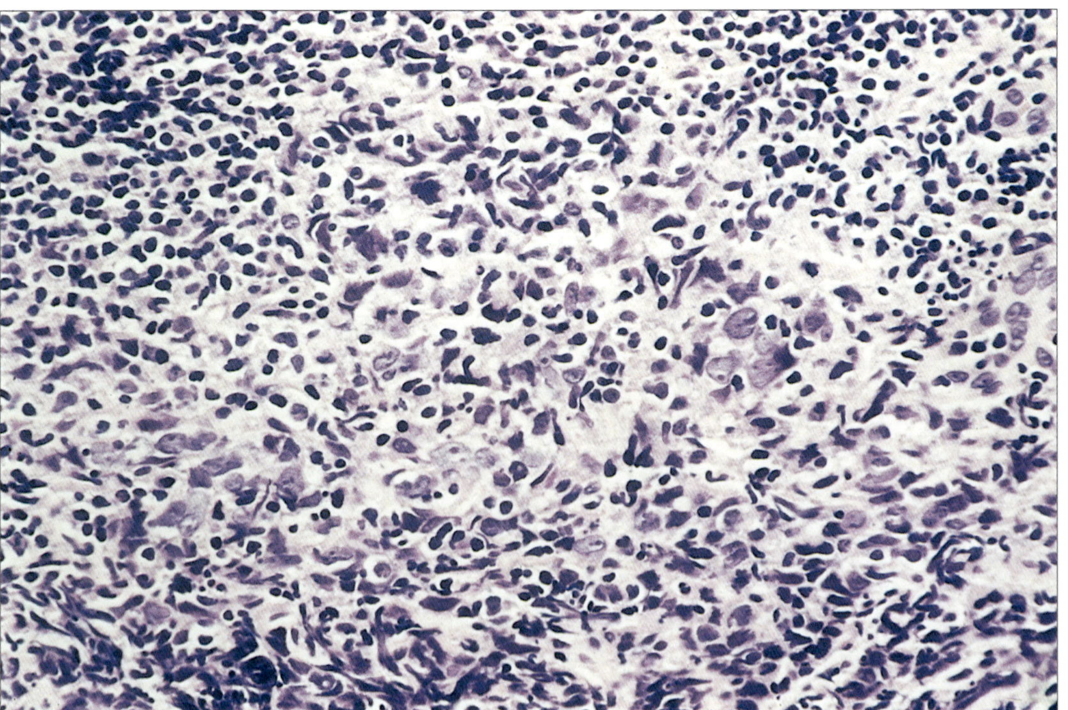

Figure 2. Slightly traumatized biopsy illustrating the Schmincke pattern. There are a few inconspicuous tumour cells surrounded by lymphocytes. (PWH reference 97.9413).

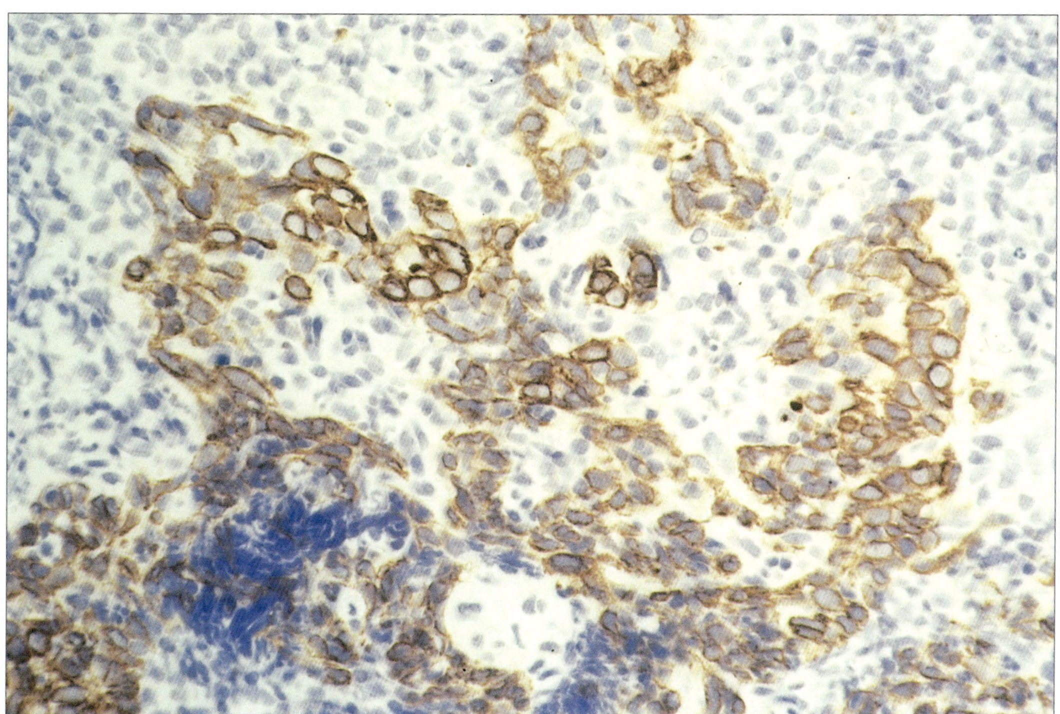

Figure 3. AE1/AE3 immunohistochemical preparation of the Schmincke tumour pattern. The tumour cells stain brown, indicating the presence of cytokeratin within the cells. This stain distinguishes lymphoepithelial carcinoma cells from immature lymphocytes. (PWH reference 97.10190; same case as *Figures 15* and *16*).

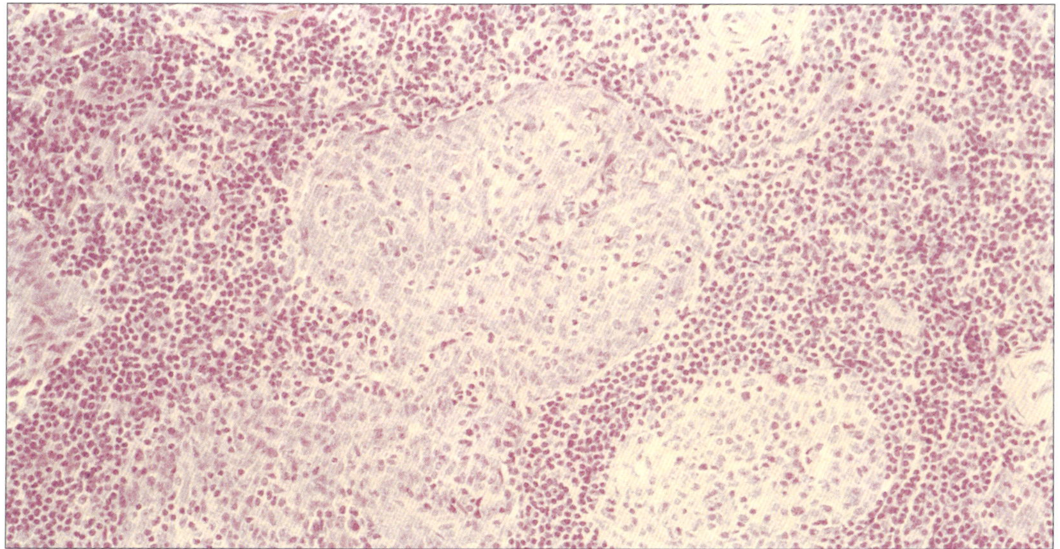

Figure 4. Regaud pattern of undifferentiated (lymphoepithelial) nasopharyngeal carcinoma.

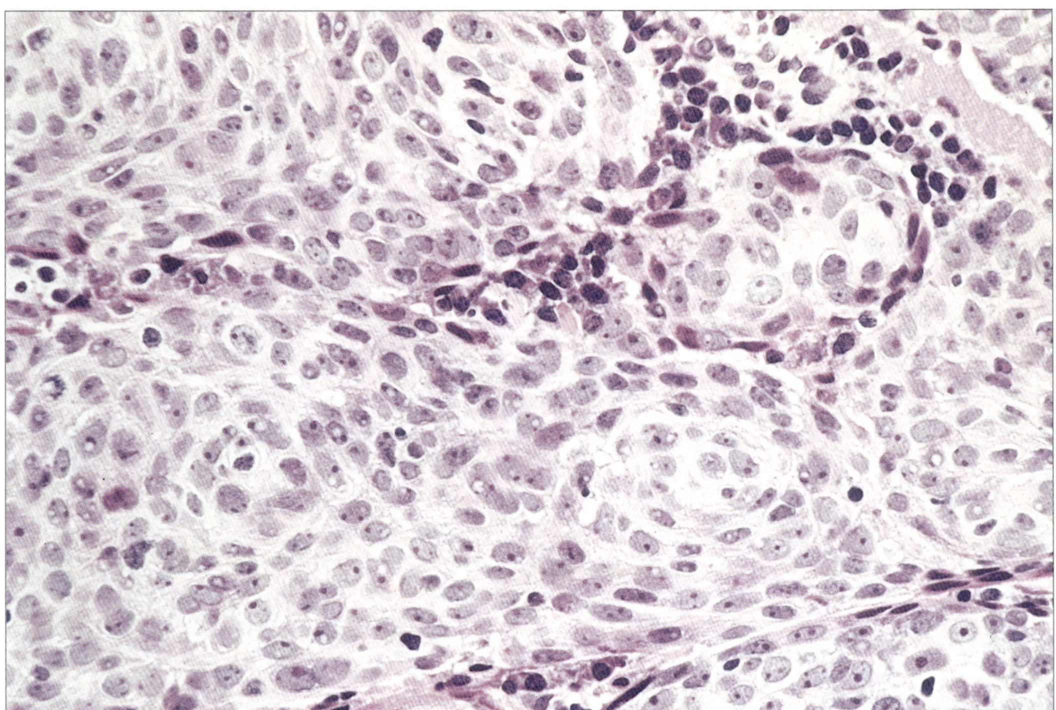

Figure 5. Regaud pattern of lymphoepithelial carcinoma showing trabeculae of tumour with visible cell borders and a tendency to whirl. This whirling should not be interpreted as the pearls of squamous cell carcinoma, although the pattern doubtless indicates the basic squamous epithelial nature of lymphoepithelial carcinoma. (PWH reference 97.15623).

carcinoma, the keratin positivity apparent in immunohistochemical stains and the desmosomes and tonofilaments seen on electron microscopy are certainly squamous features but they should not be taken to indicate the kind of squamous differentiation, the epidemiological features and the clinical behaviour of the uncommon squamous cell carcinoma of the nasopharynx, which is biologically a different tumour from lymphoepithelial carcinoma. *Figures 5, 7 and 8* illustrate appearances that are sometimes wrongly interpreted as proof that lymphoepithelial carcinoma is merely a variant of squamous cell carcinoma. In my opinion, these appearances indicate either abortive and incomplete attempts towards squamous differentiation, as one would expect from the electron microscopic characteristics, or degenerative and artefactual changes. More convincing squamous differentiation is sometimes seen in recurrent tumours that have previously been treated with radiotherapy or chemotherapy.

In addition to these features which are apparent in hematoxylin and eosin (H and E) stained sections, at least one of the two following additional criteria should be fulfilled before a diagnosis of lymphoepithelial carcinoma of the nasopharyngeal type can be accepted.

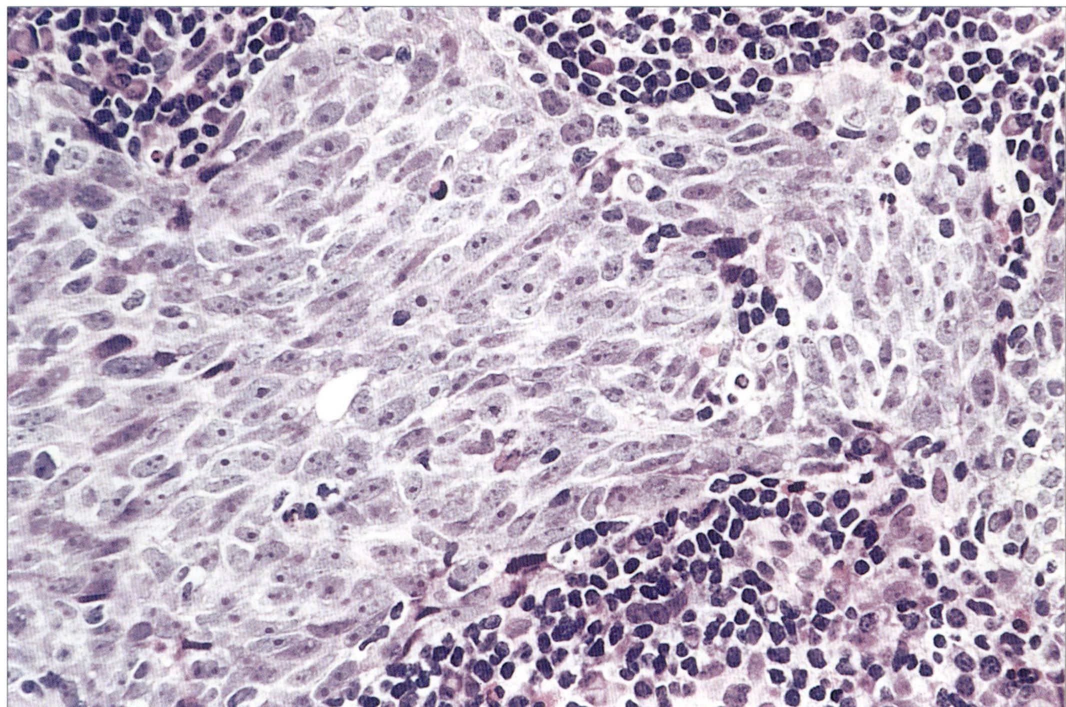

Figure 6. Higher power view of the tumour illustrated in *Figure 5* showing the prominent nucleoli and lack of intercellular bridges. (PWH reference 97.9413).

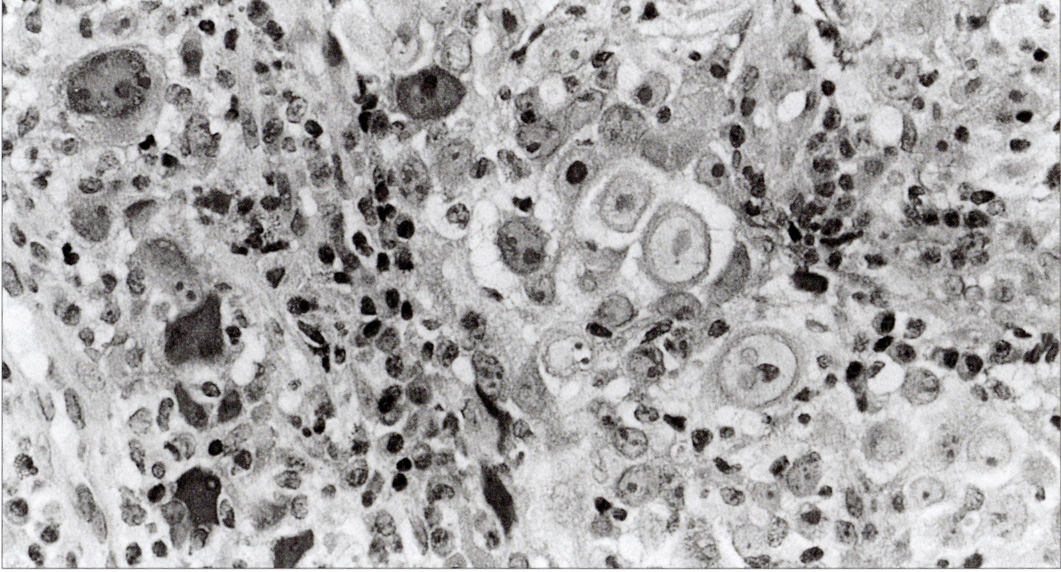

Figure 7. Lymphoepithelial carcinoma of the nasopharynx with vacuolar degenerative changes and shrinkage of some of the cells. In the past, the linear edges of the vacuoles have been misinterpreted as intercellular bridges.

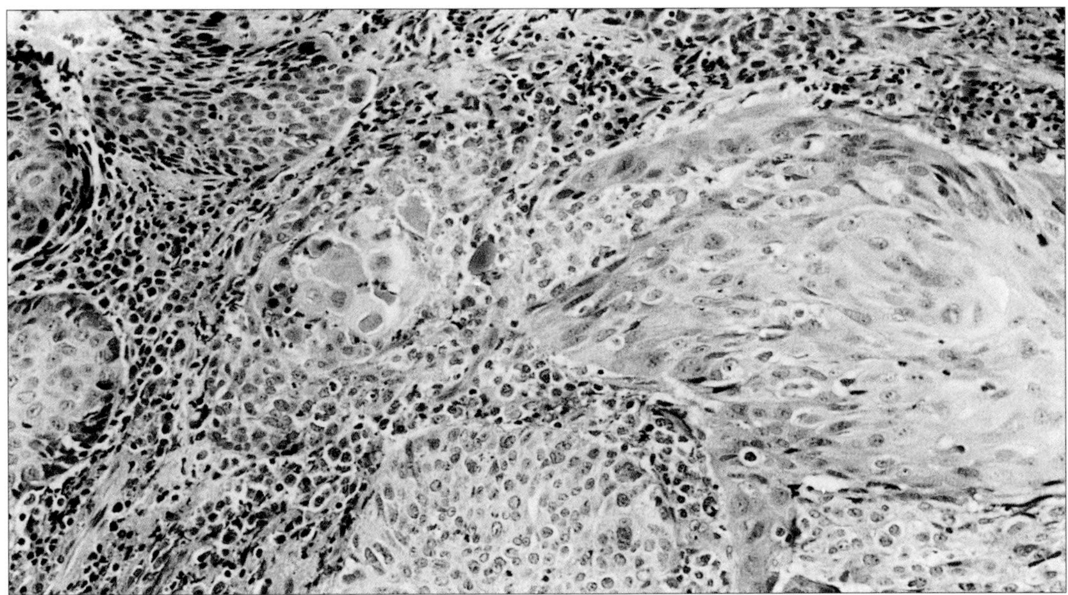

Figure 8. Discohesive cells impart a so-called pavement appearance to this lymphoepithelial carcinoma of the nasopharynx. The pavement appearance is not diagnostic of a squamous cell carcinoma.

2. *Location.* The tumour should be centered either in the region of the fossa of Rosenmüller or on the vault or posterior wall of the nasopharynx. The location should be verified by organ imaging. This criterion is second in importance only to the histology.

or

3. *The EB virus status.* The patient's EB virus serology should be raised or, if it is normal, EB virus moieties must be demonstrated in tumour cells by in situ hybridization for EB Virus-encoded RNAs (EBER). The two most reliable serological markers are the IgA antibodies against Epstein-Barr viral capsid antigen (IgA VCA), which is sensitive but relatively non specific and the IgA early intracellular antigen (IgA EA), which is more specific but less sensitive (Chapter 9). Both are produced when cells infected with Epstein-Barr virus enter a lytic cycle. In Hong Kong, more than 90% of patients with lymphoepithelial nasopharyngeal carcinoma have raised IgA VCA titers, while the figure for IgA EA is around 80%.[9] The patients with true lymphoepithelial carcinomas located outside the nasopharynx who have normal EB virus serology can only be correctly diagnosed by demonstrating EBER in the tumour cells.

These combined criteria permit a diagnosis of lymphoepithelial carcinoma of the nasopharyngeal type located outside the usual nasopharyngeal areas, even if the EB virus serology is not raised. They also allow for the diagnosis of the occasional serologically negative nasopharyngeal lymphoepithelial carcinomas without perfoming EBER stains, provided that the tumours are in a typical location and are not keratinized. Serological tests are proposed as the initial virological criteria instead of the more sophisticated and complex in situ hybridization or molecular biology procedures for demonstrating EB virus genomes because they are cheaper, are widely available, and are easily performed.

In a few cases, it is impossible to be certain from sections of a small biopsy if a nasopharyngeal tumour is a lymphoepithelial carcinoma or an anaplastic squamous carcinoma. In those cases, the location and the serology, and as a last resort, the EBER status should be taken into account when deciding how to classify the tumour.

The distinction is of some importance. Lymphoepithelial carcinoma has a characteristic geographical and racial incidence; it is apparently always associated with EB virus genomes in the tumour cells; it is more radiosensitive and has a better prognosis than squamous cell carcinoma.[10]

Proportion of Lymphoepithelial Carcinomas Found in All Types of Nasopharyngeal Cancer in Hong Kong

In a series of 261 nasopharyngeal malignancies of all kinds seen at the Prince of Wales Hospital, Hong Kong from January 1986 to September 1987, McGuire and Lee[11] classified 236 (90%) as nasopharyngeal lymphoepithelial carcinomas (my terminology). Of the 236 lymphoepithelial carcinomas, 215 (91%) exhibited the Schmincke pattern (World Health Organization classification III) and 21 (9%) the Regaud pattern (World Health Organization classification II). Amongst the 261 nasopharyngeal malignancies of all kinds, there were 7 (2.7%) squamous carcinomas, 13 (5%) malignant lymphomas and single examples of adenocarcinoma, granulocytic sarcoma, sinonasal undifferentiated carcinoma, olfactory neuroblastoma and embryonal rhabdomyosarcoma.

Light Microscopic Appearances

The primary tumour tissue that a pathologist now sees is likely to have been obtained by endoscopic biopsy. Specimens nearly always measure less than 3 mm in maximum dimensions, are frequently fragmented and are sometimes severely traumatized. The covering squamous or respiratory epithelium is usually normal or mildly inflamed, unlike the findings in small punch biopsies of squamous carcinoma of the cervix uteri, where intraepithelial squamous carcinoma is often seen.

The tumour cells are nearly always located in the submucosal lymphoid and loose connective tissue, usually separate from the overlying epithelium (*Figures 9 and 10*). Only rarely do tumour cells merge with or invade the benign epithelium of the overlying mucosa (*Figure 11*) or with deep epithelial crypts. The tumour cells exhibit either the Schmincke (*Figures 1, 2 and 3*) or the Regaud patterns (*Figures 4, 5 and 6*), although

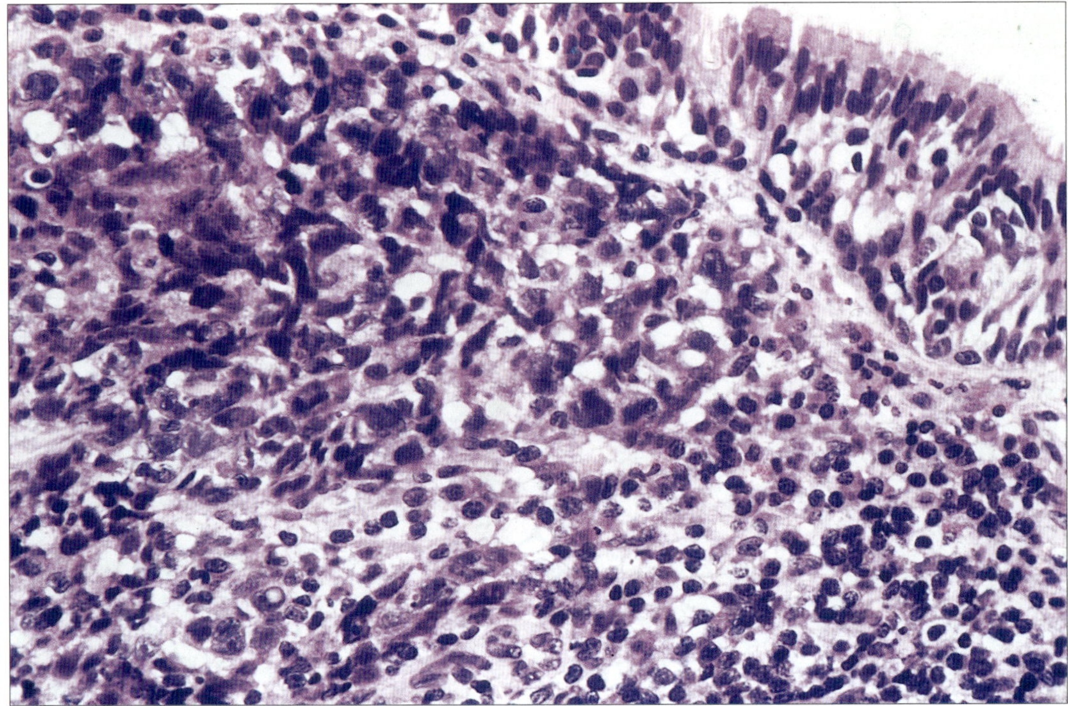

Figure 9. Slightly traumatized lymphoepithelial nasopharyngeal carcinoma in a typical submucosal location. The malignant cells are separate from the overlying respiratory mucosa, which shows no sign of any cellular atypia. The very dark, compressed, almost spindle shaped cells in the clump of submucosal tumour cells are the result of crushing artefact caused by the biopsy instrument. (PWH reference 97.14802).

sometimes, both patterns are apparent in the one tumour. Mixed forms are quite common, although the proportions of each pattern found in different series can be affected by the individual interpretations of different pathologists. The nuclei of the tumour cells are similar in both patterns. They are large, round to oval in shape, with well defined nuclear membranes and one or more prominent, large, eosinophilic nucleoli which are visible in almost every cell (*Figures 1, 4, 5, and 6*). These large nucleoli impart a superficially uniform appearance to the tumour cells, particularly at low power, but on more careful inspection at a higher power, the nuclei are seen to vary considerably in both shape and size (*Figure 6*). Mitoses are easily found and there is coarse, irregular clumping of the chromatin with intervening paler areas imparting all the histological characteristics of malignancy. The cells' cytoplasm is pale pink in both patterns.

In the Schmincke pattern (*Figures 1 and 2*), the cell borders are poorly defined, resulting in a syncytial appearance and sheets of tumour are infiltrated by numerous lymphocytes, predominantly T cells,[12,13,14] as well as scattered plasma cells. These

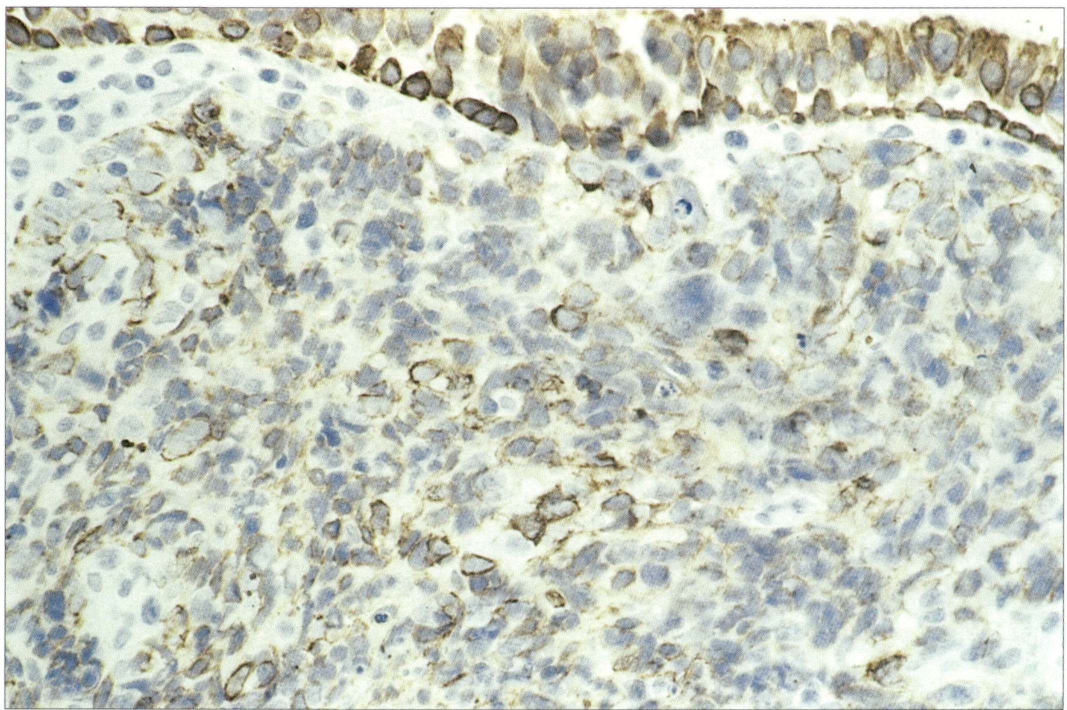

Figure 10. AE1/AE3 (cytokeratin) immunohistochemical stain of the area illustrated in *Figure 9*. The tumour cells stain less darkly and less regularly than the overlying normal respiratory epithelium. (PWH reference 97.14802).

lymphoid cells are inflammatory rather than neoplastic and are a part of the host's reaction to the tumour.

The tumour cells' borders are better defined in the Regaud pattern. The cells are more cohesive and clump together in trabeculae, columns or nests (*Figures 4, 5 and 6*). The groups of cells are separated by varying proportions of loose connective tissue, lymphocytes and plasma cells. Occasionally, there may be a vague whirling pattern suggestive of early or abortive pearl formation (*Figure 5*) but convincing pearls are not seen. Shrinkage and vacuolation in some cells may result in linear edges of the vacuoles being misinterpreted as the intercellular bridges of a squamous carcinoma (*Figure 7*). The trabecular columns seen in the Regaud pattern together with the whirls or vague "pearls", unconvincing "intercellular bridges" and the EM findings formed the basis for the belief that lymphoepithelial nasopharyngeal carcinoma was the same biological entity as squamous cell carcinoma.

Other histological features occasionally seen in the primary tumour include tumour cells with clear vacuolated cytoplasm, tissue eosinophilia, which does not seem to be associated with a better prognosis,[15] amyloid stroma[16,17] (*Figure 12*) and non-caseating epithelioid granulomas with giant cells[18] (*Figure 13*).

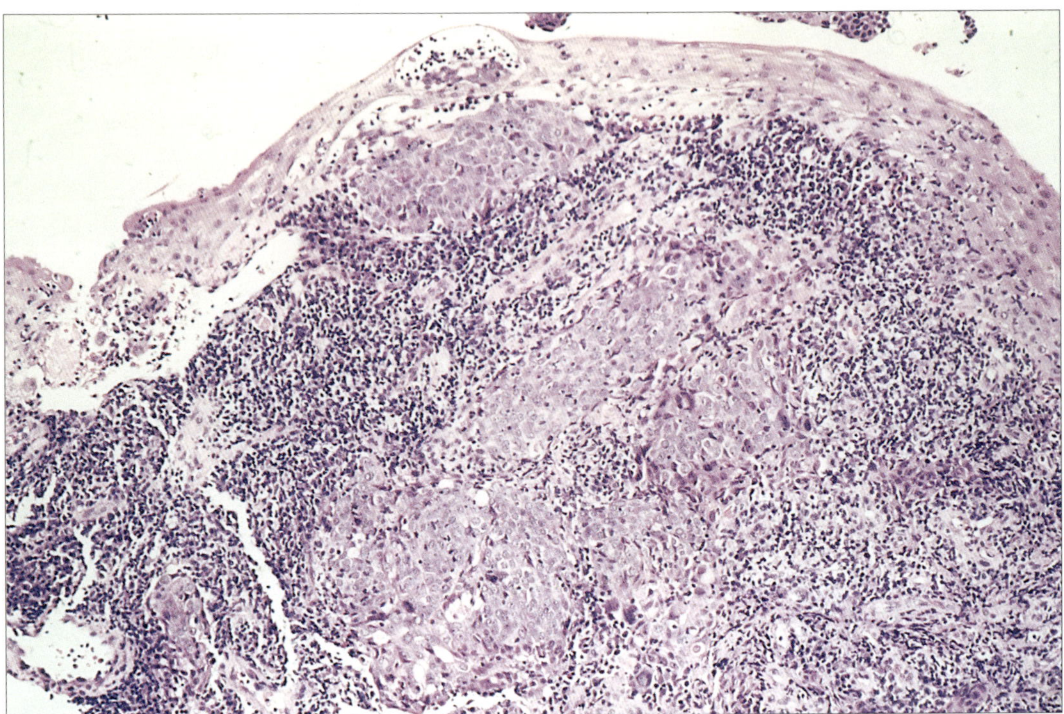

Figure 11. Submucosal lymphoepithelial nasopharyngeal carcinoma which is just starting to invade the overlying squamous mucosa. The contrast between the histologically benign surface squamous cells and the cytologically atypical malignant cells is readily apparent. Intraepithelial spread with maturation of cells as they approach the surface such as is seen in carcinoma in situ of the cervix is not found in nasopharyngeal lymphoepithelial carcinoma, although it is often found in squamous cell carcinomas of the upper respiratory tract. (PWH reference 97.11113).

Immunohistochemical Findings

In our hands, lymphoepithelial carcinoma cells virtually always stain positively with the broad spectrum IgG1 monoclonal mouse anti-keratin AE1/AE3 immunohistochemical stain (*Figures 3 and 10*), which binds to a spectrum of keratin classes from 40 to 60 kD. This consistent staining for keratin has been well known for more than 10 years, with Shi *et al.* reporting 100% positive staining in 121 cases of nasopharyngeal carcinoma, using commercial antibodies against the 40 kD, 50 kD and 56.5 kD members of the acidic keratin subfamily.[19] Similarly, Madri *et al.*,[20] Miettinen *et al.*,[21] Ziegels-Weissmann *et al.*[22] and Taxy *et al.*[23] all reported 100% positive staining for various keratins in smaller series. On the other hand, Oppedal *et al.*[24] found one cytokeratin negative tumour in a series of 66 cases (98% positive) while Kamino and associates[25] reported a lower positive rate of 24/26 (92%) for nasopharyngeal carcinomas using several stains for keratin in the 40 kD to 63 kD range. They noted that stains for high molecular weight keratins and involucrin were more likely to be negative in lymphoepitheliomas. The reason for this comparatively low positive rate is not clear.

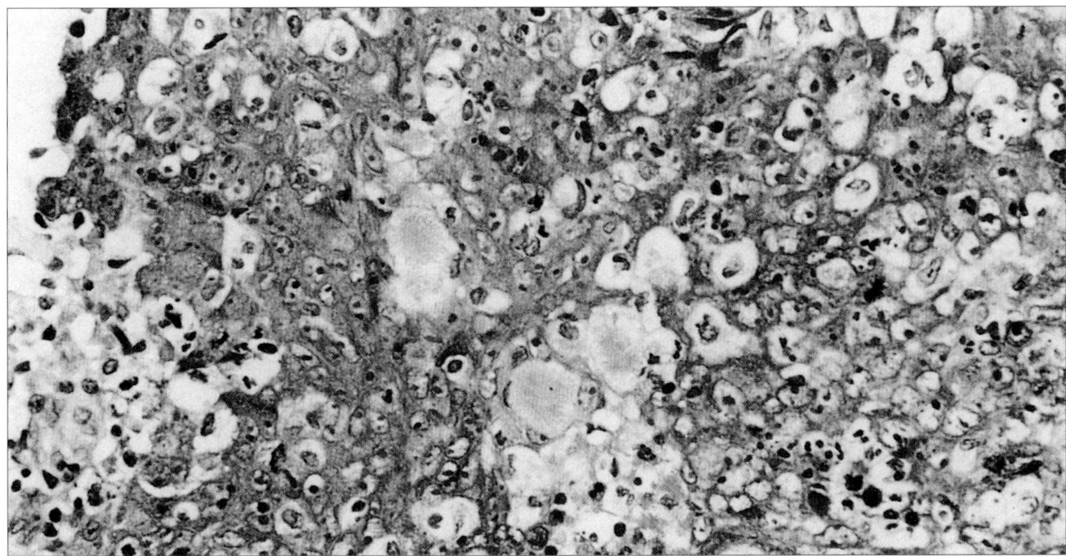

Figure 12. Primary lymphoepithelial carcinoma of the nasopharynx with clumps of pale, homogeneous amyloid material lying between tumour cells.

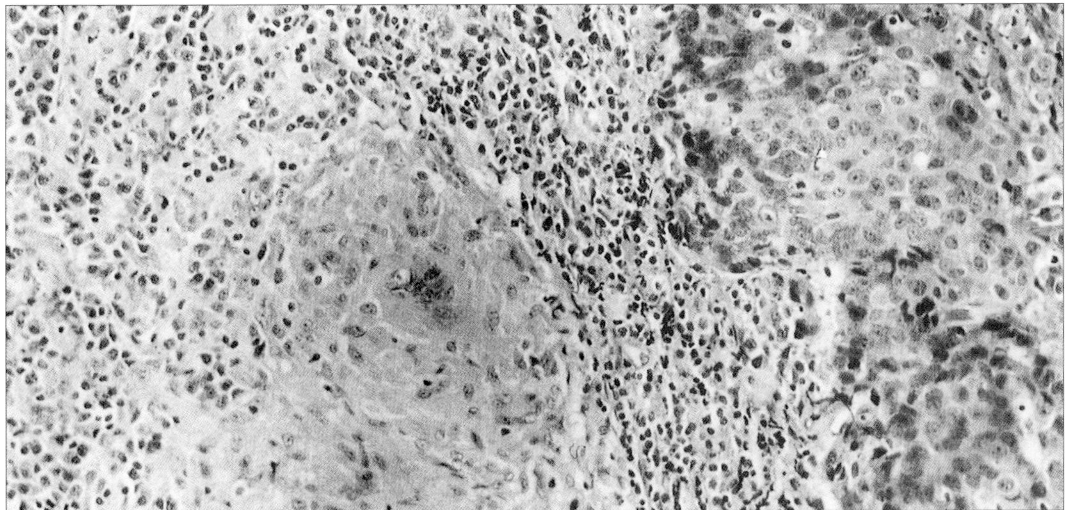

Figure 13. (Right side) Primary lymphoepithelial carcinoma of the nasopharynx with an adjacent non-caseating epithelioid granuloma, including a giant cell. This appearance usually indicates a peculiar host reaction to the tumour. It is hardly ever due to coincidental tuberculosis. Nevertheless, patients with such granulomas should be screened clinically for tuberculosis and the sections should be stained for acid fast bacilli.

Other epithelial markers which are usually positive include Cam 5.2, PKK1 and epithelial membrane antigen.

The tumour cells are S100 negative, but S100 positive Langerhans cells may be numerous amongst the lymphocytes. One study of 40 cases[26] reported no prognostic significance in these cells while another more recent analysis of 119 cases[27] found that patients with a dense infiltration of Langerhans cells survived for a statistically longer period than those without such an infiltrate, a finding similar to results published by Giannini *et al.*[28] Lai *et al.*[29] studied the immunohistochemical characteristics of the infiltrating lymphoid cells and the expression of HLA class I and II antigens in 50 pre-treatment nasopharyngeal carcinomas. The majority of lymphoid cells were activated lymphocytes expressing thymocyte OKT10 marker. T-helper/inducer CD4+ cells markedly outnumbered CD8+ cells (T-suppressor/cytotoxic). The pan-B lymphocyte CD22+ cells were scanty in the peri-tumoral areas and were absent in 29 out of 50 biopsies. A moderate number of cells expressing CD15 (monocytes/macrophages) were also detected. CD16+ cells (natural killer cells) were found to be sparse or absent. Expression of HLA class I and II antigens on the tumour cells in 35 biopsies was variable. HLA-ABC staining was intense in 6, reduced in 13 and partially lost in 16, whereas staining of HLA-DR was intense in 7, reduced in 11 and partially lost in 17. Full expression of both antigens was demonstrable in only 2 biopsy samples. The expression of HLA antigens in the tumour had no relationship to the type or degree of lymphocytic infiltration or staging of the tumour. The tumour cells were negative for all lymphoid markers, a helpful point in the differentiation of lymphoepithelial carcinoma from malignant lymphomas.

Immunohistochemical stains of nasopharyngeal lymphoepithelial carcinoma have also demonstrated over expression of p53 protein,[30] bcl-2 protein,[31] MDM-2 protein,[32] Epstein-Barr virus encoded latent membrane protein (LMP1),[33] Ki67 antigen and epidermal growth factor receptor,[34] beta-2-microglobulin and Hla-DR proteins,[35] the intercellular adhesion molecules (ICAM-1) and the blood vessel adhesion molecules (VCAM-1)[36,37] and c-myc and ras oncogenes.[38] The practical significance and correct interpretation of all these observations are unclear.

Immunofluorescence Findings

As this technique requires frozen tissue rather than formalin fixed, paraffin embedded tissue, its use is generally limited to research projects, but Epstein-Barr nuclear antigens (EBNAs) and latent membrane protein (LMP) have been demonstrated by this technique in nasopharyngeal carcinomas using monoclonal mouse antibodies.[39]

Electron microscopic Findings

Desmosomes and tonofilaments were observed in lymphoepithelial carcinoma as early as 1969[40] and were subsequently confirmed by others.[5,23] As discussed previously, this indicates squamous differentiation but does not justify the belief that the tumour is merely a variant of the kind of squamous cell carcinoma that occurs in the lung or cervix. Desmosomes are found in tumours as diverse as thymoma and mucoepidermoid carcinoma. They are not pathognomonic of a single pathological entity.

In Situ Hybridization and Polymerase Chain Reaction Studies

In addition to staining for latent membrane proteins by immunohistochemical methods, EB virus moieties in tumour cells can be demonstrated by in situ hybridization for EB virus-encoded RNAs (EBER),[41] by Southern blotting for various portions of the viral genome,[42] by pulse field gel electrophoresis,[43] by restriction fragment length polymorphism and by polymerase chain reaction on paraffin embedded formalin fixed tissues.[44–47]

Whatever the method used, EB virus genome or products seem to be present in 100% of lymphoepithelial nasopharyngeal carcinomas, as established more than 20 years ago.[48,49] However, their exact role in the pathogenesis of the neoplastic transformation is not clear. As benign, non neoplastic cells may also harbour EB virus products,[50] positive results from these tests are not diagnostic of malignancy, as is sometimes claimed.[51]

Cytogenetic Findings

Many cytogenetic abnormalities have been described in lymphoepithelial nasopharyngeal carcinoma[52–55]. Findings include non-random structural abnormalities of chromosomes 1, 3, 8, and 17[52], a consistent deletion at two specific loci of the short arm of chromosome 3[55] and allelic deletion of chromosome 9[54].

The Cell of Origin

The cell of origin of lymphoepithelial carcinoma is not known. Candidates include the basal cells of epithelial crypts, epithelial cells of minor salivary glands and basal cells of the covering mucosa. Whatever their origin, malignant cells invade the lamina propria early in the disease and spread extensively in the lamina propria before invading (*Figure 11*) and ulcerating the overlying mucosa.

Diagnostic Difficulties

1. *Unfixed autolytic specimens resulting from collection of research material.* In a University Teaching Hospital, there are likely to be several research projects requiring fresh, viable, unfixed tumour cells. To supply this need, surgeons may routinely leave biopsy material unfixed with instructions that it be transported to the researchers. If tissue intended for diagnostic light microscopy is left unfixed for more than a short period, it undergoes autolysis, the sections may be unreadable and the biopsy must then be repeated. For

that reason, the gathering of tissue for research purposes should have second priority to the handling and processing of tissues essential for diagnosis and treatment. In many countries, such research procedures require informed patient consent.

At the Prince of Wales Hospital, tumour tissue for research purposes is only taken after clinically adequate material has been obtained for histology. Additional tissue usually about 3 mm in size is then taken after adequate tissue has been placed in formalin. The tissue for research is divided into two or three pieces, depending on the size of the specimen. One piece is stored in liquid nitrogen, another is placed in cryostat mounting medium and stored at −80 degrees Celsius, and any remaining material is blocked in paraffin for additional conventional light microscopy sections.

2. *False negatives.* The commonest cause is a non representative biopsy. As lymphoepithelial carcinoma is essentially a submucosal disease, small superficial biopsies are often negative, even in advanced cases. The surgeon should always aim to take a deep biopsy.

Another important cause is the failure to recognize individual malignant cells or small, inconspicuous clumps of tumour (*Figure 14*), which may be overlooked in the H

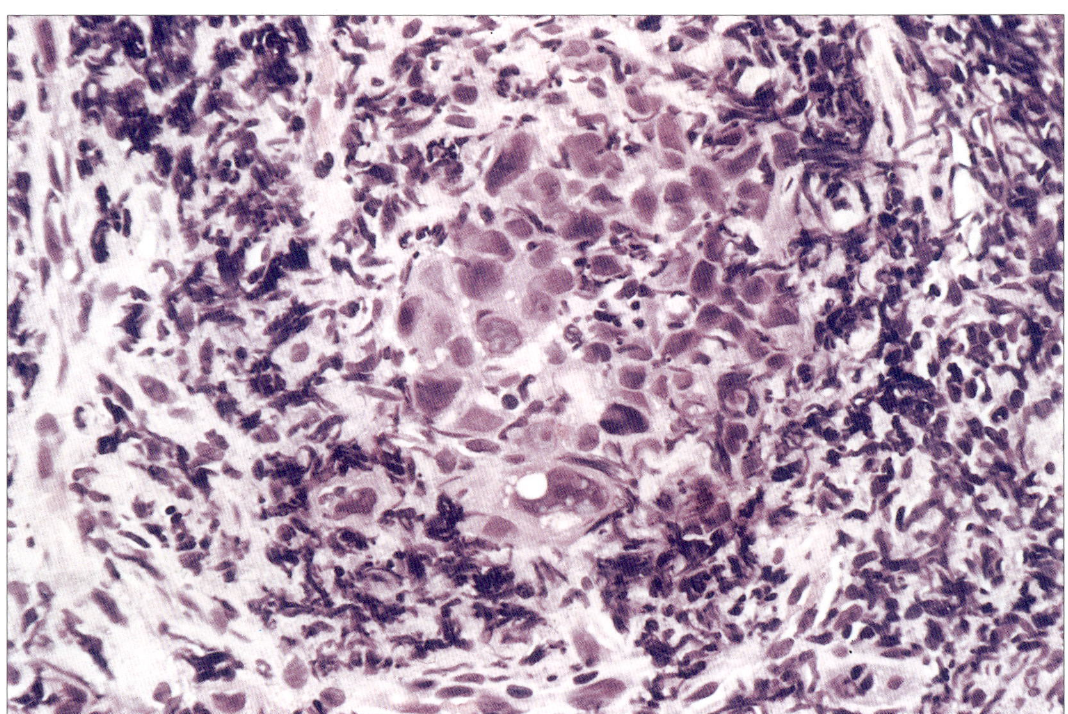

Figure 14. A small island of lymphoepithelial carcinoma cells is surrounded by traumatised cells which are presumably lymphocytes. Such small clusters of malignant cells can be easily overlooked. They can be highlighted by a cytokeratin stain. (PWH reference 97.2388).

and E stain or misintepreted as germinal centres of lymphoid follicles (*Figs. 15 and 16*). If there is a strong clinical suspicion of nasopharyngeal carcinoma and several biopsies have been interpreted as negative, review of the sections and staining of additional slides for cytokeratin may occasionally highlight tumour cells that have been initially "missed" in the H and E stain. If there is considerable crushing artefact, tumour cells may be so severely distorted that they can be almost indistinguishable from lymphocytes. Once again, the cytokeratin stain is helpful in distinguishing the two.

3. *False positives.* Falsely positive reports result from the misinterpretation of benign germinal centers of lymphoid follicles as tumour; the overcalling of swollen benign proliferating endothelial cells (*Figure 17*) or plasma cells (*Figure 18*) particularly after radiotherapy; the misdiagnosis of benign, radiation induced atypical superficial squamous cells as squamous cell carcinoma (*Figure 19*) and the failure to recognize benign epithelial or lymphoid cells distorted by crushing artefact.

Reactive germinal centres and endothelial cells are both negative for cytokeratin and are easily distinguished from carcinoma with this special stain. However, the

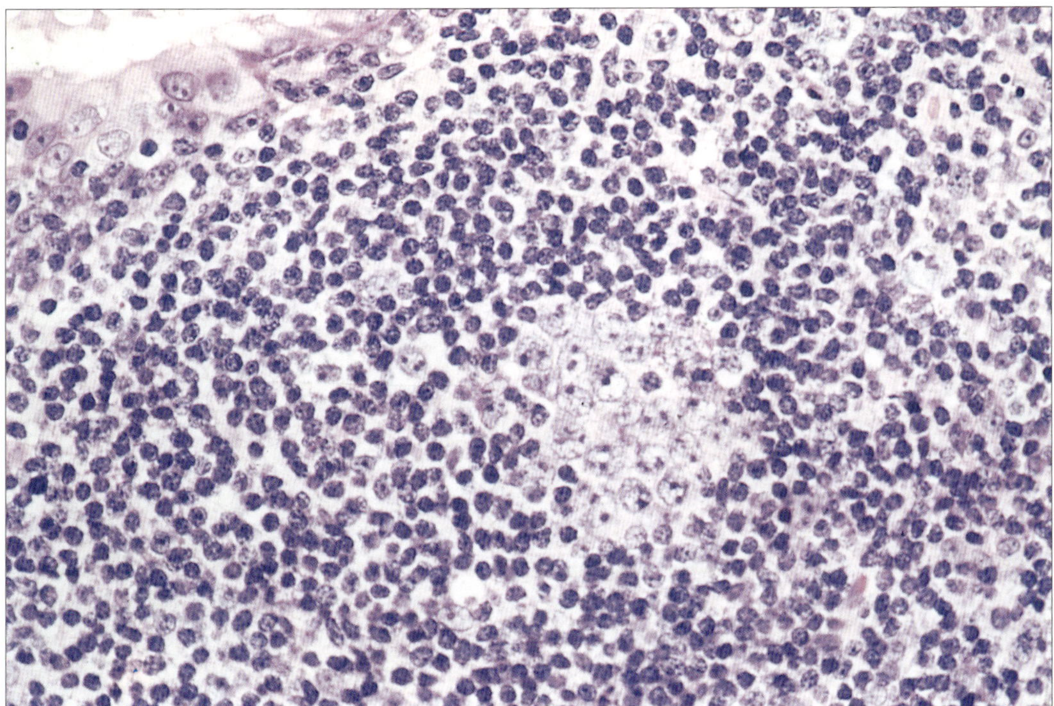

Figure 15. A small group of tumour cells closely resembling the germinal centre of a lymphoid follicle. It can be impossible to reliably differentiate the two in an H and E stain, but tumour cells stain with cytokeratin while the lymphoid cells in a germinal centre are keratin negative. (PWH reference 97.10190; same case as illustrated in *Figures 3 and 16*).

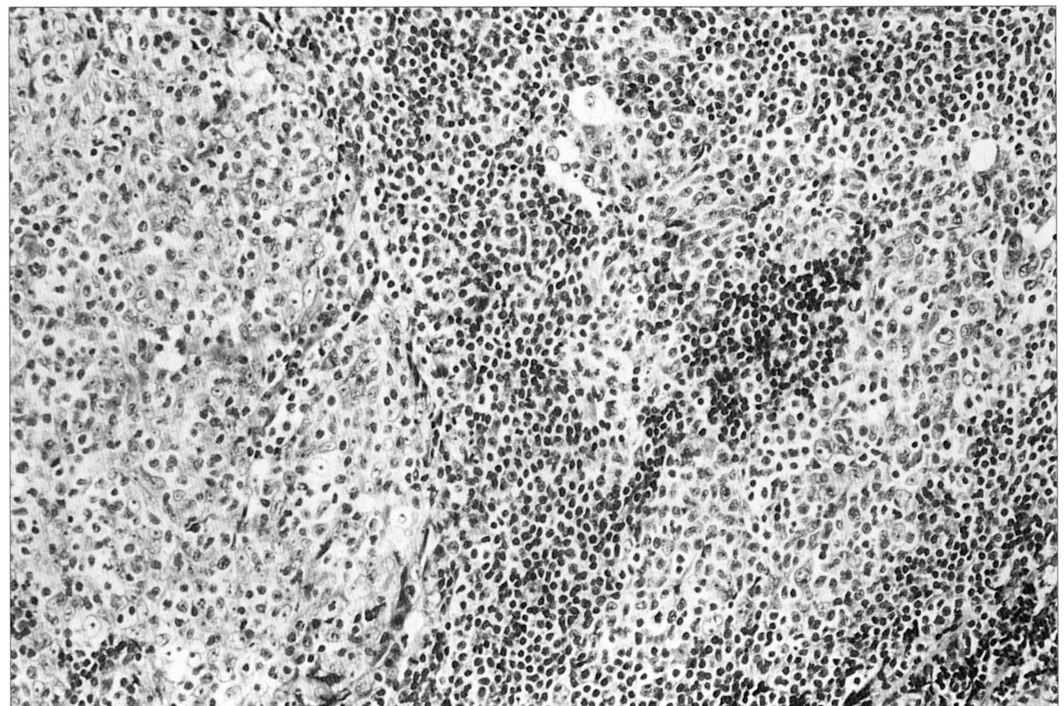

Figure 16. There is a germinal centre on the right and a clump of tumour cells infiltrated with lymphocytes (the Schmincke pattern) on the left. The slightly more pronounced eosinophilia of the tumour cells' cytoplasm provides the best clue in the H and E stain. A cytokeratin stain puts the differences beyond a shadow of doubt. (PWH reference 97.10190; same case as illustrated in *Figures 3 and 15*).

submucosal epithelial crypts which are normally present in nasopharyngeal biopsies are strongly positive for cytokeratin. Unfortunately, there is no special stain that will distinguish benign from malignant epithelial cells. The decision in that situation must be based on the morphology of the nuclei in the H&E stain.

In biopsies after recent radiotherapy, benign squamous mucosal cells may become extremely atypical and are occasionally misdiagnosed as squamous cell carcinoma. Genuine squamous differentiation is not seen in untreated lymphoepithelial carcinoma. In addition to the atypical squamous cells, the numerous plasma cells seen in nasopharyngeal biopsies taken after radiotherapy may be hyperchromatic and multinucleate and are, on rare occasions, misdiagnosed as malignant cells. These cells are cytokeratin negative.

Severe crushing artefact of benign epithelial crypts may be confused with malignancy. The cytokeratin stain is of no help in resolving this difficulty. The decision must be made on the H and E stain. A malignant diagnosis should not be made unless some of the tumour cells are well preserved and can be recognized as carcinoma, without the

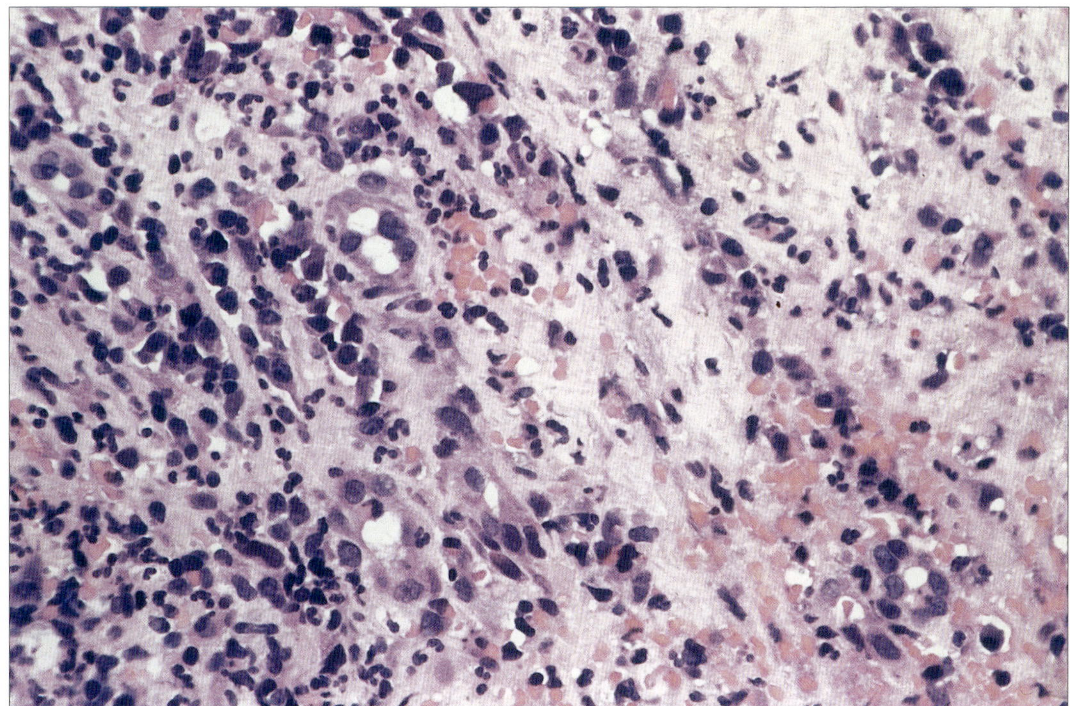

Figure 17. Swollen endothelial cells one month after radiotherapy. These should not be misinterpreted as tumour. They are cytokeratin negative and stain with endothelial immunohistochemical markers. (PWH reference 97.17301; same case as *Figures 18 and 19*).

slightest possibility of error. Malignancy should never be diagnosed if there is even a remote chance that the atypical cells in question are benign.

Differential Diagnosis

Malignant lymphoma may be extremely difficult to differentiate from a lymphoepithelial carcinoma on the basis of the H and E section of a small biopsy. The only hint is the absence of any cytoplasmic eosinophilia in most lymphomas. The slight cytoplasmic eosinophilia in lymphoepithelial carcinoma is probably due to intracytoplasmic intermediate filaments of keratin, which are clearly displayed by electron microscopy or by immunohistochemical stains. Cytokeratin stains separate lymphomas from carcinomas immediately and reliably. Lymphomas are negative for keratins and positive for lymphoid markers, particularly the leukocyte common antigen whereas lymphoepithelial carcinoma is positive for low molecular weight keratins but is negative for leukocyte common antigen.

Poorly differentiated or dedifferentiating squamous cell carcinomas may mimic a lymphoepithelial carcinoma (*Figure 20*), particularly in a small biopsy but more adequate

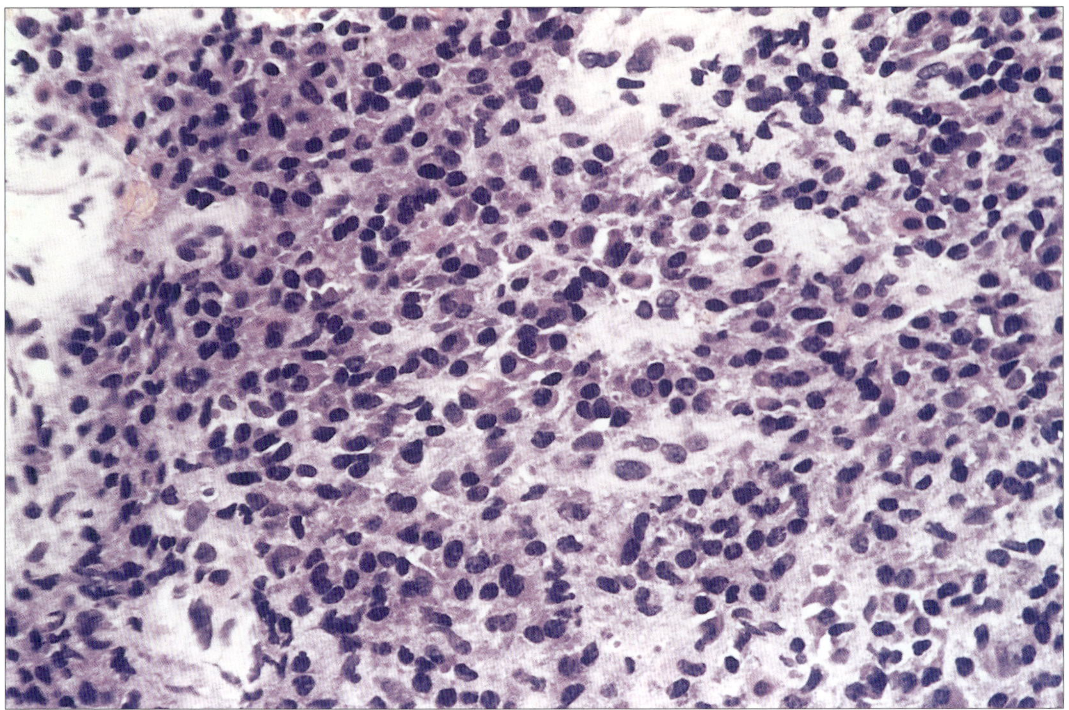

Figure 18. Reactive plasma cells one month after radiotherapy. They should not be misinterpreted as residual tumour. (PWH reference 97.17301; same case as *Figures 17 and 19*).

sampling usually reveals unequivocal keratin pearls, definite inter-cellular bridges or individual cell keratinization. In addition, the Epstein-Bar virus serology is usually negative and the tumour is likely to arise outside the usual confines of a nasopharyngeal lymphoepithelial carcinoma.

Malignant melanoma hardly ever involves the fossa of Rosenmüller. This uncommon tumour most commonly arises in the nose or the mouth and the tumour cells are nearly always S100 positive, as opposed to the tumour cells of lymphoepithelial carcinoma, which are negative. Malignant melanoma is generally more pleomorphic than lymphoepithelial carcinoma and often features multinucleate tumour cells, which are hardly ever seen in lymphoepithelial carcinoma.

The sinonasal region, as opposed to the nasopharynx, may be the site of a variety of poorly differentiated tumours from small cell (neuroendocrine) carcinoma to olfactory neuroblastoma and rhabdomyosarcoma. These tumours do not usually arise in the fossa of Rosenmüller.

Pituitary tumours, including adenomas and craniopharyngiomas as well as chordomas may infiltrate the midline submucosa in the roof of the nasopharynx but they are all better differentiated than lymphoepithelial carcinoma and their radiological features differ.

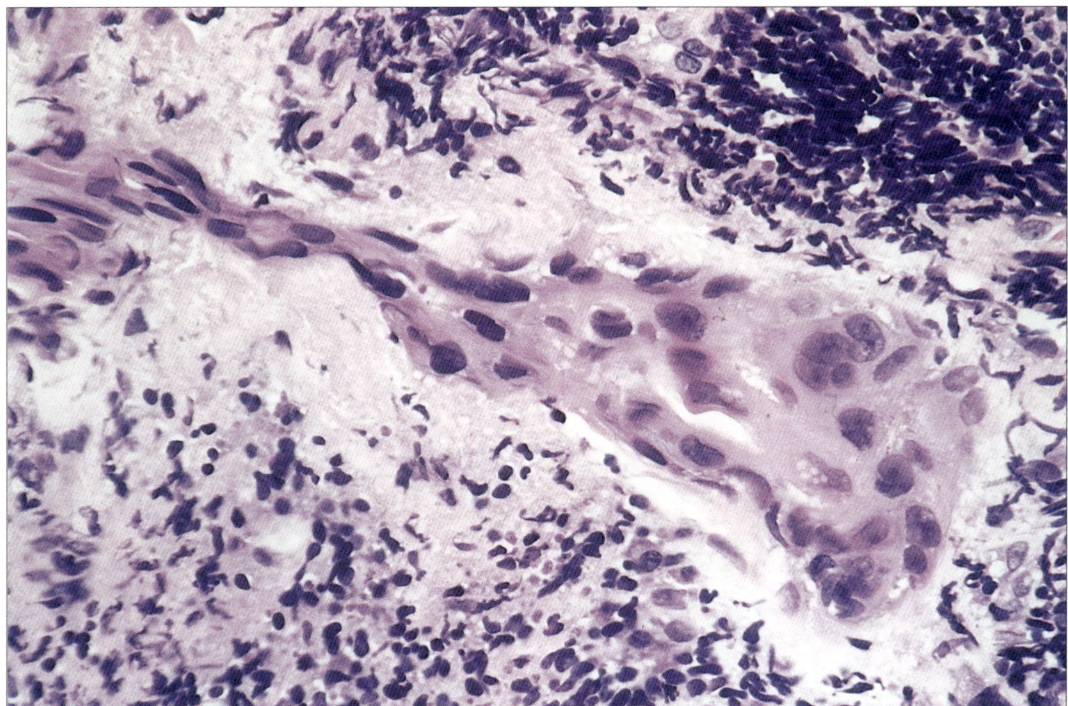

Figure 19. Radiation induced atypia of benign tonsillar crypt cells one month after radiotherapy. There is a suggestion of squamous differentiation and this group of cells appears to be in continuity with the overlying mucosa at the edge of the illustration. In some cases, it may be impossible to be sure that such cells are not residual degenerating tumour. They can be distinguished from lymphoepithelial carcinoma cells by their superficial location or their continuity with surface mucosa or tonsillar crypts. Individual cell keratinization and definite intercellular bridges in superficial cells one month after radiotherapy and the presence of numerous plasma cells elsewhere in the section are points in favour of benign radiation induced changes. Stains for cytokeratin are of no help in distinguishing the two. Benign epithelial cells are cytokeratin positive. (PWH reference 97.17301; same case as *Figures 17 and 18*).

Familial Nasopharyngeal Carcinoma

The tendency for nasopharyngeal carcinoma to run in Chinese families is well known. Familial clustering of nasopharyngeal carcinoma has also been observed in non-Chinese[56] and in Greenland natives and familial clustering has been observed in both nasopharyngeal carcinoma and in Eskimos.[57]

Association with Other Malignancies [Excluding Radiation Induced Sarcoma]

Cooper *et al.*[58] reported a 4.1% incidence of second malignancies in a series of 121 patients with cancer in the nasopharynx treated by radiotherapy alone. It is not clear how many

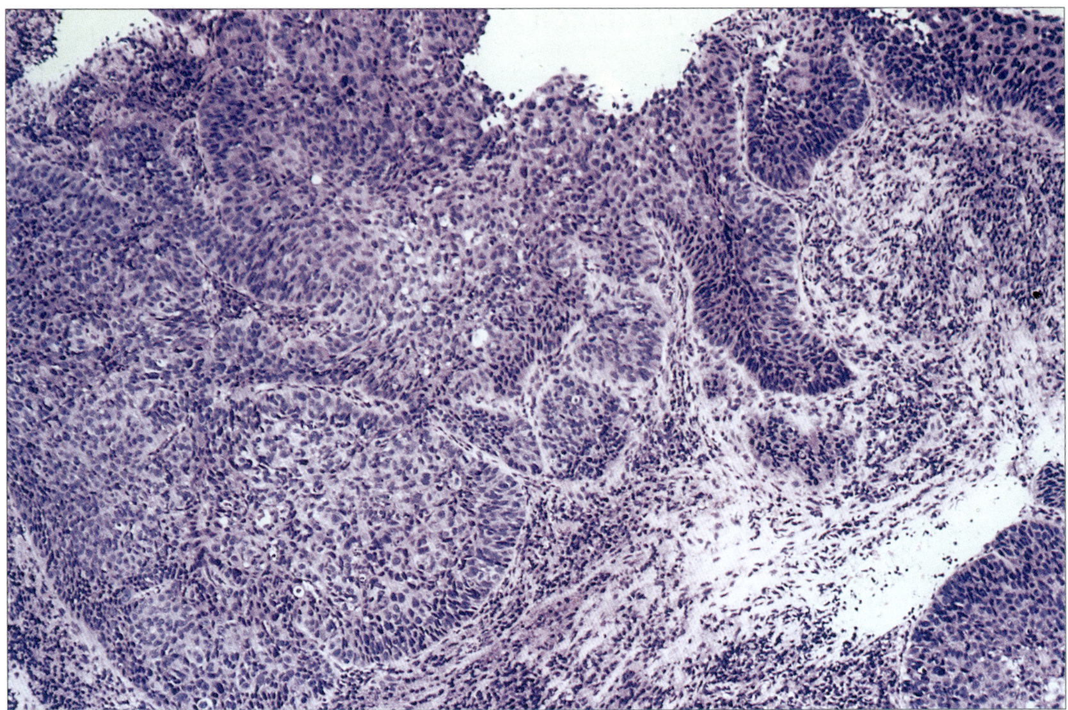

Figure 20. Biopsy of a tumour originally said to have come from the nasopharynx. The invasive tumour on the left side of the illustration resembles the Regaud variant of a lymphoepithelial carcinoma but on the right, there is intra-epithelial spread (carcinoma in situ) with individual cell keratinization as the cells approach the surface, a feature which rules out untreated lymphoepithelial carcinoma and indicates squamous cell carcinoma. Further enquiry revealed that the tumour was centered in the vallecula and was not in the usual position for a nasopharyngeal lymphoepithelial carcinoma. (PWH reference 97.15574).

of those patients, who were apparently resident in Philadelphia, had lymphoepithelial carcinoma rather than squamous cell carcinoma nor how many of the second malignancies were radiation induced.

In my experience, second malignancies that are not radiation induced do not seem to occur at a higher rate than in the general population. However, there is one Prince of Wales Hospital patient with multiple endocrine neoplasia type II, manifested by medullary carcinoma of the thyroid and unilateral adrenal pheochromocytoma, who developed lymphoepithelial nasopharyngeal carcinoma which metastasized to deep cervical lymph nodes. This seems to be a unique case.

While multiple primary squamous cell carcinomas occur in 2.4% of Hong Kong patients with squamous cell carcinoma of the oral cavity, oropharynx, hypopharynx and larynx,[59] there is no significant association between squamous cell carcinoma of the head and neck and lymphoepithelial carcinoma of the nasopharynx. Choy and associates[59] reported only one nasopharyngeal carcinoma developing in 573 Hong Kong patients with head and neck squamous cell carcinoma followed for 4.5 years (0.17%).

Malignancies Induced by Radiation Therapy

Cahan *et al.*[60] proposed that three requirements should be satisfied before a malignancy should be considered to be radiation induced.

(1) The tumour must arise in an irradiated area.
(2) The tumour must be histologically different from the patient's previous tumours.
(3) There must be a latent interval between the time that the radiation is given and the time that the tumour appears.

The length of the latent interval can be as short as two years or as long as 40 years.[61] The latent interval is shorter in those patients treated with megavoltage radiotherapy. The commonest histological type of radiation induced sarcoma is malignant fibrous histiocytoma followed by extraskeletal osteosarcoma, fibrosarcoma, malignant Schwannoma, extraskeletal chondrosarcoma and angiosarcoma.[61]

Ko and associates[62] found that the prevalence of radiation-induced malignant fibrous histiocytoma in long-term survivors of nasopharyngeal carcinoma was 0.38%. Most sarcomas arose in the maxillary sinus. The mean interval between radiotherapy and the appearance of malignant fibrous histiocytoma was 121 months. Local recurrences developed in all cases within 9 months after surgery. Six patients died of disease without distant metastasis within 30 months. Two patients were alive with disease at 20 and 32 months.

The average latent interval for sarcomas is about 10 years. This means that almost as many sarcomas arise before the 10 years interval as after. The prognosis of radiation induced sarcoma at all sites is very poor. The two year survival rate in Laskin's series was 32%. The survival rate for sarcomas arising after treatment of nasopharyngeal carcinoma seems to be worse. In Ko's series of eight patients,[62] the eventual mortality rate is likely to be 100%.

At the Prince of Wales Hospital, we have accumulated some 10 patients who developed squamous carcinoma of the tongue after radiotherapy for nasopharyngeal carcinoma. Many of the patients were women and most were non smokers with no other apparent risk factors for squamous carcinoma. These tumours all fulfilled Cahan's requirements so it seems highly likely that they were radiation induced. We have also seen radiation induced squamous cell carcinoma of the middle ear ten years after treatment for nasopharyngeal carcinoma (*Figure 21*).

Association with Dermatomyositis

An association has been noted between dermatomyositis and nasopharyngeal carcinoma in endemic areas.[63,64] Peng and associates[63] found that 27 (26%) of 104 patients with dermatomyositis had an associated malignancy. Twelve had a nasopharyngeal carcinoma, either before or after the diagnosis of dermatomyositis. They suggested

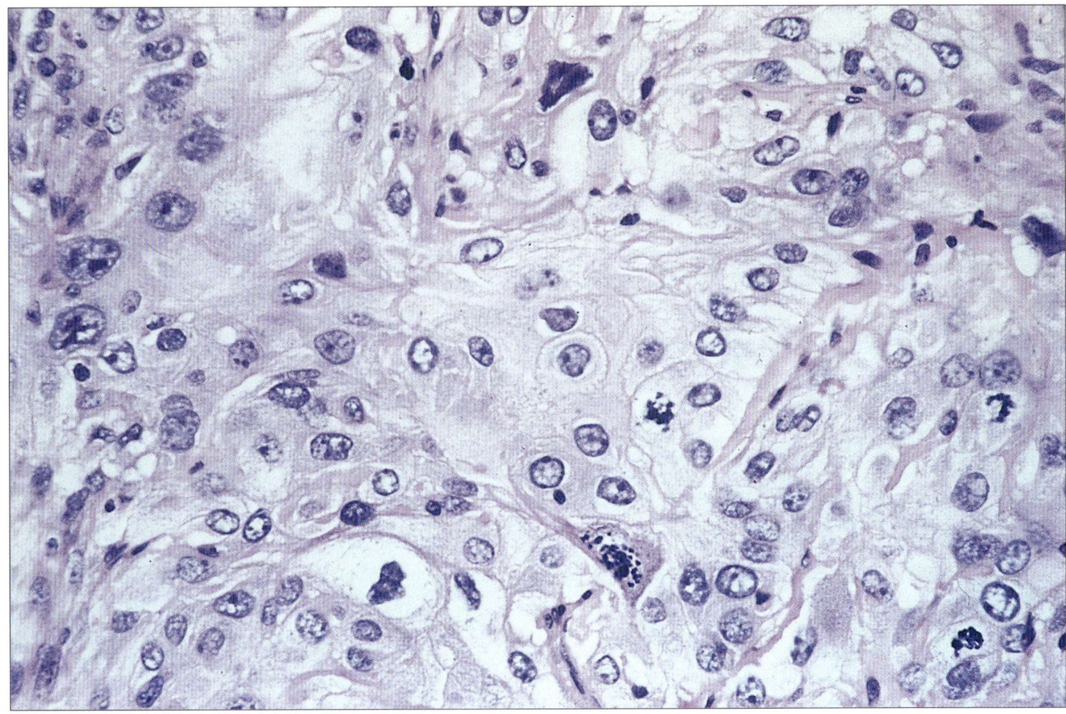

Figure 21. Radiation induced squamous cell carcinoma of the middle ear which appeared ten years after radiotherapy for nasopharyngeal carcinoma. Owing to the unavailability of modern machines, the patient had received a higher dose of radiotherapy to the mastoid bone than is now customary. In addition to the squamous carcinoma, he also suffered from radiation induced temporal lobe necrosis of the brain. However, there were no metastases nor was there any residual tumour in the nasopharynx. The illustrated middle ear tumour is a moderately well differentiated squamous cell carcinoma, histologically different from a lymphoepithelial carcinoma. It was widely separate from the nasopharynx. All of Cahan's requirements for radiation induced malignancy were fulfilled in this case. (PWH reference 97.16504).

that in endemic areas, patients with dermatomyositis should be screened for nasopharyngeal carcinoma.

Lymphoepithelial Carcinomas Outside the Nasopharynx

Lymphoepithelial carcinomas histologically identical to the nasopharyngeal tumour have been described in the salivary glands[65–68] (*Figures 22 and 23*), stomach,[69–71] base of tongue,[72] lung,[73] upper aerodigestive tract excluding the nasopharynx,[74] larynx,[75] thyroid,[76] skin,[77–80] vulva,[81] vagina,[82] uterine cervix,[83,84] urinary bladder,[85–87] breast,[88] rectum[89] and thymus,[90,91] but most of these tumours do not harbour the EB viral genomes.

The Epstein-Barr virus is said to be consistently associated with lymphoepithelial carcinoma in only four anatomical sites, namely stomach, salivary gland, lung, and

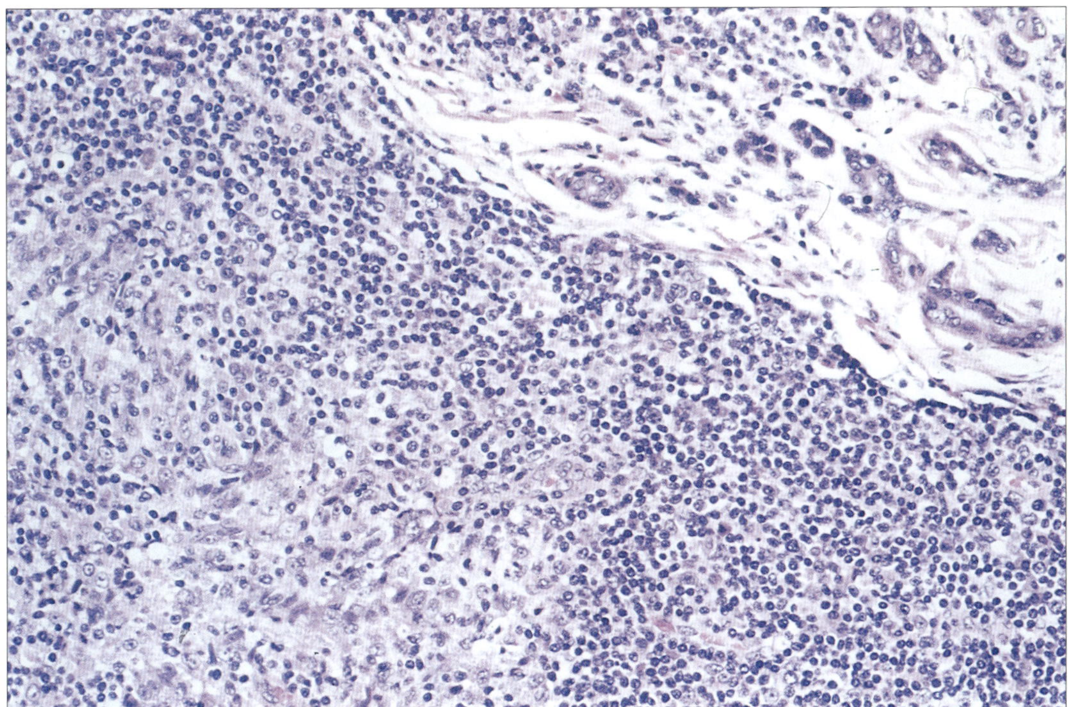

Figure 22. Eskimoma (lymphoepithelial carcinoma) of the parotid gland. Section of a large right parotid tumour from a Hong Kong Chinese male aged 27 years who presented with what was initially thought to be an enlarged right upper cervical lymph node. A fine needle aspiration was strongly suggestive of metastatic lymphoepithelial nasopharyngeal carcinoma. No other tissues apart from tumour and lymphocytes were present in the smear. The Epstein-Barr virus serology was markedly raised. Repeated biopsies of both sides and the center of the nasopharynx were all benign. A CT scan showed a normal nasopharynx but there was a tumour in the right parotid salivary gland. All the surrounding lymph nodes were of normal size and were radiologically normal. The illustration shows parotid ducts and tumour indistinguishable from the Schmincke variant of lymphoepithelial carcinoma. (PWH reference 96.515; same case as *Figure 23*).

thymus,[92] although in Hong Kong, we have seen at least one genuine, EBER positive primary lymphoepithelial carcinoma of the nasal cavity with no tumour in the nasopharynx (*Figure 24*). Racial or geographical factors seem to influence these associations. Thus, the EB virus association with tumours of the salivary glands, lung and the nasal cavity is apparently restricted to Asian patients and Eskimos, whereas the association with gastric and thymic lymphoepithelial carcinomas is independent of race.[92] The presence or absence of EB virus does not appear to be prognostically important.

Lymphoepithelial carcinoma of the parotid (Eskimoma) (*Figures 22 and 23*) is of some practical importance in Hong Kong. We see approximately two new cases per year in the Prince of Wales Hospital. The Epstein-Barr serology is raised and the tumour can easily be misinterpreted as metastatic nasopharyngeal carcinoma in parotid lymph

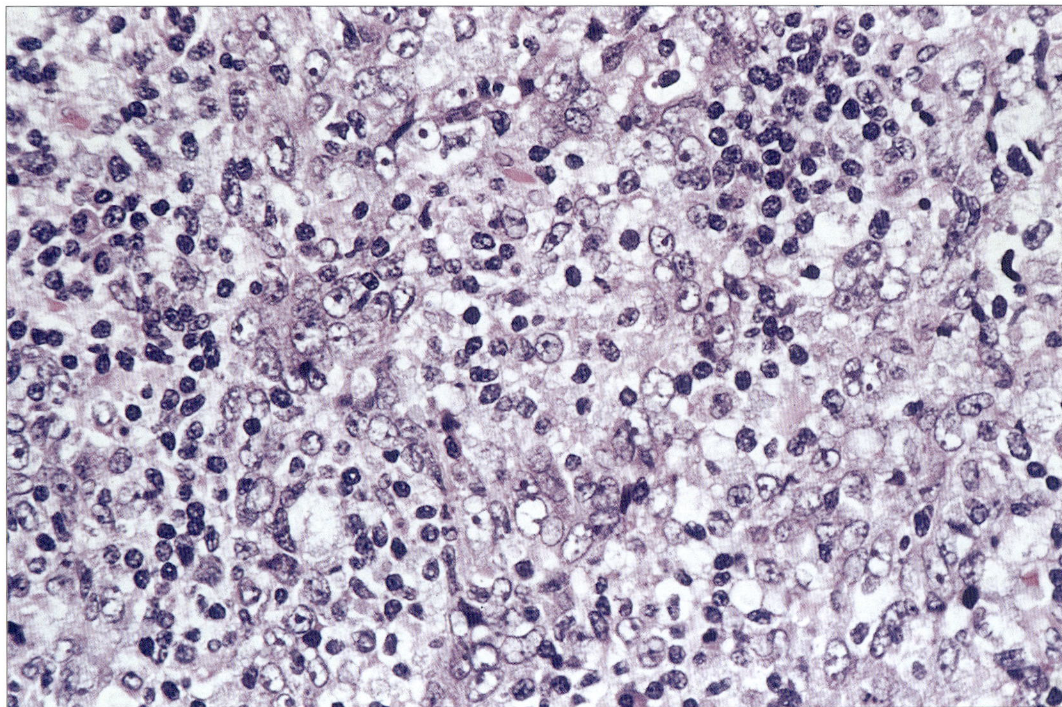

Figure 23. Higher power view of the parotid tumour illustrated in *Figure 22* showing a tumour indistinguishable from the Schmincke variant of lymphoepithelial carcinoma. (PWH reference 96.515, same case as *Figure 22*).

nodes with extension into the adjacent parotid. Organ imaging usually indicates the correct diagnosis because the nasopharynx is radiologically normal while the main tumour mass is centered in the parotid rather than in parotid nodes or in deep cervical lymph nodes. The deep cervical nodes are usually the first to be involved with metastases from a nasopharyngeal primary but are not usually involved in the early stages of an Eskimoma.

Epstein Barr Virus in Other Tumours

The finding of EB virus genomes in a tumour is not diagnostic of a lymphoepithelial carcinoma. In addition to Burkitt's lymphoma, varying concentrations of the virus or viral related products can be found in many other unrelated tumours and proliferative lesions. These include a percentage of nasopharyngeal squamous cell carcinomas,[43,93,94] oral hairy leukoplakia,[95–97] basaloid-squamous carcinoma of the nasopharynx,[98] squamous cell carcinomas of the larynx,[99] inverted (Schneiderian) papilloma of the nose,[100] gastric adenocarcinomas,[101] Castleman's disease,[102] various lymphomas other than Burkitt's lymphoma[103–106] and pulmonary lymphomatoid granulomatosis.[107]

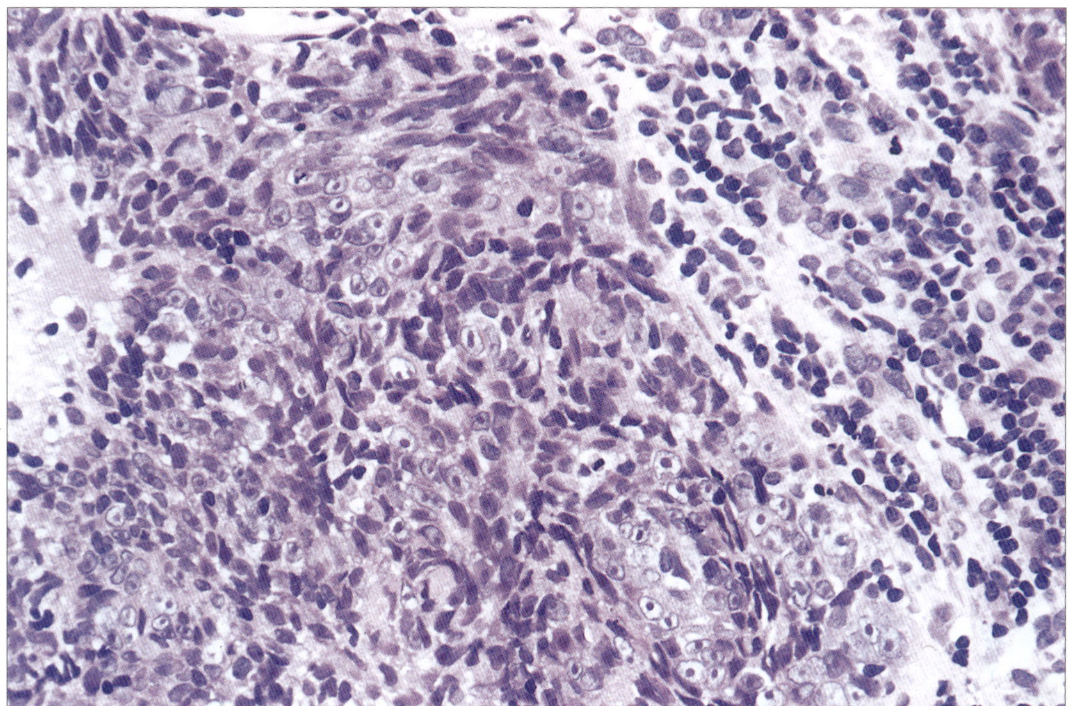

Figure 24. Primary lymphoepithelial carcinoma of the inferior nasal turbinate of a Hong Kong Chinese male aged 51 years. The tumour is histologically identical to a primary lymphoepithelial carcinoma of the nasopharynx. The patient's nasopharynx was clinically and radiologically normal, his EB serology was raised and the EBER stain was positive in the tumour cells, thus fulfilling the requirements for a genuine lymphoepithelial carcinoma located outside the nasopharynx. (PWH reference 97.16372).

By itself, the EB virus is not diagnostic of any one particular clinicopathological entity.

Metastases

The deep cervical lymph nodes are the first site for metastases and enlarged cervical nodes are one of the commonest presenting symptoms. In a recent series published by Huang *et al.*,[108] metastases distant from the cervical lymph nodes appearing after radiotherapy to the primary nasopharyngeal carcinoma occurred in 125 out of 629 patients (20%). Metastases were located in bone (75%), lung (46%), liver (38%), and retroperitoneal lymph nodes (10%). Multiple organ involvement occurred in 57%. Ninety five percent of the distant metastases appeared within 3 years after completion of the initial radiotherapy, 52% in the first year, 23% in the second year and 20% in the third year. The median survival time from the discovery of distant metastasis was 11.2 months for bone metastases, 16.3 months for pulmonary metastases, and 3.2 months for hepatic metastases. Those who presented with distant metastases had a significantly shorter survival than those who developed metastases after primary radiotherapy. The presence of hepatic metastases, short metastasis free interval, and older age at presentation were associated with reduced survival after the diagnosis of distant metastasis.[109]

Surgeons are generally reluctant to perform an open biopsy on enlarged cervical lymph nodes when metastatic lymphoepithelial carcinoma is suspected. In my experience, fine needle aspiration cytology of enlarged cervical nodes performed and interpreted by well trained, experienced personnel with adequate organ imaging facilities and technical support for the preparation, staining and assessment of the adequacy of the smears gives very reliable results (Chapter 8). However, if these requirements are not met, the results can be unreliable.

The histological appearances of the tumour obtained from open biopsies of cervical nodes is generally identical to the primary tumour. Occasionally, the tumour provokes a granulomatous reaction, with epithelioid cells and giant cells[110] (*Figure 25*), which may prompt an erroneous diagnosis of tuberculosis. As acid fast bacilli are often not found in sections from genuine cases of tuberculosis, a Ziehl Nielsen stain is only helpful

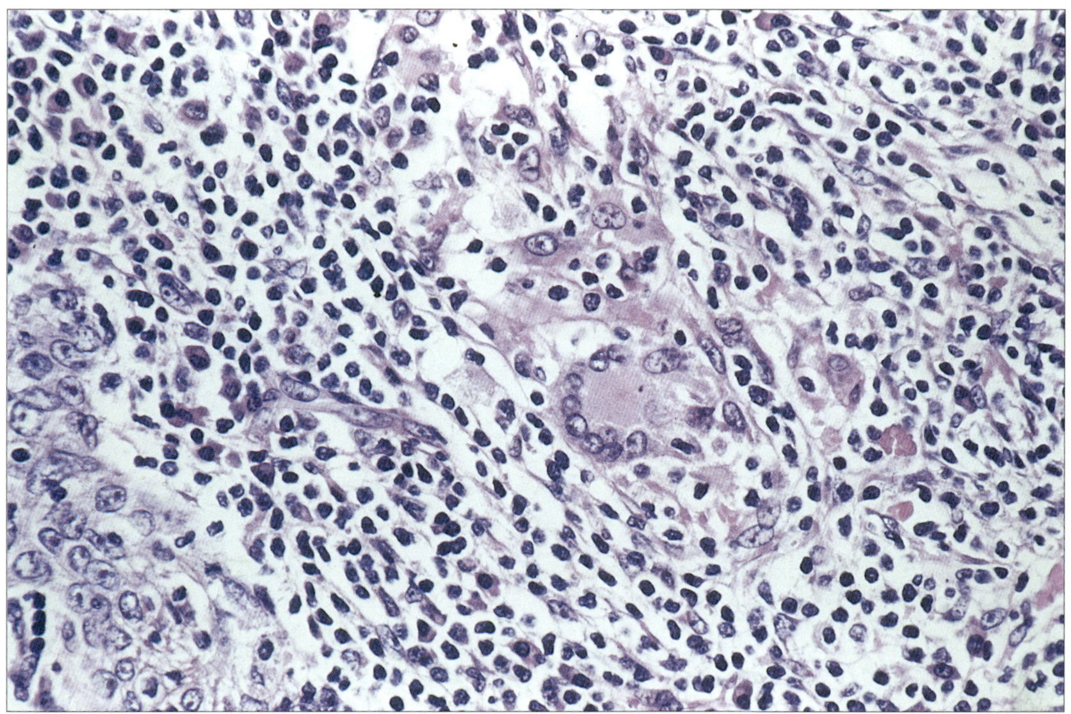

Figure 25. Granulomatous reaction with a Langhans giant cell in a cervical lymph node associated with metastatic lymphoepithelial carcinoma from a primary nasopharyngeal carcinoma. The metastatic tumour can be seen at the lower left hand corner. There was no clinical evidence of tuberculosis and acid fast stains were negative. The granulomatous reaction is an unusual host response to the carcinoma. (PWH reference 95.9330).

if it is positive. If there is no clinical support for a diagnosis of tuberculosis and if acid fast stains are negative, it is best to withhold anti-tuberculous therapy and to regard such granulomas as a host response to the tumour until there is better evidence of tuberculous infection.

Summary

1. Lymphoepithelial nasopharyngeal carcinoma is a distinct clinicopathological entity which is different from squamous cell carcinoma, although it stains for keratins and exhibits some squamous features on electron microscopic examination. This view is contrary to the concept implicit in the World Health Organization classification of nasopharyngeal carcinomas.
2. The diagnosis cannot be made without knowledge of the site. The diagnostic criteria should be expanded to include the location (usually in the fossa of Rosenmüller) and the serum EB virus antibody levels in addition to the histological features.
3. The EB virus is intimately involved in the pathogenesis and EB viral genomes can be found in lymphoepithelial carcinoma cells in 100% of cases.
4. The cell of origin of lymphoepithelial carcinoma is not known. Candidates include the basal cells of epithelial crypts, epithelial cells of minor salivary glands and basal cells of the covering mucosa. Whatever their origin, the malignant cells invade the submucosal tissues early in the disease and spread extensively in the lamina propria, usually without involving the overlying mucosa.

References

1. Rosai, J. 1996. In: *Ackerman's Surgical Pathology*, 8th ed. St. Louis: Mosby-Year Book Inc., 296.
2. Choa, A., Gibb, A.G. 1991. In: *Nasopharyngeal Carcinoma*, eds. van Hasselt, C.A., Gibb, G.A. Hong Kong: The Chinese University Press, 6.
3. Ash, J.E., Beck, M.R., Wilkes, J.D. 1964. *Tumours of the Upper Respiratory Tract and Ear*. Washington, D.C.: Armed Forces Institute of Pathology, 37.
4. Shanmugaratnam, K., Sobin, L.H. 1978. International histological classification of tumours, No. 19. Histological typing of upper respiratory tract tumours. Geneva: World Health Organization.
5. Hyams, V.J., Batsakis, J.G., Michaels, L. 1988. *Tumours of the Upper Respiratory Tract*. Washington D.C.: Armed Forces Institute of Pathology, 62–66.
6. Hsu, H.C., Chen, C.L., Hsu, M.M., Lynn, T.C., Tu, S.M., Huang, S.C. 1987. Pathology of nasopharyngeal carcinoma: proposal of a new histologic classification correlated with prognosis. *Cancer*; 59:945–951.
7. Michau, C., de Thé, G., Orofiamma, B., *et al.* 1981. Practical value of classifying NPC in two major microscopical types. In: *Cancer Campaign: Nasopharyngeal Carcinoma*, Vol 5, eds. Grundman, E., Krueger, G.R.F., Ablashi, D.V. Stuttgart, Germany: Gustave Fisher Verlag, 51–56.
8. Krueger, G.R., Wustrow, J. 1981. Current histological classification of nasopharyngeal carcinoma at Cologne University. In: *Cancer Campaign: Nasopharyngeal Carcinoma*, Vol 5, eds. Grundman, E., Krueger, G.R.F., Ablashi, D.V. Stuttgart, Germany: Gustave Fisher Verlag, 11–15.

9. Tam, J.S. 1991. In *Nasopharyngeal Carcinoma*, eds. van Hasselt, C.A., Gibb, G.A. Hong Kong: The Chinese University Press, 148–151.
10. Reddy, S.P., Raslan, W.F., Gooneratne, S., Kathuria, S., Marks, J.E. 1995. Prognostic significance of keratinization in nasopharyngeal carcinoma. *Am. J. Otolaryngol.*; 16:103–108.
11. McGuire, L.J., Lee, J.C.K. 1990. The histopathologic diagnosis of nasopharyngeal carcinoma. *Ear Nose Throat J.*; 69:229–236.
12. Busson, P., Braham, K., Clausse, B., Tursz, T. 1988. Constitutive expression of HLA class II antigens on EBV positive malignant cells from nasopharyngeal carcinoma: possible involvement in T cell infiltration. *Cancer Detect. Prev.*; 12:363–368,
13. Herait, P., Ganem, G., Lipinski, M., Carlu, C., Micheau, C., Schwaab, G., de Thé, G., Tursz, T. 1987. Lymphocyte subsets in tumour of patients with undifferentiated nasopharyngeal carcinoma: presence of lymphocytes with the phenotype of activated T cells. *Brit. J. Cancer*; 55:135–139.
14. Hsu, M.M. 1990. Local infiltration of T-lymphocyte subsets as a prognostic indicator in patients with nasopharyngeal carcinoma. *Ear Nose Throat J.*; 69:543–547.
15. Leighton, S.E., Teo, J.G., Leung, S.F., Cheung, A.Y., Lee, J.C., van Hasselt, C.A. 1996. Prevalence and prognostic significance of tumour-associated tissue eosinophilia in nasopharyngeal carcinoma. *Cancer*; 77:436–440.
16. Chan, K.M., McGuire, L.J., Lee, J.C.K. 1988. Cytology of amyloidosis in smears of nasopharyngeal carcinoma (letter). *Acta Cytol.*; 32:377–380.
17. Prathap, K., Looi, L.M., Prasad, U. 1984. Localized amyloidosis in nasopharyngeal carcinoma. *Histopathology*; 8:27–34.
18. McGuire, L.J., Lee, J.C.K. 1990. The histopathologic diagnosis of nasopharyngeal carcinoma. *Ear Nose Throat J.*; 69:229–236.
19. Shi, S.R., Goodman, M.L., Bhan, K. 1984. Immunohistochemical study of nasopharyngeal carcinoma with monoclonal keratin antibodies. *Am. J. Pathol.*; 117:53–63.
20. Madri, J.A., Barwick, K.W. 1982. An immunohistochemical study of nasopharyngeal neoplasms using keratin antibodies. Epithelial versus non-epithelial neoplasms. *Am. J. Surg. Pathol.*; 6:143–149.
21. Miettinen, M., Lehto, V.P., Virtanen, I. 1982. Nasopharyngeal lymphoepithelioma. Histologic diagnosis as aided by immunohistochemical demonstration of keratin. *Virchows Arch. B Cell Pathol.*; 40:163–169.
22. Ziegels-Weissmann, J., Nadji, M., Penneys, N.S., Morales, A.R. 1984. Prekeratin immunohistochemistry in the diagnosis of undifferentiated carcinoma of the nasopharyngeal type. *Arch. Path. Lab. Med.*; 108:588–589.
23. Taxy, J.B., Hidvegi, D.F., Battifora, H. 1985. Nasopharyngeal carcinoma. Antikeratin immunohistochemistry and electron microscopy. *Am. J. Clin. Pathol.*; 83:320–325.
24. Oppedal, B.R., Bohler, P.J., Marton, P.F., Brandtzaeg, P. 1987. Carcinoma of the nasopharynx. Histopathological examination with supplementary immunohistochemistry. *Histopathology*; 11:1161–1169.
25. Kamino, H., Huang, S.J., Fu, Y.S. 1988. Keratin and involucrin immunohistochemistry of nasopharyngeal carcinoma. *Cancer*; 61:1142–1148.
26. Vera-Sempere, F.J., Micheau, C., Llombart-Bosch, A. 1987. S-100 protein positive cells in nasopharyngeal carcinoma (NPC): absence of prognostic significance. A clinicopathological and immunohistochemical study of 40 cases. *Virchows Arch.*; 411:233–237.
27. Ma, C.X., Jia, T.C., Li, X.R., Zhand, Z.F., Yiao, C.B. 1995. Langerhans cells in nasopharyngeal carcinoma in relation to prognosis. *In Vivo*; 9:225–229.
28. Giannini, A., Bianchi, S., Messerini, L., Gallo, O., Gallina, E., Asprella-Libonati, G., Olmi, P., Zampi, G. 1991. Prognostic significance of accessory cells and lymphocytes in nasopharyngeal carcinoma. *Path. Res. Pract.*; 187:496–502.
29. Lai, F., M-M., Cheng, P.N.M., Tsao, S.Y., Lai, K.N. 1990. Immunohistochemical characteristics of the infiltrating lymphoid cells and expression of HLA class I and II antigens in nasopharyngeal carcinoma. *Virchows Arch. A Pathol. Anat. Histopathol.*; 417:347–352.

30. Sheu, L.F., Chen, A., Tseng, H.H., Leu, F.J., Lin, J.K., Ho, K.C., Meng, C.L. 1995. Assessment of p53 expression in nasopharyngeal carcinoma. *Human Path.*; 26:380–386.
31. Kouvidou, C.H., Kanavaros, P., Papaioannou, D., Stathopoulos, E., Sotsiou, F., Datseris, G., Tzardi, M., Kittas, C., Delides, G. 1995. Expression of bcl-2 and p53 proteins in nasopharyngeal carcinoma. Absence of correlation with the presence of EBV encoded EBER1-2 transcripts and latent membrane protein-1. *J. Clin. Pathol. Clin. Mol. Pathol.*; 48:17–22.
32. Kanavaros, P., Kouvidou, C., Dai, Y., Tzardi, M., Datseris, G., Darivianaki, K., Rontogianni, D., Delides, G. 1995. MDM-2 protein expression in nasopharyngeal carcinomas. Comparative study with p53 protein expression. *J. Clin. Pathol. Clin. Mol. Pathol.*; 48:322–325.
33. Vera-Sempere, F.J., Burgos, J.S., Botella, M.S., Cordoba, J., Gobernado, M. 1996. Immunohistochemical expression of Epstein-Barr virus-encoded latent membrane protein (LMP-1) in paraffin sections of EBV-associated nasopharyngeal carcinoma in Spanish patients. *Eur. J. Cancer, Part B, Oral Oncol.*; 32:163–168.
34. Zheng, X., Hu, L., Chen, F., Christensson, B. 1994. Expression of Ki67 antigen, epidermal growth factor receptor and Epstein-Barr virus encoded latent membrane protein (LMP1) in nasopharyngeal carcinoma. *Eur. J. Cancer, Part B, Oral Oncol.*; 30:290–295.
35. Kouvidou, Ch., Rontogianni, D., Tzardi, M., Datseris, G., Panayiotides, I., Darivianaki, K., Karidi, E., Delides, G., Kanavaros, P. 1995. Beta-2-microglobulin and HLA-DR expression in relation to the presence of Epstein-Barr virus in nasopharyngeal carcinomas. *Pathobiology*; 63:320–327.
36. Ruco, L.P., Stoppacciaro, A., Uccini, S., Breviario, F., Dejana, E., Gallo, A., De Vincentiis, M., Pileri, S., Nicholls, J.M., Baroni, C.D. 1994. Expression of intercellular adhesion molecule-1 and vascular cell adhesion molecule-1 in undifferentiated nasopharyngeal carcinoma (lymphoepithelioma) and in malignant epithelial tumours. *Human Path.*; 25:924–928.
37. De Vincentiis, M., Gallo, A., Minni, A., Simonelli, M., Uccini, S., Ruco, L. 1996. Undifferentiated nasopharyngeal carcinoma (U-NPC): Immunohistochemical study of adhesion molecules. *Rev. Laryngol. Otol. Rhinol.*; 117:215–217.
38. Porter, M.J., Field, J.K., Leung, S.F., Lo, D., Lee, J.C., Spandidos, D.A., van Hasselt, C.A. 1994. The detection of the c-myc and ras oncogenes in nasopharyngeal carcinoma by immunohistochemistry. *Acta Otolaryngol.* (Stockh); 114:105–109.
39. Stewart, J.P., Arrand, J.R. 1993. Expression of the Epstein-Barr virus latent membrane protein in nasopharyngeal carcinoma biopsy specimens. *Human Path.*; 24:239–242.
40. Lin, H.S., Lin, C.S., Yeh, S., Tu, S.M. 1969. Fine structure of nasopharyngeal carcinoma with special reference to the anaplastic type. *Cancer*; 23:390–405.
41. Chao, T.Y., Chow, K.C., Chang, J.Y., Wang, C.C., Tsao, T.Y., Harn, H.J., Chi, K.H. 1996. Expression of Epstein-Barr virus-encoded RNAs as a marker for metastatic undifferentiated nasopharyngeal carcinoma. *Cancer*; 78:24–29.
42. Pathmanathan, R., Prasad, U., Sadler, R., Flynn, K., Raab-Traub, N. 1995. Clonal proliferations of cells infected with Epstein-Barr virus in preinvasive lesions related to nasopharyngeal carcinoma. *N. Engl. J. Med.*; 333:693–698.
43. Kripalani-Joshi, S., Law, H.Y. 1994. Identification of integrated Epstein-Barr virus in nasopharyngeal carcinoma using pulse field gel electrophoresis. *Int. J. Cancer*; 56:187–192.
44. Niemhom, S., Maeda, S., Raksakait, K., Petchclai, B. 1995. Epstein-Barr virus DNA in nasopharyngeal carcinoma in Thai patients at Ramathibodi Hospital, Bangkok. *Southeast Asian J. Trop. Med. Public Health*; 26 (Suppl. 1):325–328.
45. Della Torre, G., Pilotti, S., Donghi, R., Pasquini, G., Longoni, A., Grandi, C., Salvatori, P., Pierotti, M.A., Rilke, F. 1994. Epstein-Barr virus genomes in undifferentiated and squamous cell nasopharyngeal carcinomas in Italian patients. *Diagn. Mol. Path.*; 3:32–37.
46. Brousset, P., Butet, V., Chittal, S., Selves, J., Delsol, G. 1992. Comparison of in situ hybridization using different nonisotopic probes for detection of Epstein-Barr virus in nasopharyngeal carcinoma and

immunohistochemical correlation with anti-latent membrane protein antibody. *Lab. Invest.*; 67:457–464.

47. Choi, P.H., Suen, M.W., Huang, D.P., Lo, K.W., Lee, J.C. 1993. Nasopharyngeal carcinoma: genetic changes, Epstein-Barr virus infection, or both. A clinical and molecular study of 36 patients. *Cancer*; 72:2873–2878.
48. Zur Hausen, H., Schulte-Holthausen, H., Klein, G., *et al.* 1970. EBV DNA in biopsies of Burkitt tumours and anaplastic carcinomas of the nasopharynx. *Nature*; 228:1056–1059.
49. Nonoyama, N., Huang, C.H., Pagano, J.S., *et al.* 1973. DNA of Epstein Barr virus detected in tissue of Burkitt's lymphoma and nasopharyngeal carcinoma. *Proc. Natl. Acad. Sci. USA*; 70:3265–3268.
50. Chen, C.L., Hsu, M.M., Hsu, H.C. 1996. Differential expression of EBER1 in nontumour nasopharyngeal biopsies and nontumour component of nasopharyngeal carcinoma. *Intervirol.*; 39:230–235.
51. Nicholls, J.M., Chua, D., Chiu, P.M., Kwong, D.L. 1996. The detection of clinically occult nasopharyngeal carcinoma in patients following radiotherapy — an analysis of 69 patients. *J. Laryngol. Otol.*; 110:496–499.
52. Bernheim, A., Rousselet, G., Massaad, L., Busson, P., Tursz, T. 1993. Cytogenetic studies in three xenografted nasopharyngeal carcinomas. *Cancer Genet. Cytogenet.*; 66:11–15.
53. Waghray, M., Parhar, R.S., Taibah, K., Al-Sedairy, S. 1992. Rearrangements of chromosome arm 3q in poorly differentiated nasopharyngeal carcinoma. *Genes Chromosomes Cancer*; 4:326–330.
54. Huang, D.P., Lo, K.W., van Hasselt, C.A., Woo, J.K., Choi, P.H., Leung, S.F., Cheung, S.T., Cairns, P., Sidransky, D., Lee, J.C. 1994. A region of homozygous deletion on chromosome 9p21–22 in primary nasopharyngeal carcinoma. *Cancer Res.*; 54:4003–4006.
55. Choi, P.H., Suen, M.W., Huang, D.P., Lo, K.W., Lee, J.C. 1993. Nasopharyngeal carcinoma: genetic changes, Epstein-Barr virus infection, or both. A clinical and molecular study of 36 patients. *Cancer*; 72:2873–2878.
56. Levine, P.H., Pocinki, A.G., Madigan, P. Bale, S. 1992. Familial nasopharyngeal carcinoma in patients who are not Chinese. *Cancer*; 70:1024–1029.
57. Albeck, H., Bentzen, J., Ockelmann, H.H., Nielsen, N.H., Bretlau, P., Hansen, H.S. 1993. Familial clusters of nasopharyngeal carcinoma and salivary gland carcinomas in Greenland natives. *Cancer*; 72:196–200.
58. Cooper, J.S., Scott, C., Marcial, V., Griffin, T., Fazekas, J., Laramore, G., Hoffman, A. 1991. The relationship of nasopharyngeal carcinomas and second independent malignancies based on the Radiation Therapy Oncology Group experience. *Cancer*; 67:1673–1677.
59. Choy, A.T.K., van Hasselt, C.A., Chisholm, E.M., Williams, S.R., King, W.W.K., Li, A.K.C. 1992. Multiple primary cancers in Hong Kong Chinese patients with squamous cell cancer of the head and neck. *Cancer*; 70:815–820.
60. Cahan, W.G., Woodard, H.Q., Higinbotham, N.L., Stewart, F.W., Coley, B.L. 1948. Sarcoma arising in irradiated bone: report of eleven cases. *Cancer*; 1:3–29.
61. Laskin, W.B., Silverman, A., Enzinger, F.M. 1988. Postradiation soft tissue sarcomas: an analysis of 53 cases. *Cancer*; 62:2330–2340.
62. Ko, J.Y., Chen, C.L., Lui, L.T., Hsu, M.M. 1996. Radiation-induced malignant fibrous histiocytoma in patients with nasopharyngeal carcinoma. *Arch. Otolaryngol. Head Neck Surg.*; 122:535–538.
63. Peng, J.C., Sheen, T.S., Hsu, M.M. 1995. Nasopharyngeal carcinoma with dermatomyositis. Analysis of 12 cases. *Arch. Otolaryngol. Head Neck Surg.*; 121:1298–1301.
64. Hu, W.J., Chen, D.L., Min, H.Q. 1996. Study of 45 cases of nasopharyngeal carcinoma with dermatomyositis. *Am. J. Clin. Oncol.*; 19:35–38.
65. Cleary, K.R., Batsakis, J.G. 1990. Undifferentiated carcinoma with lymphoid stroma of the major salivary glands. *Ann. Otol. Rhinol. Laryngol.*; 99:236–238.
66. Hamilton-Dutoit, S.J., Therkildsen, M.H., Nielsen, N.H., Jensen, H., Hansen, J.P.H., Pallesen, G. 1991. Undifferentiated carcinoma of the salivary gland in Greenlandic Eskimos: demonstration of Epstein-Barr virus DNA by in situ nucleic acid hybridization. *Human Path.*; 22:811–815.

67. Kountakis, S.E., SooHoo, W., Maillard, A. 1995. Lymphoepithelial carcinoma of the parotid gland. *Head Neck*; 17:445–450.
68. Tsai, C.C., Chen, C.L., Hsu, H.C. 1996. Expression of Epstein-Barr virus in carcinomas of major salivary glands: a strong association with lymphoepithelioma-like carcinoma. *Human Path.*; 27:258–262.
69. Burke, A.P., Yen, T.S.B., Shekita, K.M., Sobin, L.H. 1990. Lymphoepithelial carcinoma of the stomach with Epstein-Barr virus demonstrated by polymerase chain reaction. *Mod. Path.*; 3:377–380.
70. Shibata, D., Tokumaga, M., Uemura, Y., *et al.* 1991. Association of Epstein-Barr virus with undifferentiated gastric carcinoma with intense lymphoid infiltration. *Am. J. Pathol.*; 139:469–474.
71. Min, K., Holmquist, S., Peiper, S.C., O'Leary, T.J. 1991. Poorly differentiated adenocarcinoma with lymphoid stroma (lymphoepithelioma-like carcinoma) of stomach. Report of three cases with Epstein-Barr virus genome demonstrated by polymerase chain reaction. *Am. J. Clin. Pathol.*; 96:219–227.
72. Morais, D., Blasco, M.J., Benito, J.I., Mateos, J.J., Miyar, V. 1996. Undifferentiated carcinoma, or lymphoepithelioma, of the base of the tongue. *Acta Otorrinolaringol. Esp.*; 47:75–77.
73. Chan, J.K., Hui, P.K., Tsang, W.Y., Law, C.K., Ma, C.C., Yip, T.T., Poon, Y.F. 1995. Primary lymphoepithelioma-like carcinoma of the lung. A clinicopathologic study of 11 cases. *Cancer*; 76:413–422.
74. Frank, D.K., Cheron, F., Cho, H., Di Costanzo, D., Sclafani, AP. 1995. Nonnasopharyngeal lymphoepitheliomas (undifferentiated carcinomas) of the upper aerodigestive tract. *Ann. Otol. Rhinol. Laryngol.*; 104(4 Pt 1):305–310.
75. Andryk, J., Freije, J.E., Schultz, C.J., Campbell, B.H., Komorowski, R.A. 1996. Lymphoepithelioma of the larynx. *Am. J. Otolaryngol.*; 17:61–63.
76. Jochum, W., Padberg, B.C., Schroder, S. 1994. Lymphoepithelial carcinoma of the thyroid gland. A thyroid gland carcinoma with thymus-like differentiation. *Pathologe*; 15:361–365.
77. Carr, K.A., Bulengo-Ransby, S.M., Weiss, L.M., Nickoloff, B.J., Bulengo, S. 1992. Lymphoepitheliomalike carcinoma of the skin. A case report with immunophenotypic analysis and in situ hybridization for Epstein-Barr viral genome. *Am. J. Surg. Pathol.*; 16:909–913.
78. Takayasu, S., Yoshiyama, M., Kurata, S., Terashi, H. 1996. Lymphoepithelioma-like carcinoma of the skin. *J. Dermatol.*; 23:472–475.
79. Leung, E.Y., Yik, Y.H., Chan, J.K. 1995. Lack of demonstrable EBV in Asian lymphoepithelioma-like carcinoma of skin [letter]. *Am. J. Surg. Pathol.*; 19:974–976.
80. Jimenez, F., Clark, R.E., Buchanan, M.D., Kamino, H. 1995. Lymphoepithelioma-like carcinoma of the skin treated with Mohs micrographic surgery in combination with immune staining for cytokeratins. *J. Am. Acad. Dermatol.*; 32(5 Pt 2):878–881.
81. Axelsen, S.M., Stamp, I.M. 1995. Lymphoepithelioma-like carcinoma of the vulvar region. *Histopathology*; 27:281–283.
82. Dietl, J., Horny, H.P., Kaiserling, E. 1994. Lymphoepithelioma-like carcinoma of the vagina: a case report with special reference to the immunophenotype of the tumour cells and tumour-infiltrating lymphoreticular cells. *Int. J. Gynecol. Path.*; 13:186–189.
83. Walsh, C.B., Kay, E., Prendiville, W., Turner, M., Leader, M. 1993. Lymphoepithelioma-like carcinoma of the uterine cervix with c-erbB-2, p53 oncoprotein expression and DNA quantification. *Histopathology*; 23:592–593.
84. Weinberg, E., Hoisington, S., Eastman, A.Y., Rice, D.K., Malfetano, J., Ross, J.S. 1993. Uterine cervical lymphoepithelial-like carcinoma. Absence of Epstein-Barr virus genomes. *Am. J. Clin. Pathol.*; 99:195–199.
85. Amin, M.B., Ro, J.Y., Lee, K.M., Ordonez, N.G., Dinney, C.P., Gulley, M.L., Ayala, A.G. 1994. Lymphoepithelioma-like carcinoma of the urinary bladder. *Am. J. Surg. Pathol.*; 18:466–473.
86. Dinney, C.P., Ro, J.Y., Babaian, R.J., Johnson, D.E. 1993. Lymphoepithelioma of the bladder: a clinicopathological study of 3 cases. *J. Urol.*; 149:840–841.
87. Gulley, M.L., Amin, M.B., Nicholls, J.M., Banks, P.M., Ayala, A.G., Srigley, J.R., Eagan, P.A., Ro, J.Y. 1995. Epstein-Barr virus is detected in undifferentiated nasopharyngeal carcinoma but not in lymphoepithelioma-like carcinoma of the urinary bladder. *Human Path.*; 26:1207–1214.

88. Kumar, S., Kumar, D. 1994. Lymphoepithelioma-like carcinoma of the breast. *Mod. Path.*; 7:129–131.
89. Palazzo, J.P., Mittal, K.R. 1996. Lymphoepithelioma-like carcinoma of the rectum in a patient with ulcerative colitis. *Am. J. Gastroenterol.*; 91:398–399.
90. Dimery, I.W., Lee, J.S., Blick, M., *et al.* 1988. Association of the Epstein-Barr virus with lymphoepithelioma of the thymus. *Cancer*; 61:2475–2480.
91. Matsuno, Y., Mukai, K., Uhara, H., *et al.* 1992. Detection of Epstein-Barr virus DNA in a Japanese case of Lymphoepithelioma-like thymic carcinoma. *Jpn. J. Cancer Res.*; 83:127–130.
92. Iezzoni, J.C., Gaffey, M.J., Weiss, L.M. 1995. The role of Epstein-Barr virus in lymphoepithelioma-like carcinomas. *Am. J. Clin. Pathol.*; 103:308–315.
93. Horiuchi, K., Mishima, K., Ichijima, K., Sugimura, M., Ishida, T., Kirita, T. 1995. Epstein-Barr virus in the proliferative diseases of squamous epithelium in the oral cavity. *Oral Surg. Oral Med. Oral Pathol. Oral Radiol. Endod.*; 79:57–63.
94. Della, Torre, G., Pilotti, S., Donghi, R., Pasquini, G., Longoni, A., Grandi, C., Salvatori, P., Pierotti, M.A., Rilke, F. 1994. Epstein-Barr virus genomes in undifferentiated and squamous cell nasopharyngeal carcinomas in Italian patients. *Diagn. Mol. Path.*; 3:32–37.
95. Palefsky, J.M., Berline, J., Penaranda, M.E., Lennette, E.T., Greenspan, D., Greenspan, J.S. 1996. Sequence variation of latent membrane protein-1 of Epstein-Barr virus strains associated with hairy leukoplakia. *J. Infect. Dis.*; 173:710–714.
96. Murray, P.G., Niedobitek, G., Kremmer, E., Grasser, F., Reynolds, G.M., Cruchley, A., Williams, D.M., Muller-Lantzsch, N., Young, L.S. 1996. In situ detection of the Epstein-Barr virus-encoded nuclear antigen 1 in oral hairy leukoplakia and virus-associated carcinomas. *J. Pathol.*; 178:44–47.
97. Lau, R., Middeldorp, J., Farrell, P.J. 1993. Epstein-Barr virus gene expression in oral hairy leukoplakia. *Virology*; 195:463–474.
98. Wan, S.K., Chan, J.K., Lau, W.H., Yip, T.T. 1995. Basaloid-squamous carcinoma of the nasopharynx. An Epstein-Barr virus-associated neoplasm compared with morphologically identical tumours occurring in other sites. *Cancer*; 76:1689–1693.
99. Kiaris, H., Ergazaki, M., Segas, J., Spandidos, D.A. 1995. Detection of Epstein-Barr virus genome in squamous cell carcinomas of the larynx. *Int. J. Biol. Markers*; 10:211–215.
100. Macdonald, M.R., Le, K.T., Freeman, J., Hui, M.F., Cheung, R.K., Dosch, H.M. 1995. A majority of inverted sinonasal papillomas carries Epstein-Barr virus genomes. *Cancer*; 75:2307–2312.
101. Harn, H.J., Chang, J.Y., Wang, M.W., Ho, L.I., Lee, H.S., Chiang, J.H., Lee, W.H. 1995. Epstein-Barr virus-associated gastric adenocarcinoma in Taiwan. *Human Path.*; 26:267–271.
102. Murray, P.G., Deacon, E., Young, L.S., Barletta, J.M., Mann, R.B., Ambinder, R.F., Rowlands, D.C., Jones, E.L., Ramsay, A.D., Crocker, J. 1995. Localization of Epstein-Barr virus in Castleman's disease by in situ hybridization and immunohistochemistry. *Hematol. Path.*; 9:17–26.
103. Kumar, S., Kingma, D.W., Weiss, W.B., Raffeld, M., Jaffe, E.S. 1996. Primary cutaneous Hodgkin's disease with evolution to systemic disease. Association with the Epstein-Barr virus. *Am. J. Surg. Pathol.*; 20:754–759.
104. Nakamura, S., Sasajima, Y., Koshikawa, T., Kitoh, K., Kato, M., Ueda, R., Mori, S., Suchi, T. 1995. Ki-1 (CD30) positive anaplastic large cell lymphoma of T-cell phenotype developing in association with long-standing tuberculous pyothorax: report of a case with detection of Epstein-Barr virus genome in the tumour cells. *Human Path.*; 26:1382–1385.
105. Medeiros, L.J., Jaffe, E.S., Chen, Y.Y., Weiss, L.M. 1992. Localization of Epstein-Barr viral genomes in angiocentric immunoproliferative lesions. *Am. J. Surg. Pathol.*; 16:439–447.
106. Chen, C.L., Sadler, R.H., Walling, D.M., Su, I.J., Hsieh, H.C., Raab-Traub, N. 1993. Epstein-Barr virus (EBV) gene expression in EBV-positive peripheral T-cell lymphomas. *J. Virol.*; 67:6303–6308.
107. Guinee, D. Jr., Jaffe, E., Kingma, D., Fishback, N., Wallberg, K., Krishnan, J., Frizzera, G., Travis, W., Koss, M. 1994. Pulmonary lymphomatoid granulomatosis. Evidence for a proliferation of Epstein-

Barr virus infected B-lymphocytes with a prominent T-cell component and vasculitis. *Am. J. Surg. Pathol.*; 18:753–764.

108. Huang, C.J., Leung, S.W., Lian, S.L., Wang, C.J., Fang, F.M., Ho, Y.H. 1996. Patterns of distant metastases in nasopharyngeal carcinoma. *Kao Hsiung I Hsueh Ko Hsueh Tsa Chih*; 12:229–234.
109. Teo, P.M., Kwan, W.H., Lee, W.Y., Leung, S.F., Johnson, P.J. 1996. Prognosticators determining survival subsequent to distant metastasis from nasopharyngeal carcinoma. *Cancer*; 77:2423–2431.
110. Wockel, W., Wernert, M. 1986. Excessive epithelioid cell granulomatous reaction associated with a lymphoepithelial carcinoma (Schmincke-Regaud). *Path. Res. Pract.*; 181:349–356.

CHAPTER 6

Clinical Picture

C. Andrew van Hasselt and *Sing Fai Leung*

The presenting complaints of patients with nasopharyngeal carcinoma (NPC) can often be deceptive and confusing until the tumour reaches a relatively advanced stage. These difficulties, combined with the problems of examining the nasopharynx, present a diagnostic challenge to the clinician. The symptoms are closely related to the position of the tumour in the nasopharynx and the degree of direct and regional spread which may have occurred. Early symptoms are often minimal in nature and thus liable to be ignored or misinterpreted by both doctor and patient.[1]

NPC affects a relatively younger group of the population than almost any other head and neck neoplasm and the examining physician should not dismiss the possibility of this disease in young adults. In endemic regions the peak age incidence is in the 40–60 years age range with at least 60% of patients being under 50 years of age.[1] This age distribution applies to both sexes almost equally.

Mode of Presentation[1]

The relative frequency of the presenting complaint, based on a series of 437 patients, is outlined in *Table 1*. By far the commonest complaint prompting the patient to seek medical advice was the presence of a mass in the neck, which accounted for the initial attendance of almost half the patients. Nasal complaints were encountered in almost one third of patients, but aural symptoms, perhaps surprisingly, were less common (17%). Neurological complaints were even less common and tended to occur relatively late in the disease. It is rare to find patients with NPC who are totally asymptomatic, the few cases encountered usually being relatives of patients discovered at family screening clinics.

Analysis of Presenting Symptoms and Signs

Neck Mass

This is the most common symptom prompting the patient to seek medical advice. The vast majority of cases have unilateral cervical lymphadenopathy at the time of presentation. Nodal enlargements are normally painless. In almost all cases the superior

Table 1. Main presenting complaints.

Complaint	Percentage frequency
NECK MASS	**43**
Unilateral	36
Bilateral	6
NASAL	**30**
Blood stained discharge	18
Unilateral obstruction	5
Bilateral obstruction	4
Post-nasal drip	2
Moderate/severe epistaxis	<1
Nasal discomfort	<1
AURAL	**17**
Unilateral deafness	12
Tinnitus	3
Bilateral deafness	1
Otalgia	<1
Otorrhoea	<1
OTHER SYMPTOMS	**9**
Headache	4
Diplopia	1
Throat pain	1
Facial parasthesiae	<1
Facial palsy	<1
Hoarseness	<1
Dysphagia	<1
Shoulder weakness	<1
Tongue changes	<1
Blindness	<1
Trismus	<1
Vertigo	<1
Symptoms from distant metastases	**1**

cervical nodes are the first group to be affected, followed by enlargement of the mid and lower cervical nodes. Upper cervical nodes are also more bulky than lower cervical nodes, reflecting an orderly pattern of spread in a cephalad-caudal direction.[2] Bilateral neck involvement is not uncommon and when present, the nodes are often very bulky.

Nasal Symptoms

Nasal symptoms, in order of frequency, include a blood-stained nasal discharge, unilateral nasal obstruction, bilateral nasal obstruction, posterior nasal discharge often blood stained and frequently associated with continuous clearing of the throat. Epistaxis is seldom severe. Many of these symptoms can also be caused by rhinitis and sinusitis. The presence of blood in the nasal or post-nasal discharge is a hallmark symptom of NPC. Tuberculosis affecting the nasopharynx is a rare condition, but can give rise to all of the above symptoms.

Aural Symptoms

Symptoms related to the ear include hearing loss, tinnitus, otalgia and otorrhoea, all of which are usually unilateral. Of these, hearing loss is the most common. It is almost exclusively conductive in nature and due to middle ear effusion caused by malfunction of the eustachian tube. This is initially due to infiltration of the tubal musculature by the tumour and intermittent interference with the opening mechanism.[3] Tubal dysfunction may become more persistent as the tumour spreads into the surrounding spaces and structures. Since adult-onset serous otitis media, due to causes other than nasopharyngeal carcinoma is relatively uncommon, this is a warning sign for early recognition of the cancer.[4] In the assessment of tubal function, tympanometry is of paramount importance, supplemented by the recording of pure tone audiometric thresholds.

Tinnitus occurs in approximately one third of patients with NPC and can be particularly troublesome and difficult to treat.[5] Otalgia is surprisingly rare in view of the marked tendency of the tumour to infiltrate the parapharyngeal region and erode the skull base. Severe pain may result from infiltration of the glossopharyngeal nerve, which carries sensory nerve fibres to the middle ear, as it courses from the jugular foramen to the oropharyngeal region.

Neurological Symptoms

Neurological complaints comprise headaches or cranical nerve symptoms and are indicative of advanced local disease. Headache is the most common neurological symptom, occurring in almost 20% of patients.[1]

The incidence of cranial nerve palsy varies greatly between studies. These can occur as isolated or multiple palsies. The distribution of involvement is illustrated in *Figure 1*. Neel[6] in an analysis of 182 cases and Stillwagon[7] in 36 cases, reported incidences of 20% and 50% respectively. Our own study of 437 cases carried out in an endemic area showed the palsy rate to be lower at 12%.[1,8] CT scanning has confirmed that tumour infiltration (either intra- or extra-cranial) is responsible for the cranial nerve palsies.

Nerves V and VI are the most commonly affected resulting in altered facial sensation and diplopia. This is due to their relative proximity to the roof of the nasopharynx as they course through the cavernous sinus. Nerves III and VII may rarely be involved in more advanced cases, but these nerves are never involved alone, a point useful to the general practitioner in differential diagnosis.[8] Involvement of nerves IX to XII is an indication of advanced disease. Horner's syndrome occurs in 3% of all patients[1] and is invariably accompanied by a paresis of one or more of the last four cranial nerves. The syndrome is encountered in rare instances as a separate entity due to involvement

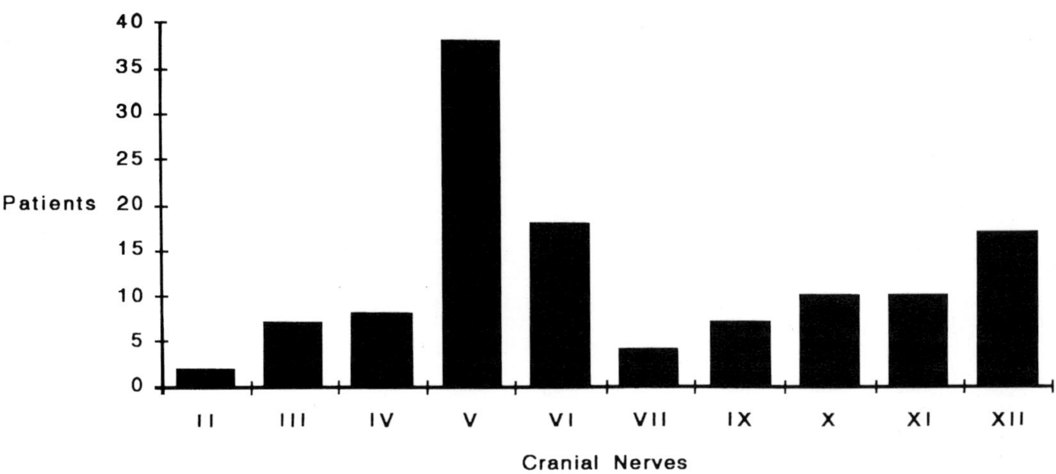

Figure 1. Distribution of cranial nerve palsies due to NPC.[1]

of the sympathetic plexus surrounding the internal carotid artery within the carotid canal.

Other Symptoms

These symptoms include trismus and other complaints, such as those from distant metastases.

Trismus is found when the primary tumour infiltrates the pterygoid muscles, thus restricting the degree of jaw opening. As a symptom of NPC on presentation it is rare. More frequently it is a sequel of radiotherapy, where fibrosis of the pterygoid muscles cause restriction of jaw movement.

Symptoms related to distant metastases are extremely uncommon on presentation. The most frequent symptom is bone pain, the skeleton being the most common site affected by distant metastases. Most studies suggest that 5% of patients have distant metastases at the time of first presentation and one in five of these has multi-organ deposits. These patients tend to be in the older age groups. The brain appears to be immune from haematogenous spread, but occasionally hypopituitarism, due to direct extension by the primary tumour, may occur.

Young Patients

In Hong Kong and other parts of southern China, NPC occasionally occurs under the age of 21 years. In the second decade it forms the fourth most common malignancy in males and the fifth most common in females. The histological appearances are the same as those found in adults although in children sarcomas account for one in four cases.[9,10]

In general, the range of symptoms is similar to that encountered among the older age group, but multiple symptoms are more frequent. Despite the fact that the mean duration of symptoms at presentation is slightly shorter than in adults, most patients are at an advanced stage on presentation. However, the response to treatment, the pattern of survival and relapse rates are similar to those of adult patients.[9,10]

Delay in Diagnosis

The stage at which the disease first presents is of great importance in determining the prognosis. Early tumours have an excellent prospect of cure but only one in five patients has Stage I tumour (Ho's[11] and UICC[12] Stage-Classifications) at the time of diagnosis, while three quarters have regional lymph node deposits palpable within the neck. The patients in the latter group have a less favourable prognosis.

In a study carried out in Hong Kong,[1] half of the patients had attended their doctor within 3 months of the onset of significant symptoms, over three quarters within 6 months, while only a very small number had failed to seek medical advice within a year. Those patients who presented with a neck mass had, on average, been aware of it for at least 4 months before seeking medical advice, while 15%, although aware of a swelling, did not even mention it to the doctor.

Symptoms related to the nose are often dismissed as unimportant initially by both the attending physician and the patient. This is not surprising as these symptoms are commonly present in simple upper respiratory tract infections, in allergic and other non-specific rhinitis and in acute and chronic sinusitis. Consequently the mean duration of nasal symptoms prior to first attendance is predictably longer than for other complaints.[1]

Sociological Aspects

A study of the social and educational background of a group of patients with NPC in an endemic region showed that only half had completed a primary education and one third a secondary education. Two thirds of the patients were aware of NPC as a disease entity, but none had acquired the information at school and less than one third by means of the media. In the vast majority of patients, information was derived from discussions with friends or relatives. Only one in six patients actually suspected the diagnosis at the first visit to the doctor.

It would seem, therefore, that an important factor in delayed diagnosis is lack of awareness on the part of the general public. However, other factors almost certainly play a role, including trivialisation of symptoms, fear of doctors and failure or procrastination in arriving at a diagnosis by the attending physician.

References

1. Skinner, D.W., van Hasselt, C.A., Tsao, S.Y. 1991. Nasopharyngeal carcinoma: a study of the modes of presentation. *Ann. Otol. Rhinol. Laryngol.*; 100:541–551.

2. Sham, J.S., Choy, D., Wei, W.I. 1990. Nasopharyngeal carcinoma: orderly neck node spread. *Int. J. Radiat. Oncol. Biol. Phys.*; 4:929–933.
3. Su, T.Y., Juan, K.H. 1985. Eustachian tube function in patients with nasopharyngeal carcinoma. *Kaohsiung J. Med. Sci.*; 1:53–62.
4. Sham J.S., Wei, W.I., Lau, S.K., Yau, C.C., Choy, D. 1992. Serous Otitis Media. An opportunity for early recognition of nasopharyngeal carcinoma. *Arch. Otolarynol. Head Neck Surg.*; 8:794–797.
5. Chowdhury, C.R., Ho, J.H.C., Wright, A., Tsao, S.Y., Au, G.K.H., Tung, Y. 1988. Prospective study of the effects of ventilation tubes on hearing after radiotherapy for carcinoma of the nasopharynx. *Ann. Otol. Rhinol. Laryngol.*; 97:142–145.
6. Neel, H.B. 1986. A prospective evaluation of patients with nasopharyngeal carcinoma: an overview. *J. Otolaryngol.*; 92:137–140.
7. Stillwagon, G.B., Lee, D.J., Moses, H., Kashima, H., Harris, A., John, M. 1986. Response of cranial nerve abnormalities in nasopharyngeal carcinoma to radiation therapy. *Cancer*; 57:2272–2274.
8. Leung, S.F., Tsao, S.Y., Teo, P., Foo, W. 1990. Cranial nerve involvement by nasopharyngeal carcinoma: response to treatment and clinical significance. *Clin. Oncol.*; 2:138–141.
9. Sham, J.S.T., Poon, Y.F., Wei, W.I., Choy, D. 1990. Nasopharyngeal carcinoma in young patients. *Cancer*; 65:2606–2610.
10. Huang, T.B. 1990. Cancer of the nasopharynx in childhood. *Cancer*; 66:968–971.
11. Ho, J.H.C. 1978. Stage classification of nasopharyngeal carcinoma: a review. In: *Nasopharyngeal Carcinoma: Etiology and Control*, eds. de Thé, G., Ito, Y. International Agency for Research on Cancer (IARC) Scientific Publications No. 20. New York: World Health Organization, 99–113.
12. International Union against Cancer. 1987. *TNM Classification of Malignant Tumors*. Berlin: Springer-Verlag.

CHAPTER 7

Clinical Diagnosis

John K.S. Woo

Introduction

An understanding of the epidemiology (Chapter 3) of nasopharyngeal carcinoma (NPC) and of its presenting features (Chapter 6) is necessary to alert the clinician to those patients who are particularly prone to develop this type of tumour. The presenting symptoms are diverse and, in a considerable proportion of patients, tend to be vague and non-specific. Careful examination of the nasopharynx must therefore be regarded as mandatory in all suspicious patients. However, a normal looking nasopharynx does not necessarily exclude a tumour, as the primary growth may be submucosal or too small to be identified. In suspicious cases, therefore, a biopsy is essential to provide tissue, on which a definitive diagnosis is based irrespective of the appearance of the nasopharynx.

History

The symptoms of nasopharyngeal carcinoma vary tremendously from one patient to another. As these are discussed in depth elsewhere, reference here will be brief. In the early phase of the disease, symptoms, if present, are usually related to the ear, the nose or both. These include hearing loss, tinnitus, nasal obstruction and blood stained nasal or post-nasal discharge. These symptoms should always be of concern to the clinician if unexplained, especially if unilateral. If the disease is advanced, the above symptoms may be more clear-cut or the patient may complain of a neck lump or symptoms of cranial nerve abnormalities or distant metastases.

Examination

A full head and neck examination is essential in all cases. Particular care is taken to look for serous otitis media, cranial nerve lesions and cervical lymphadenopathy. When nodes are palpable, their site and size must be carefully assessed as part of the staging process. Here, the neck is divided into three levels (1 to 3) from top downwards by two skin creases, one passing through the thyroid notch and the other passing through the sterno-clavicular joint. The lower the neck node involvement, the more advanced is the disease spread and the higher the neck staging.

The nasopharynx is one of the most difficult areas of the head and neck to examine using conventional techniques. The traditional method of indirect examination with a mirror, although adequate in many patients, is limited by variations in anatomy and the sensitivity of the gag reflex. In difficult cases, direct nasopharyngoscopy[1] may become necessary. This is preferably performed under topical anaesthesia both for the patient's comfort and to enable a biopsy to be taken if necessary.

A narrow end-viewing flexible fibrescope is ideal for this examination. It gives an undistorted view (*Figures 1 and 2*) and provides the flexibility required to inspect the area in detail. The excellent optics, narrow diameter and flexible tip of the fibrescope allow accurate assessment of the entire nasopharynx, enabling small lesions to be detected and large lesions to be accurately assessed. Mastery of the instrument is relatively simple to achieve with instruction and practice.

Alternatively rigid 0º and 30º Hopkins rod endoscopes are also suitable for direct inspection of the nose and nasopharynx.[1] In some cases, however, anatomical variations, such as a severely deviated nasal septum or pathological abnormalities, prevent the instrument being advanced through the nose into the nasopharynx. In these instances, a retrograde view of the nasopharynx can be obtained by passing a 90º endoscope through the mouth.[1] This provides a paramount wide-angled and centred view of the

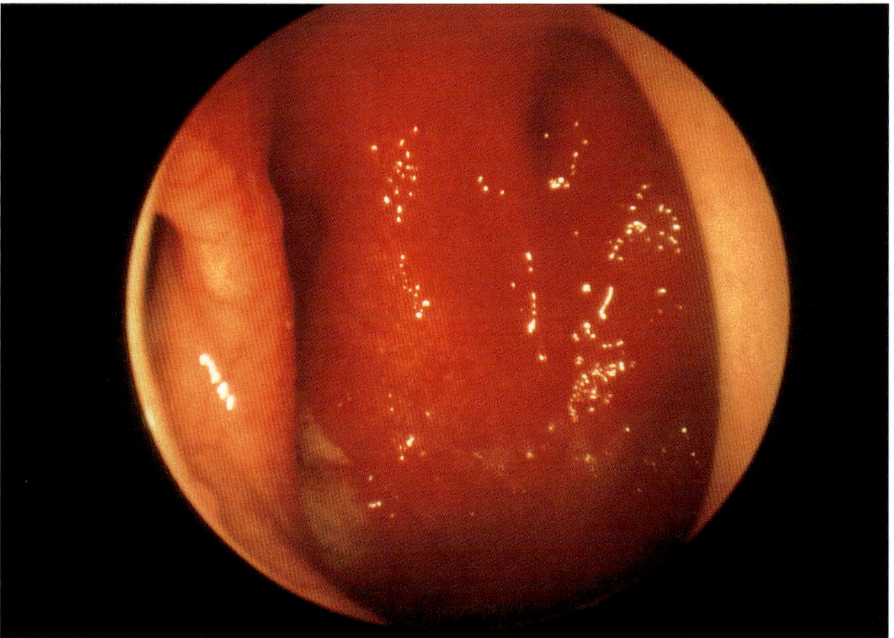

Figure 1. Normal nasopharynx viewed end-on through the right nostril.

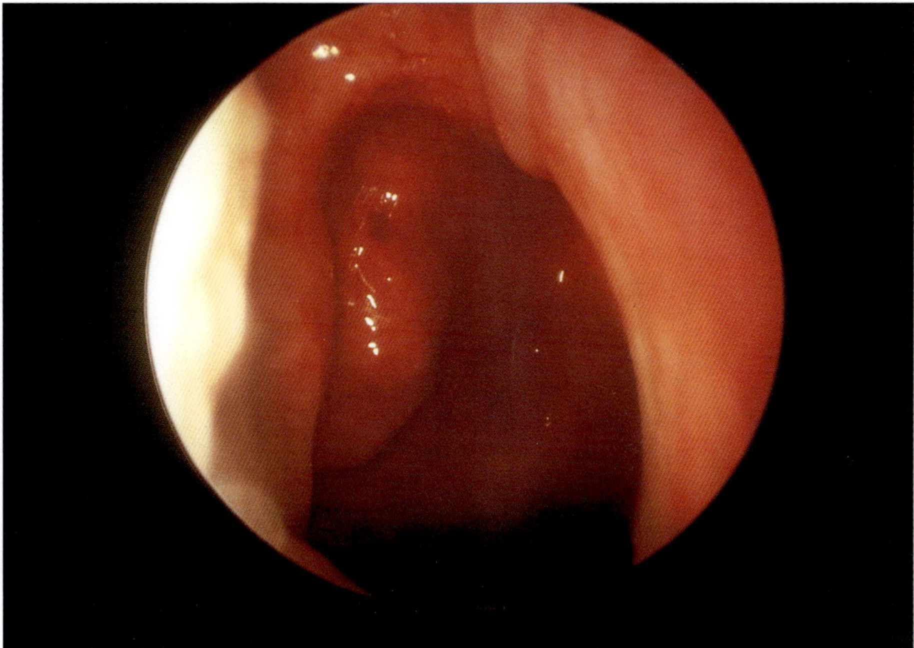

Figure 2. Early NPC viewed end-on through the right nostril.

entire nasopharynx with superb clarity of detail, which is invaluable in detecting even minute degrees of asymmetry. Furthermore, it is a great asset in photographic documentation (*Figure 3*). The extra effort expended in a meticulous examination is especially relevant in endemic areas, particularly as early tumours (*Figure 4*) may be identified by this means from time to time.

Gross Appearance

Although there may be considerable variation in appearance of the primary tumour depending on its size and the presence or absence of ulceration, familiarity with its usual features is important in reaching a clinical diagnosis. Tumours almost always arise laterally in the region of the fossa of Rosenmüller. Due to wide variations in the configuration of the fossa (Chapter 2), in certain instances an early tumour may be obscured so that it cannot be detected even by an experienced observer. As the growth enlarges, it usually encroaches on the Eustachian cushion (*Figure 5*). In a small number of cases, the tumour may arise from the vault or posterior wall of the nasopharynx where it is seen as a raised, well circumscribed mass, the surface of which is frequently ulcerated. Alternatively it may take the form of an irregular ulcer with raised edges. More advanced tumours appear as large masses with no clear indication as to their precise site of origin. The tumour is generally pale in colour and moderately vascular. Contact bleeding is common if the tumour is touched by the examining endoscope.

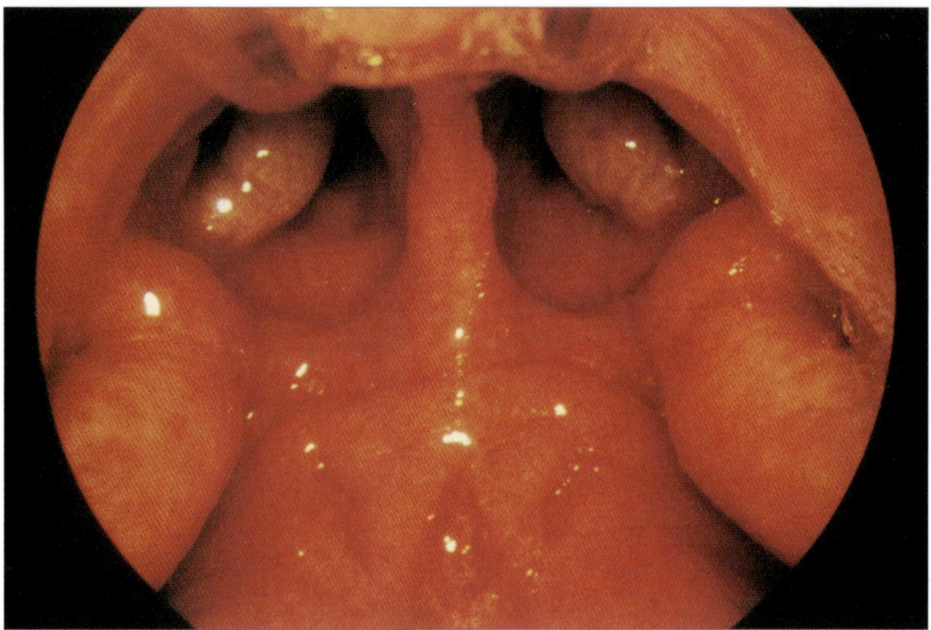

Figure 3. Normal nasopharynx viewed from the oropharynx through a 90º Hopkins telescope.

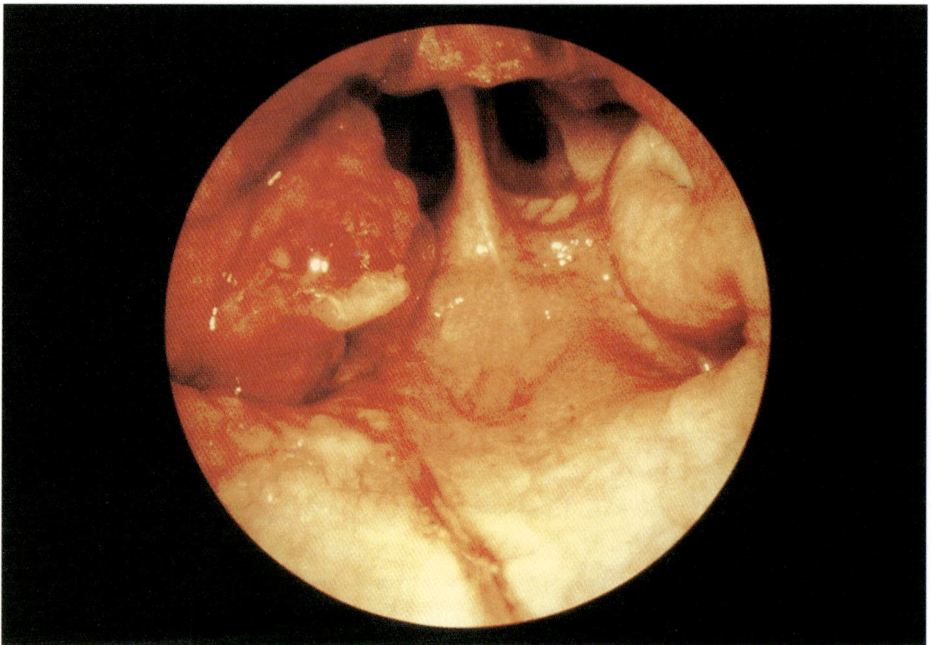

Figure 4. Early NPC on the right Eustachian cushion viewed through a 90º Hopkins telescope.

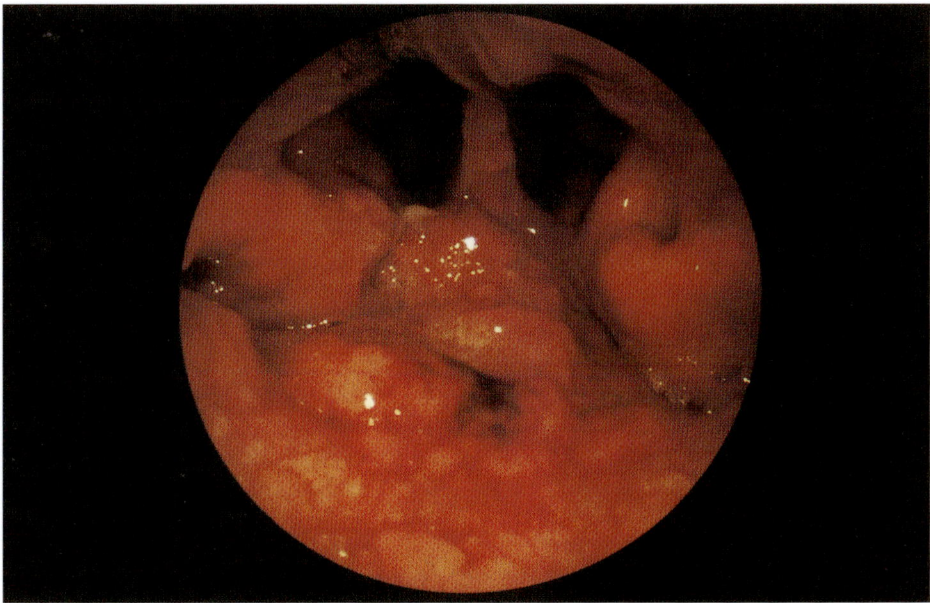

Figure 5. An ulcerated NPC. Note its relation to the eustachian cushion.

Tissue obtained by biopsy is typically soft and friable and is generally of pale grey or beige colour.

The observer should be constantly aware of the possible existence of submucosal disease which is often associated with a normal looking nasopharynx or a very mild degree of asymmetry. The latter may provide the only clue to the diagnosis.

The gross appearance of the tumour within the nasopharynx in no way indicates the extent of infiltration of the disease process.

Investigations

Biopsy of the nasopharynx

Biopsy of the nasopharynx is the definitive diagnostic investigation for patients suspected of having NPC if a visible tumour is present. Ideally, the biopsy should be taken at the out-patient clinic on the first visit. Additional investigations are only required in cases where no lesion is detected on clinical examination or for staging of the tumour.

With the availability of modern equipment, representative biopsies should be obtained from suspicious areas under direct endoscopic visual control. A blind biopsy is no longer acceptable, as the tumour may be missed and a negative biopsy may well impart a false sense of security to both the patient and the clinician, thus delaying the diagnosis.

The biopsy procedure is carried out under topical anaesthesia, with the patient either sitting or supine (*Figure 6*). The endoscope is passed through the side of the nose

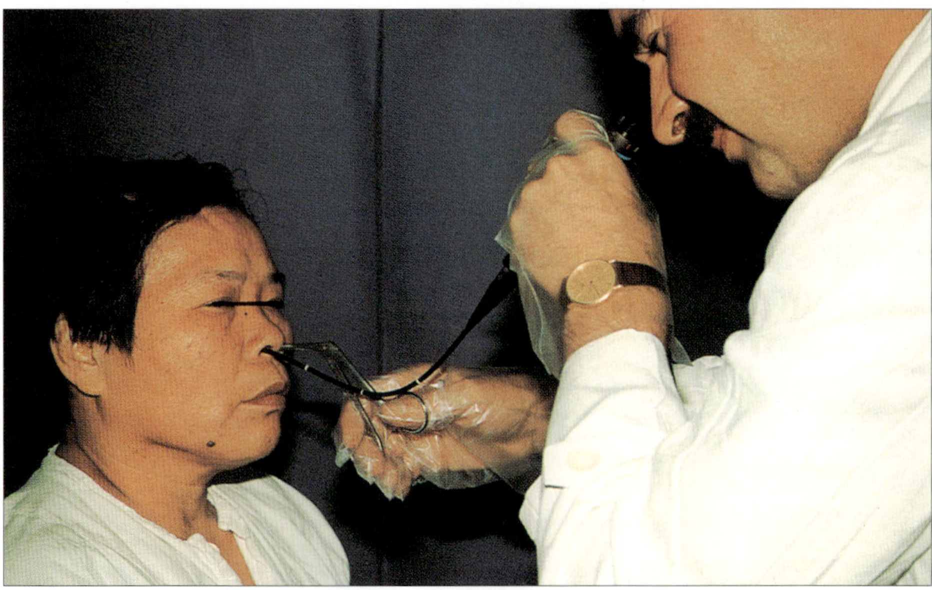

Figure 6. Biopsy of the nasopharynx in the out-patient clinic.

opposite to the suspected tumour site, leaving the ipsilateral side clear for the passage of the biopsy forceps (*Figures 6 and 7*). This arrangement of instruments provides the greatest flexibility and widest view possible from the endoscope, while reserving the most direct route for the passage of the biopsy forceps. A cupped biopsy forceps of

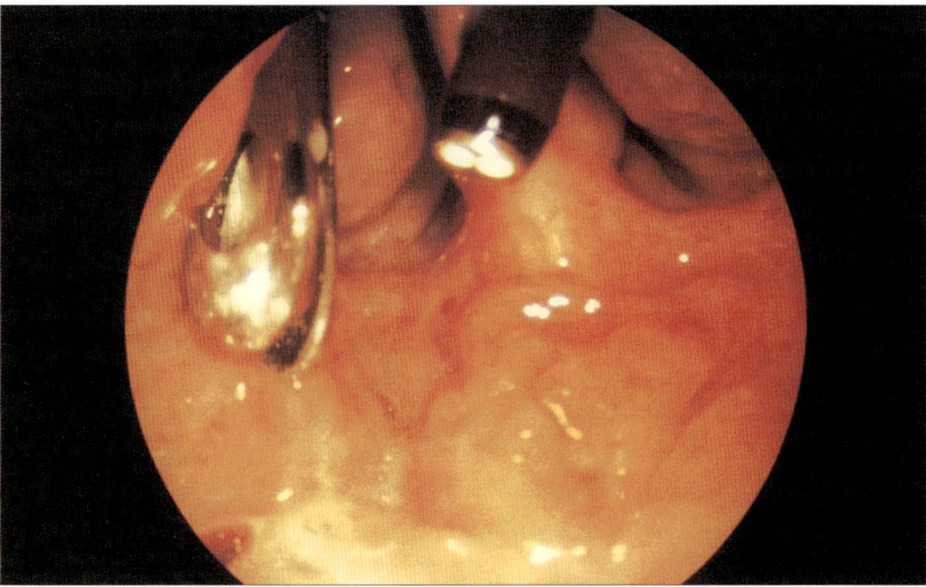

Figure 7. Biopsy of the nasopharynx under direct vision using a flexible endoscope.

adequate size is favoured to ensure that sufficient tissue is obtained. Either a flexible or a wide-angled 0º rigid Hopkins rod endoscope can be used for this procedure. The latter technique gives a better picture when video or photographic documentation is required. Biopsies taken through the operating channel in the flexible endoscope are discouraged as the tiny forceps provides an inadequate tissue sample. The higher risk of unrepresentative biopsies and false negative results leads us to strongly recommend the use of an independent biopsy forceps of suitable size. All specimens, after prior arrangement with the pathologists, should be sent fresh for histological examination. Fresh material may be required if special staining is indicated to assist diagnosis in doubtful cases.

The biopsy procedure is relatively painless as the tumour is friable and insensitive. However, if a biopsy is taken from a normal area, some discomfort may be experienced by the patient. Although some bleeding is to be expected, significant post-biopsy epistaxis is infrequent.[1,2,3]

In patients with clinical suspicion of NPC but with no visible tumour, or in cases where a biopsy under local anaesthesia has proved negative, the nasopharynx should be re-examined and biopsied under general anaesthesia. A Yankauer speculum is introduced through the open mouth, lifting the soft palate forward to enable the beak of the speculum to be placed behind the Eustachian cushion to expose the depths of the fossa of Rosenmüller. This is the only area of the nasopharynx, which, on account of anatomical diversity, may not be adequately visualised on endoscopic examination under local anaesthesia. Multiple deep biopsies are then taken from both fossae of Rosenmüller and from the posterior wall and vault of the nasopharynx. A definitive diagnosis can thus be established in virtually all cases. Repeated biopsies under general anaesthesia and, less commonly, nasopharyngeal curettage are rarely required to establish the diagnosis. Bleeding is normally controlled by packing the nasopharynx for a few minutes, but occasionally diathermy is required.

The technique as described using local anaesthesia has been found to have diagnostic sensitivity comparable to that obtained by direct examination and biopsy under general anaesthesia[3] and, in view of the fact that it is more convenient, time-saving and cost-effective, we consider this to be the method of choice.

Other investigations

In the majority of cases, the only investigation necessary to reach a diagnosis is biopsy combined with histological examination. In atypical cases however, especially where the disease is submucosal or biopsies are negative, additional investigations are indicated.

Serology

The detection of IgA antibodies to Epstein-Barr virus specific antigens is helpful in the diagnosis of NPC.[4] The IgA anti-viral capsid antigen (VCA) titre is a highly sensitive indicator of NPC although lacking in specificity, especially at low levels. The IgA anti-early antigen (EA) titre on the other hand is a less sensitive test. Indeed its level may even drop back to normal during the later phase of the disease. However, its specificity is high, a raised titre being an almost certain indicator of NPC. These tests, especially in combination, are useful to general practitioners in endemic areas, as they may provide guidelines for referral to specialists if titres are raised. They may also serve to alert the specialist to the possibility of NPC, especially in patients in which clinical examination is normal.

Imaging

Plain x-ray of the nasopharynx and base of skull may show a soft tissue shadow in the nasopharynx or bone erosion of the base of skull or cervical vertebrae. However, in the well equipped modern hospital, it is now obsolete as an aid to the early diagnosis of NPC, having been superceded by modern imaging techniques.[5]

CT scanning of the nasopharynx and base of skull, in addition to demonstrating the same features as plain radiographs, carries the added advantage of clearly defining soft tissue planes. It is especially useful in demonstrating the less common submucosal type of disease (*Figure 8*). It is the gold standard for staging of local and regional disease and is indispensable in radiotherapy planning.

MRI of the nasopharynx is more accurate than CT in detecting and staging nasopharyngeal carcinoma.[6,7] Nevertheless its value is limited by its relative lack of bone detail and high cost. However, MRI is much more sensitive than CT in detecting marrow involvement by tumour. It is especially useful in detecting or defining perineural

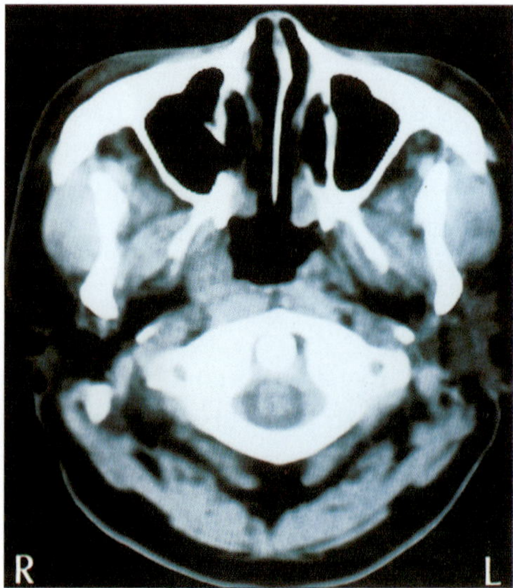

Figure 8. CT scan of the nasopharynx showing submucosal spread of tumour into the right parapharyngeal space. Note that the nasopharynx is smooth and almost symmetrical.

and intracranial tumour extension. Its ability to differentiate tissue densities renders it invaluable in distinguishing soft tissue abnormalities due to tumour from those of inflammation or scarring after radiotherapy.

Ultrasound examination of the primary tumour has very little use due to the difficulties of access to and application of the ultrasound probe in the nasopharynx. However, when a better designed probe becomes available, it may prove useful in detecting submucosal tumour in the nasopharynx and parapharyngeal extension of disease. Currently the use of ultrasound is confined to the diagnosis and monitoring of regional or distant metastases (Chapter 8).

Cytology

Specimens for exfoliative cytology are obtained by scraping the nasopharynx, employing different techniques such as using a brush, a cotton swab or a special applicator combined with suction (Chapter 9). The sensitivity varies widely with the method employed and the skill and experience of the cytologist. Thus far, the technique has failed to gain general acceptance as a reliable method of diagnosis.

Fine needle aspiration (FNA) of neck nodes for cytology is very useful in patients with suspicious nodal enlargement especially in the absence of a detectable primary tumour. FNA cytology readily differentiates metastatic nodal disease from tuberculosis. In NPC, the nodal disease is typically of the undifferentiated variety and can be recognized by an experienced cytologist.

Cytological smears from tissue biopsies or FNA material can be stained for the presence of Epstein-Barr virus associated nuclear antigen (EBNA) by specific monoclonal antibodies. Its presence greatly increases the likelihood of NPC.[8] On the other hand, a negative result virtually excludes NPC in endemic areas, as nearly all nasopharyngeal carcinomas are Epstein-Barr virus related. This test may prove useful in doubtful cases.

Differential Diagnosis

As outlined in the section on symptomatology (Chapter 6), nasopharyngeal carcinoma may manifest itself in a wide variety of ways.[9,10] Consequently the differential diagnosis varies according to the method of presentation. In patients attending with epistaxis, nasal obstruction or discharge, NPC may be mistaken for such common conditions as rhinitis in its various forms, sinusitis, deviated septum or nasal polypi. In non-endemic areas these symptoms arouse no suspicion, so that routine examination of the nasopharynx forms the basis of successful diagnosis and should never be omitted. A tumour causing these symptoms is almost certain to be visible on nasopharyngeal inspection.

NPC may also masquerade as serous otitis media. In any adult patient with unexplained serous otitis media, especially if unilateral and of recent onset, NPC must be suspected as a possible cause even in a non-endemic area. Great care must therefore be taken to exclude this tumour before making a definitive diagnosis of simple secretory otitis media and if no tumour is found a careful follow up is essential.

If a mass is visible in the nasopharynx, the appearance and site of the lesion should be taken into account when making a tentative diagnosis. A large mass of adenoids, which is sometimes present in the adult patient, has a smooth surface with longitudinal furrows and is centrally located. Simple cysts can be diagnosed with confidence by their small size and smooth rounded appearance. In case of cysts larger than 1 cm, particularly if they appear pulsatile, meningocele or meningo-encephalocele should be excluded by an MRI before any biopsy is attempted. Visual assessment is extremely important in the diagnosis of juvenile angiofibroma. This condition affects adolescent males and, although NPC normally presents in adults, the age incidence of the two groups does tend to overlap. Careful inspection of the tumour is vital, as biopsy of an angiofibroma should be avoided in view of the risk of torrential haemorrhage from this highly vascular lesion. The definitive diagnosis in angiofibroma is usually dependent on clinical appearance, MRI and rarely angiography. Occasionally, other diseases may present with a mass in the nasopharynx. These include tuberculosis, lymphoma, midline lethal granuloma and sino-nasal undifferentiated carcinoma. Rarely, tumours arising from embryological remnants, such as chordomas, tumours arising from Rathke's pouch and teratomas, may occur in the nasopharynx.[11] Other conditions including salivary gland tumour, fibrous tumour, giant-cell tumour, rhabdomyosarcoma and melanoma involving the nasopharynx have been reported.[12–18]

If the patient presents with a neck swelling, the diagnostic procedure is carried out in routine fashion as for any lump in the neck. Careful examination of the entire upper respiratory tract is mandatory and neck node biopsy should never be considered until all other investigations have proved negative. The conditions most likely to resemble NPC are inflammatory conditions, especially tuberculosis, lymphoma and other primary or secondary malignant tumours.

Patients presenting with cranial nerve palsies, without symptoms referred to the nose or ears, may mimic a wide range of neurological conditions. The most common palsies are those affecting the 5th and 6th cranial nerves as a result of skull base erosion by the tumour.[9,10] Occasionally patients may present with swallowing problems or hoarseness due to infiltration of the lower cranial nerves in the parapharyngeal space.[19] It is therefore important to examine the nasopharynx in all patients with unexplained cranial nerve palsies.

Diagnosis of Residual and Recurrent Disease

The diagnosis of residual and recurrent disease in the nasopharynx is much more difficult than the primary disease. After a full course of treatment, depending on the total radiation dose and the technique used, the local tissue inevitably exhibits varying degrees of reaction. Excessive crust formation and a mucosa which bleeds readily render subsequent examination and interpretation of the findings in the nasopharynx difficult and confusing. Furthermore, due to fibrosis of the pterygoid muscles, varying degrees of trismus may develop rendering throat examination difficult or even impossible. All of these post-irradiation changes may be present simultaneously, thereby compounding the diagnostic problems.

The nasopharynx may show post-irradiation changes that last for many months or even years. During the early post-radiotherapy period, regular nasal douching with saline by patients can help to minimise crust formation in the nose and nasopharynx and allow a more accurate assessment to be made. The use of a flexible endoscope with a suction channel facilitates the removal of crusts and permits a detailed inspection of the mucosa. However, unlike primary disease, residual or recurrent disease may not stand out as the whole nasopharynx may look abnormal after radiotherapy. Thus, an even higher degree of suspicion is necessary and any dubious area should be biopsied. This approach facilitates detection of small persistent or recurrent lesions, which are amenable to treatment. In case of doubt, reference to previous clinical and radiological documentation of the disease is of the utmost importance. As in the primary disease, residual or recurrent tumour may be entirely submucosal, and MRI and CT scanning of the region play an important role in the diagnosis. Under these circumstances biopsies of the nasopharynx must be deep and include the previously diseased area.

In the neck, fibrosis of the soft tissue after irradiation renders accurate examination difficult and at times impossible. The accuracy of fine needle aspiration cytology for the diagnosis of neck disease is adversely affected by irradiation. Not only is the sampling error inevitably increased because of the difficulties in the accurate placement of the needle in the post-irradiated neck, but the cytological interpretation of the aspirate is also more difficult. The latter is particularly true in the early post-treatment period as tumour cells seen in these situations are not uniformly viable. The foregoing problems multiply the chances of false positive and false negative results. Ultrasound examination of the irradiated neck is useful in detecting the presence of nodes and accurately guiding FNA in suspicious cases. The echographic features of these nodes help to distinguish post-irradiation from malignant changes (Chapter 8). In doubtful cases, close follow up and repeated aspiration biopsies are essential. Sometimes, excisional biopsy combined, where indicated, with radical neck dissection may be the only solution to this difficult diagnostic problem. However, removal of tissue for diagnostic purposes by excision, or more importantly incision of individual lymph nodes should be avoided if possible, as this may compromise the prognosis, presumably by causing dissemination of tumour cells.[20,21]

Accurate diagnosis of the presence and extent of residual or recurrent disease is of vital importance in determining the treatment strategy.

Recommended Diagnostic Procedure

We have found it advantageous to develop a routine diagnostic approach for patients suspected of having NPC. This differs according to the clinical presentation as well as to the appearance of the nasopharynx on inspection and is outlined in the flow chart (*Table 1*).[2] The principles of this approach are as follows:

Table 1. Approach to patients with suspected nasopharyngeal carcinoma.

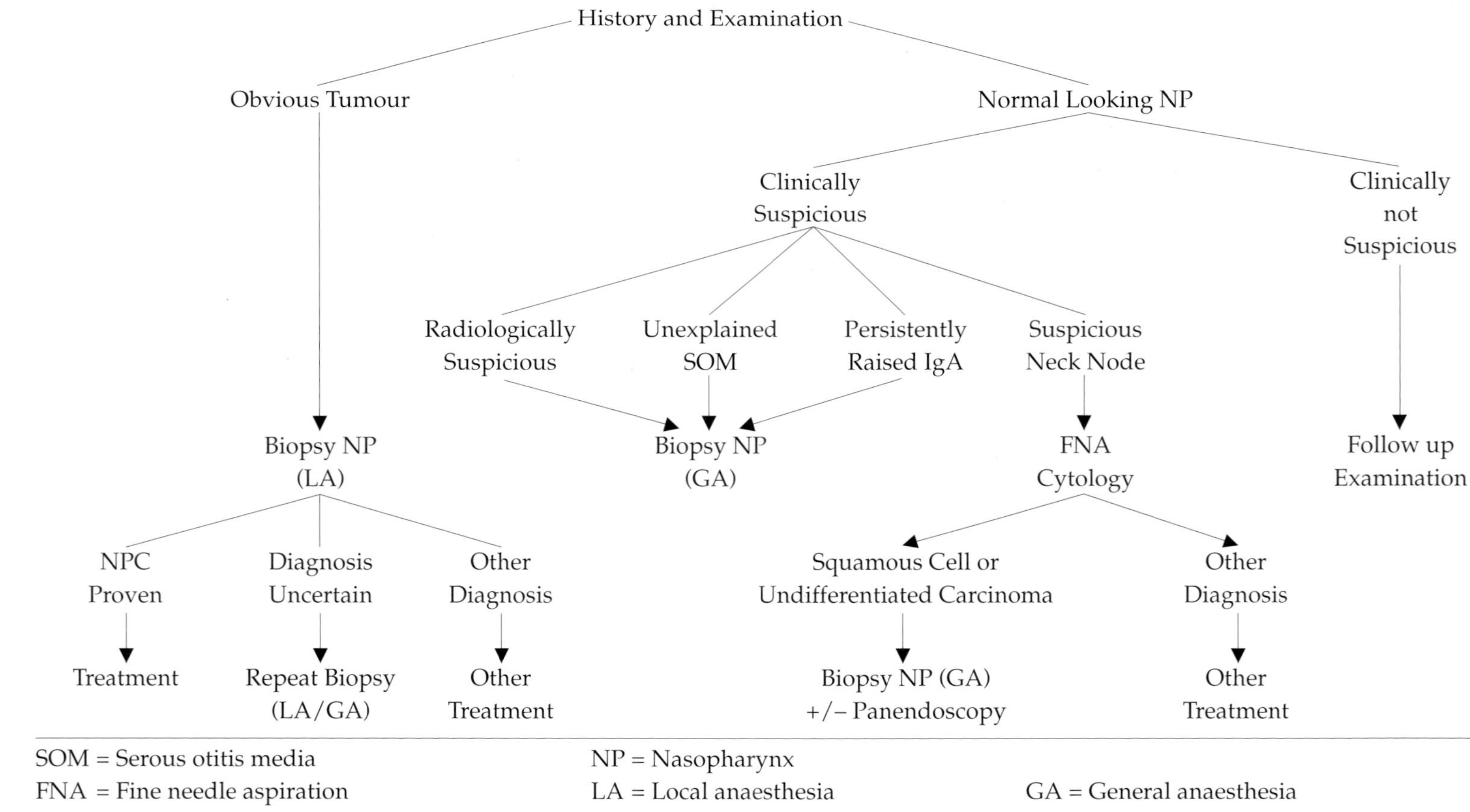

SOM = Serous otitis media
FNA = Fine needle aspiration
NP = Nasopharynx
LA = Local anaesthesia
GA = General anaesthesia

Obvious nasopharyngeal abnormality

If a nasopharyngeal mass is seen on examination, biopsy under direct vision, utilizing a flexible or rigid rod-type endoscope, is performed under local anaesthesia. When a diagnosis cannot be made in the first instance, biopsy may be repeated under either local or general anaesthesia.

Normal nasopharynx

Patients suspected clinically as having NPC but with a normal nasopharynx are examined under general anaesthesia. Deep biopsies are taken from multiple sites and these must include the fossae of Rosenmüller on both sides. The indications for this procedure include:

i. Persistent unilateral serous otitis media in an adult (especially in a high risk population)
ii. Suspected or proven metastatic nodal disease without an obvious primary, particularly if FNA cytology shows poorly differentiated squamous cell or undifferentiated carcinoma
iii. Raised IgA EA or persistently raised IgA VCA titres
iv. Radiological evidence consistent with NPC.

This diagnostic approach is both systematic and cost-effective.

Whether the nasopharynx appears normal or there is an obvious mass, there is no place for:

i. Plain x-rays
ii. Blind biopsies of the nasopharynx
iii. Open neck biopsies — especially incisional biopsies.

Diagnosis in the High Risk Group

The presence of persistently raised serological markers in any individual, particularly in association with a positive family history, is considered a significant risk factor predisposing to the formation of NPC. Such patients should be managed particularly carefully. Sometimes, serial and multiple biopsies need to be undertaken before a diagnosis can be reached. Very rarely, a definitive local diagnosis cannot be made until a systemic metastasis develops. Gene mapping, though not yet readily applicable, may prove useful in the future.

Concluding Remarks

The presence of a silent swelling in the upper half of neck should alert the physician to a possible nasopharyngeal primary tumour irrespective of race or geographical location.

Examination of the nasopharynx is mandatory and must be carried out with great care, using special equipment if necessary. Biopsy of the nasopharynx should be carried out in all suspect cases, even if no tumour is seen. The diagnosis in difficult cases may be aided by special diagnostic techniques including serology and imaging. Incisional biopsies of neck glands should be avoided. A careful planned approach to diagnosis will avoid undue delay or misdiagnosis.

References

1. Woo, J.K.S. 1997. Nasopharyngoscopy. In: *Operative Otolaryngology*, Chap. 37, eds. Bleach, N., Milford, C., van Hasselt, C.A. Oxford: Blackwell Science, 265–268.
2. Woo, J.K.S., Sham, C.L. 1990. Diagnosis of nasopharyngeal carcinoma. *Ear Nose Throat J.*; 69:241–242, 251–252.
3. Waldron, J., van Hasselt, C.A., Wong, K.Y.R. 1992. Sensitivity of biopsy using local anaesthesia in detecting nasopharyngeal carcinoma. *Head Neck*; 14(1):24–27.
4. Tam, J.S., Murray, H.G.S. 1990. Nasopharyngeal carcinoma and Epstein-Barr virus-associated serological markers. *Ear Nose Throat J.*; 69:261–266.
5. Waldron, J., Kreel, L., Metreweli, C., Woo, J.K.S., van Hasselt, C.A. 1992. Comparison of plain radiographs and computed tomographic scanning in nasopharyngeal carcinoma. *Clin. Radiol.*; 45(6):404–406.
6. Ginsberg, L.E. 1998 Radiologic and pathologic anatomy of the nasopharynx. *Proceedings of the UICC Workshop on Nasopharyngeal Cancer — Issues and Challenges*, 59–63.
7. Chong, V.F.H. 1998 Imaging issues. *Proceedings of the UICC Workshop on Nasopharyngeal Cancer — Issues and Challenges*, 64–65.
8. Huang, D.P., Ho, H.C., Henle, W., Henle, G., Saw, D., Lui, M. 1978. Presence of EBNA in nasopharyngeal carcinoma and control patient tissues related to EBV serology. *Int. J. Cancer*; 22:266–274.
9. Ho, J.H.C. 1982. Nasopharynx. In: *Treatment of Cancer*, ed. Halnan, K.E. New York: Igaku-Shoin Press, Chap. 12, 249–267.
10. Skinner, D.W., van Hasselt, C.A. 1990. Nasopharyngeal carcinoma: methods of presentation. *Ear Nose Throat J.*; 69:237–240.
11. Clifford, P.P.P. 1979. Tumours of the nasopharynx. In: *Clinical Otolaryngology*, eds. Maran, A.G.D., Stell, P.M. Oxford: Blackwell Scientific Publications, Chap. 24, 315–327.
12. Kristensen, S., Tveteras, K., Friedmann, I., Thomsen, P. 1989. Nasopharyngeal Warthin's tumour: a metaplastic lesion. *J. Laryngol. Otol.*; 103(6):616–619.
13. van Hasselt, C.A., Ng, H.K. 1991. Papillary adenocarcinoma of the nasopharynx. *J. Laryngol. Otol.*; 105(10):853–854.
14. Wang, C.C., See, L.C., Hong, J.H., Tang, S.G. 1996. Nasopharyngeal adenoid cystic carcinoma: five new cases and a literature review. *J. Otolaryngol.*; 25(6):399–403.
15. Job, A., Walter, N., David, T.M. 1991. Solitary fibrous tumour of the nasopharynx. *J. Laryngol. Otol.*; 105(3):213–214.
16. Rimmelin, A., Roth, T., George, B., Dias, P., Clouet, P.L., Dietemann, J.L. 1996. Giant-cell tumour of the sphenoid bone: case report. *Neuroradiology*; 38(7):650–653.
17. Wight, R.G., Harris, S.C., Shortland, J.R., Shaw, J.D. 1988. Rhabdomyosarcoma of the nasopharynx: a case with recurrence of tumour after 20 years. *J. Laryngol. Otol.*; 102(12):1182–1184.
18. Grewal, D.S., Lele, S.Y., Mallya, S.V., Baser, B., Bahal, N.K., Rege, J.D. 1994. Malignant melanoma of nasopharynx extending to the nose with metastasis in the neck. *Postgrad. Med.*; 40(1):31–33.
19. Choa, G. 1981. Cancer of the nasopharynx. In: *Cancer of the Head and Neck*, eds. Suen, J., Myer, E. New York, Edinburgh, Melbourne: Churchill Livingstone, Chap. 16, 393.

20. McGuirt, W.F., McCabe, B.F. 1978. Significance of lymph node biopsy before definitive treatment of cervical metastatic carcinoma. *Laryngoscope*; 88:594–597.
21. Cai, W.M., Zhang, H.X., Hu, Y.H., Gu, X.Z. 1983. Influence of biopsy on the prognosis of nasopharyngeal carcinoma — a critical study of biopsy from the nasopharynx and cervical lymph node of 649 patients. *Int. J. Radiat. Oncol. Biol. Phys.*; 9:1439–1444.

CHAPTER 8

Imaging

COMPUTED TOMOGRAPHY AND MAGNETIC RESONANCE IMAGING

Wynnie W.M. Lam and *Ann D. King*

The main role of imaging in nasopharyngeal carcinoma (NPC) is to delineate the exact extent of the tumour. This is crucial, as the majority of the primary tumours are treated by radiotherapy (RT) and the RT port must cover the entire tumour together with the immmediate lymphatic area. Imaging plays a lesser role in the establishment of the diagnosis which is essentially based on clinical history, physical examination, serological tests and biopsy of the tumour under endoscopic guidance. However imaging may be helpful in submucosal disease when endoscopy and biopsy are negative. Routine imaging to rule out distant metastases is not justified and is indicated only in the presence of clinical symptoms. Imaging also plays a major role in the follow up of patients with suspected recurrent disease.

Radiological Anatomy

Computed tomography (CT) and magnetic resonance (MR) imaging have completely superceded the plain radiograph in the staging of NPC. Our description of the radiological anatomy will therefore concentrate on these two modalities.

The nasopharynx extends from the skull base to the oropharynx, from which it is demarcated by a horizontal plane through the hard and soft palate.[1] The structures within the nasopharyngeal mucosal space are the mucosa, lymphoid tissue, the projecting posterior lip of the eustachian tube (torus tubarius) and the intra-pharyngeal portion of the levator palatini muscle. Laterally the nasopharynx widens into the deep lateral pharyngeal recess known as the fossa of Rosenmüller which is bordered anteriorly by the torus tubarius and levator palatini. The opening of the eustachian tube is thus seen anterior and medial to the fossa on axial sections (*Figure 1*), and inferior to the fossa on coronal sections.

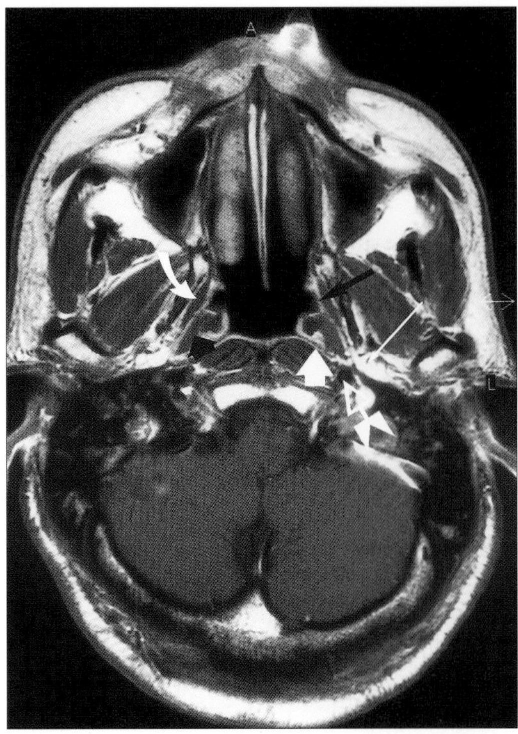

Figure 1. Axial T1-weighted contrast enhanced MR image through the nasopharynx at the level of the eustachian tube orifice (long black arrow) and fossa of Rosenmüller (white arrow head). Levator palatini (black arrow head), tensor palatini (curved white arrow), parapharyngeal fat space (long thin white arrow) and carotid artery (open white arrow) are shown.

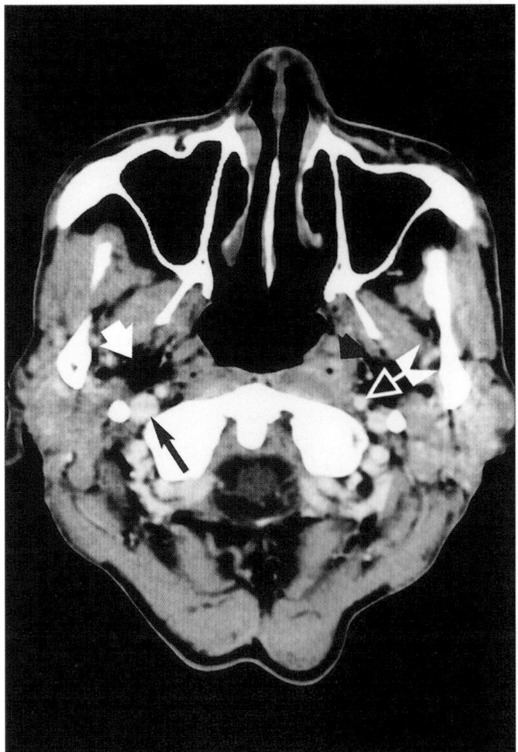

Figure 2. Axial CT image through the nasopharynx demonstrating a small tumour in the left fossa of Rosenmüller (black arrow head). Parapharyngeal fat space (white arrow head), internal jugular vein (black arrow), internal carotid artery (open white arrow).

MR imaging with its superior contrast resolution has the advantage of demonstrating the anatomical structures of the nasopharynx in more detail than CT (*Figure 2*).[2,3] The muscles are of low intermediate signal on all sequences and, as well as demonstrating the prevertebral and pterygoid muscles, the levator and tensor palatini muscles can be identified in all cases (*Figure 1*). These latter muscles are particularly well demonstrated on contrast enhanced T1- weighted images where they stand out against the high signal of the mucosa.[4] Likewise the pharyngobasilar fascia is identified on MR imaging particularly below the skull base where it is seen as a band of low signal on both T1 and T2 weighted images.

The parapharyngeal fat space is a symmetrical fatty triangle containing vessels which borders the lateral aspect of the nasopharynx. The parapharyngeal space extends from the skull base to the hyoid bone and beside the nasopharynx it is bordered laterally by the parotid space, the masticator space which contains the pterygoid muscles and posteriorly by the carotid space. It can best be appreciated on axial and coronal sections where it is identified as an area of low attenuation on CT (*Figure 2*) and high signal on T1-weighted MR sequences (*Figure 1*). The carotid artery and internal jugular vein, within the carotid sheath, are seen as tubular structures with enhancement on contrast CT and little or no signal on MR sequences due to the signal void caused by the rapid flow of blood (*Figures 1 and 2*). The normal lateral retropharyngeal nodes, measuring 4 mm or less in adults, can sometimes be identified on MR imaging.[5,6] Multiplanar imaging is especially useful in the assessment of the skull base. Coronal and axial CT with bone settings have the advantage of being able to depict small bony details especially around the neural foramina (*Figures 3 and 4*).

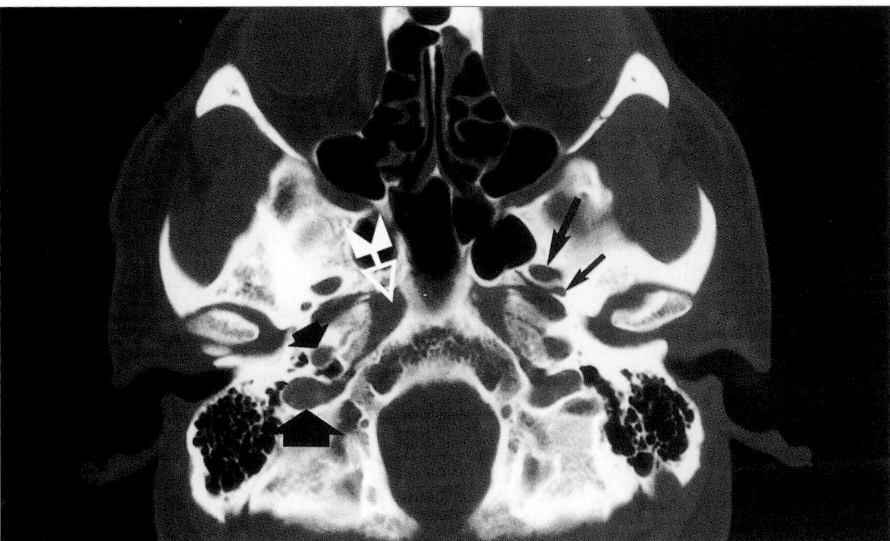

Figure 3. Axial CT image demonstrating the normal skull base foramina. Foramen ovale (black arrow), foramen spinosum (small black arrow), foramen lacerum (open white arrow), jugular fossa (large black arrow head) and vertical segment of the carotid canal (small black arrow head).

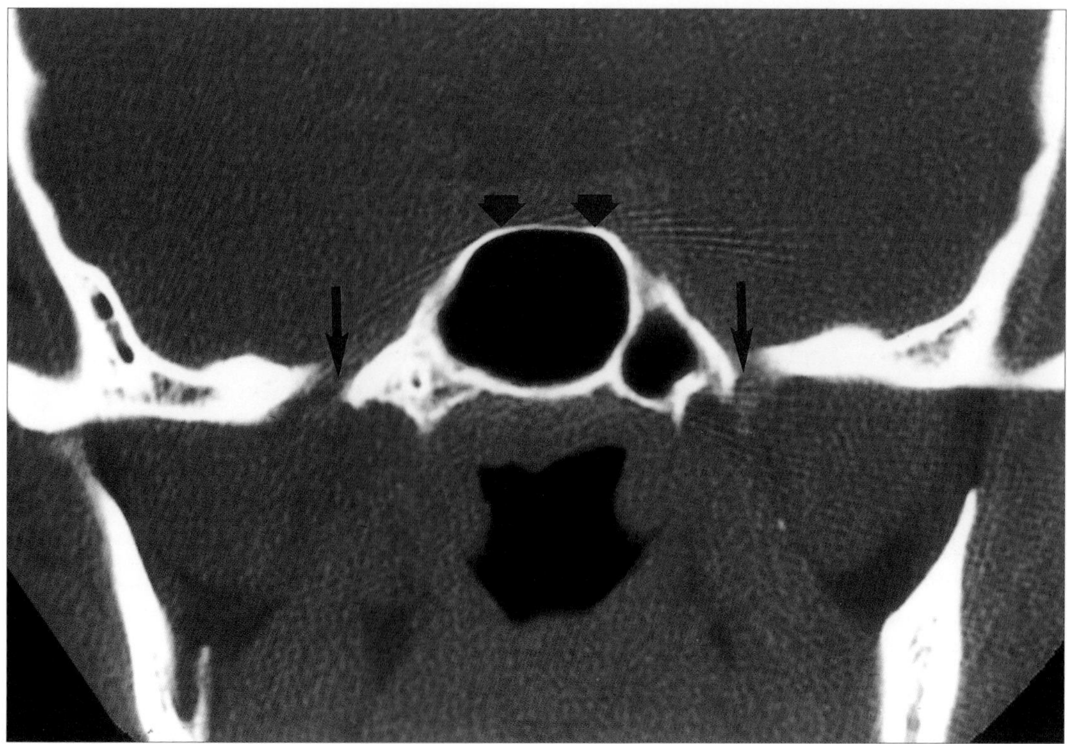

Figure 4. Coronal CT image of the skull base demonstrating the foramen ovale (black arrows) and sphenoid sinus (black arrow heads).

Staging Of The Primary Tumour

The Ho (1978) stage classification has been favoured in Hong Kong, being superior to the UICC and AJC classifications in terms of actuarial survival, disease free survival, and freedom from distant metastases. However, regardless of which system is used to stage the primary extent of tumour, the aims of imaging are similar. The emphasis is to identify tumour confined to the nasopharyngeal lumen, extension into the nasal cavity, oropharynx or paranasopharyngeal space, and invasion of the skull base and cranial nerves by more advanced disease. Computed tomography and MR imaging are the two principal modalities for evaluating the primary tumour and of these MR imaging, is more accurate in delineating the extent of disease.[4,7]

Small tumours

Less than 13% of patients with nasopharyngeal carcinoma present with disease confined to the nasopharyngeal space. The delineation of small volume disease can be difficult on imaging (*Figure 2*) and the assessment of the extent of mucosal disease without knowledge of the endoscopic findings[1] or positive biopsy sites may lead to interpretive errors. Evaluation of the symmetry of the nasopharynx on CT is notoriously difficult because of inflammatory change, secretions and lymphoid tissue within this region. This is particularly so in the fossa of Rosenmüller where minor asymmetry should not be mistaken for disease. In these cases a modified valsalva manoeuvre may open a collapsed lateral pharyngeal recess.[1] MR imaging is of advantage in this area because of its ability, on T2-weighted and contrast enhanced T1-weighted sequences, to differentiate the very high signal intensity of the mucosa from the lower signal intensity of the adjacent torus tubarius and intrapharyngeal portion of the levator palatini muscle.

The carcinoma itself has a long relaxation time and is mildly hyperintense relative to muscle on T2-weighted sequences and isointense to muscle on T1-weighted sequences. After the administration of contrast the signal intensity on T1-weighted images increases to become greater than that of muscle but less than the adjacent mucosa (*Figure 5*). T2-weighted sequences, also show good contrast between NPC and the adjacent structures in the nasopharyngeal mucosal space. The ability of MR imaging to demonstrate the pharyngobasilar fascia is a further advantage over CT in the evaluation of early stage disease.

Large tumours

As the tumour grows there is extension in all directions to involve complex anatomical structures and spaces which are described as follows:-

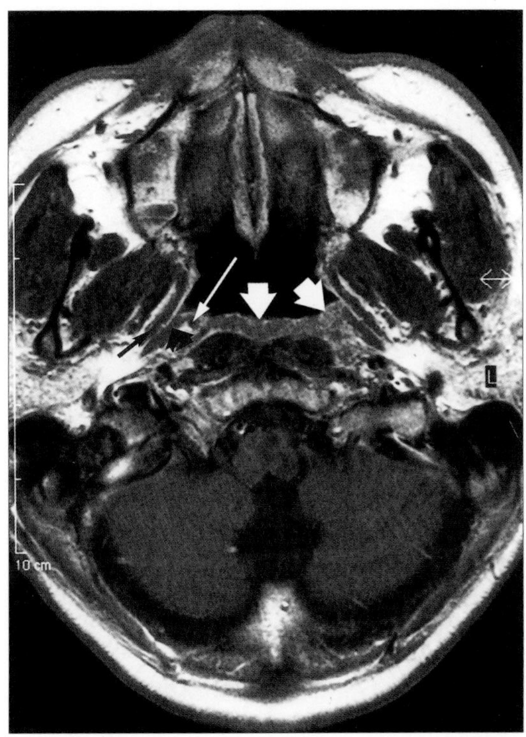

Figure 5. Axial T1-weighted contrast enhanced MR image through the nasopharynx demonstrating a small tumour in the posterior wall and left fossa of Rosenmüller (white arrow heads). Tensor palatini (black arrow), levator palatini (black arrow head) and the torus tubarius (long thin white arrow) are shown.

1) Lateral extension to involve the extrapharygneal portion of the levator palatini muscle, tensor palatini muscle, pterygoid plates, parapharyngeal fat space containing branches of cranial nerve V3, the medial pterygoid, lateral pterygoid, temporalis and masseter muscles, mandible and posterolaterally the parotid gland (*Figure 6*).
2) Posterior extension involves the prevertebral muscles, clivus, anterior portion of the foramen magnum and bodies of the C1 and C2, and posterolaterally the carotid space containing the internal carotid artery, jugular vein, cranial nerves IX to X11, the sympathetic plexus and metastasis to the retropharyngeal nodes (*Figures 6 and 7*).
3) Anterior extension to involve the pterygoid process, the nasal cavity, pterygomaxillary fissure and pterygopalatine fossa, maxillary sinus and posterior ethmoid air cells (*Figure 8*).
4) Superior extension involves the petrous temporal bone, sphenoid, foramina lacerum, ovale and rotundum, carotid canal, sphenoid sinus, cavernous sinus, cranium and orbit (*Figure 9*).
5) Inferior extension to the oropharynx (*Figure 10*).

Invasion laterally involves the extrapharyngeal portion of the levator palatini, the tensor palatini, eustachian tube and parapharyngeal fat space. The sinus of Morgagni is an opening in the pharyngobasilar fascia through which the levator palatini and

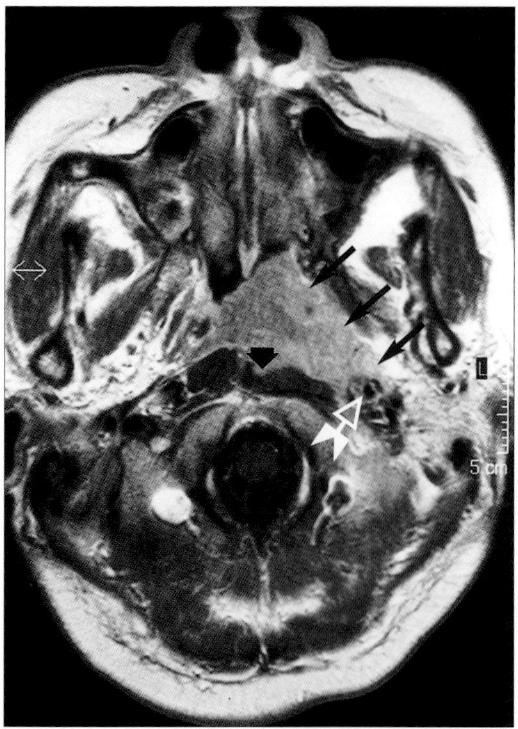

Figure 6. Axial T1-weighted contrast enhanced MR image through the nasopharynx demonstrating a large NPC with lateral invasion into the left paranasopharyngeal muscles and fat space (black arrows). There is also posterior invasion into the prevertebral muscles (black arrow head) and carotid sheath (white open arrow).

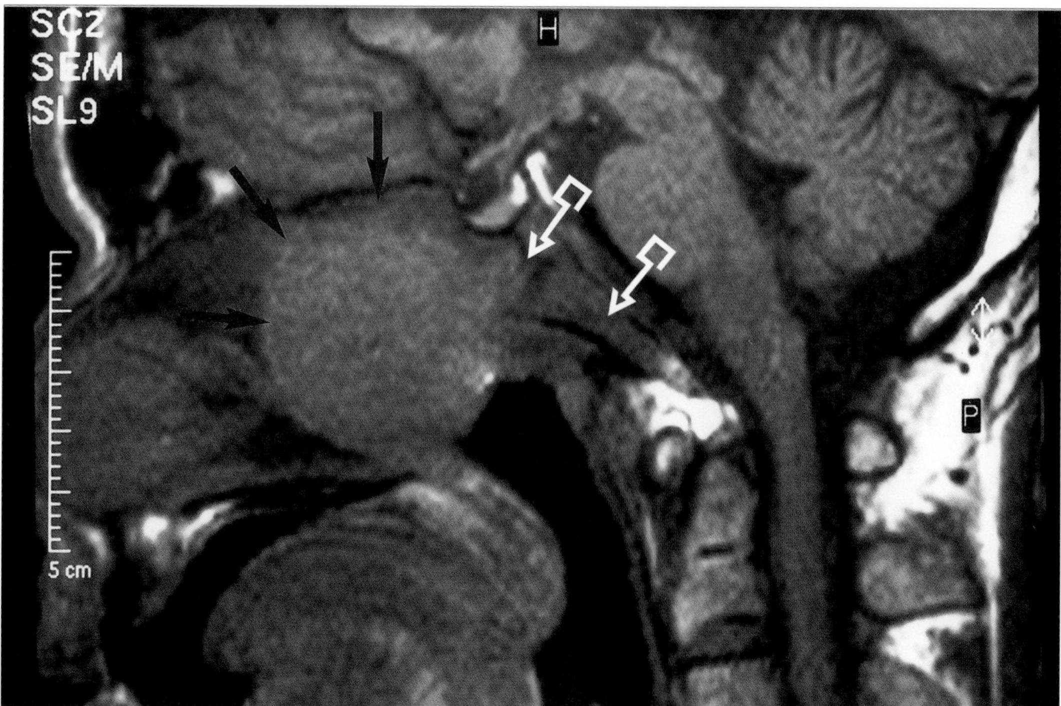

Figure 7. Sagittal T1-weighted image of the nasopharynx demonstrating a large tumour (black arrows) extending posteriorly into the clivus (white open arrows).

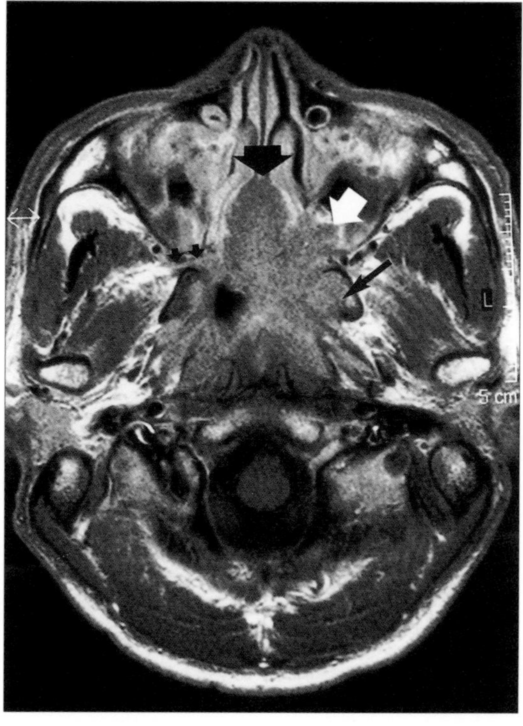

Figure 8. Axial T1-weighted contrast enhanced MR image through the nasopharynx demonstrating a large NPC with anterior invasion into the nasal cavity (large black arrow head), pterygoid process (black arrow), pterygomaxillary fissure (small black arrow heads) and left maxillary sinus (large white arrow head).

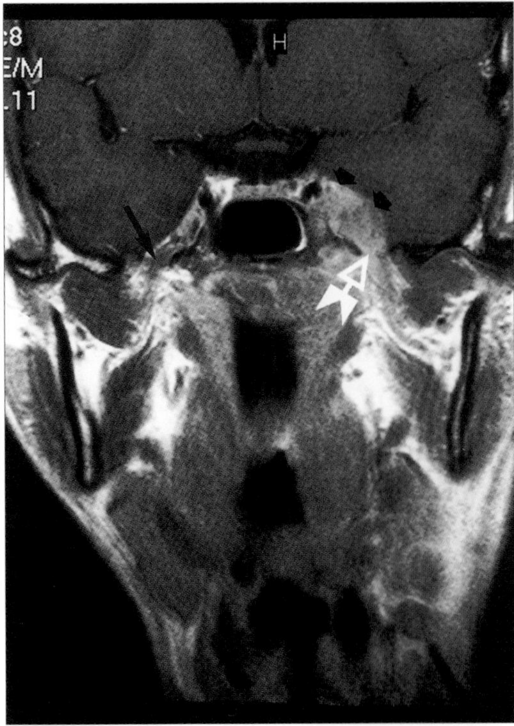

Figure 9. Coronal T1-weighted contrast enhanced MR image through the nasopharynx and skull base demonstrating a tumour in the roof and left lateral wall which extends superiorly to involve the body of the sphenoid, left foramen ovale (open white arrow) and left side of the cavernous sinus (small black arrow heads). The normal foramen ovale and mandibular nerve is shown on the right (black arrow).

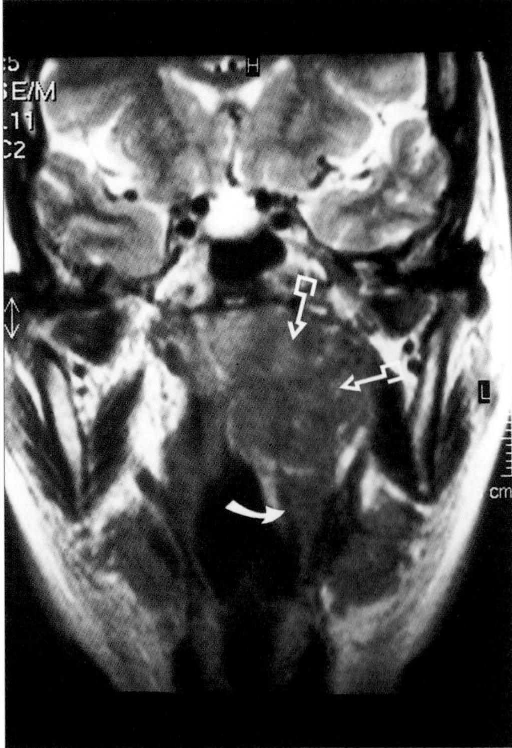

Figure 10. Coronal T2-weighted (fast spin echo) image demonstrating a large tumour of intermediate signal intensity in the nasopharynx (open white arrows) with extension into the oropharynx (curved white arrow).

eustachian tube pass to reach the nasopharyngeal mucosal space. This defect lies close to the lateral pharyngeal recess which is the commonest site for the development of NPC. Therefore it is not surprising that tumour extension frequently occurs at this point into the paranasopharyngeal space. Lateral extension into the parapharyngeal fat space is the most common region of extension seen on CT with invasion in 84% of patients.[8] This figure may ultimately prove to be slightly lower on MR imaging which has the ability to distinguish between compression by a large bulging tumour still confined within the mucosal space and direct invasion. Paranasopharyngeal extension is associated with serous otitis media.[9] The opacification of the middle ear and mastoid air cells is frequently seen and well demonstrated on both CT and MR imaging.

Disease within the nasal cavity is also well demonstrated on multiplanar MR imaging. This is especially the case around the superior meatus and sphenoethmoidal recess which can be difficult to evaluate on endoscopy. Tumour at these sites may spread into the sphenoid sinus or sphenopalatine foramen and pterygomaxillary fissure.

MR imaging is also of value in the assessment of oropharyngeal disease. Direct tumour extension can be distinguised from retropharyngeal nodes, which has implications for both treatment and staging.

Advanced tumours

Computed tomography has been the method of choice for demonstrating skull base erosion[10] (*Figure 11*). Thin section CT in the axial and coronal planes using a bone

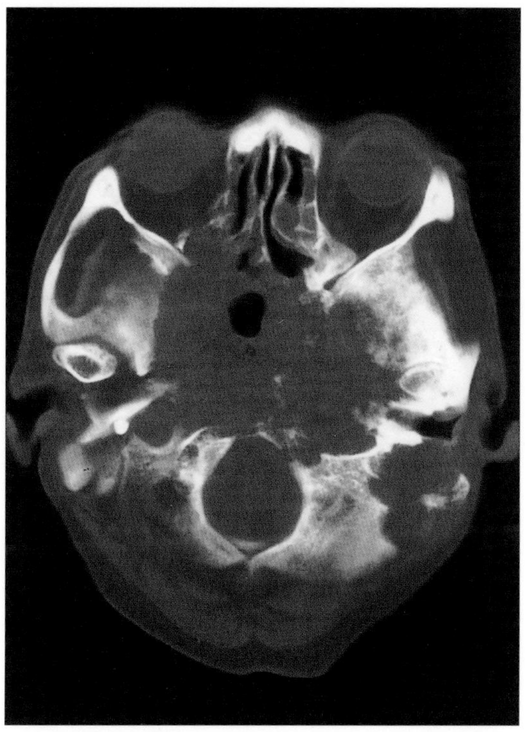

Figure 11. Axial CT image demonstrating extensive erosion of the skull base involving the body and wings of the sphenoid, pterygoid processes, petrous temporal bones, clivus and anterior margin of the foramen magnum.

algorithm is especially sensitive to early cortical bone invasion (*Figure 12*). However MR imaging already has several proven advantages over CT in evaluation of the skull base disease. MR imaging provides a sagittal plane which is invaluable in the assessment of invasion into the clivus and, once tumour has breached the cortex, it is more sensitive in evaluating the extent of marrow infiltration. In addition MR can identify perineural spread.[11,12] Recent work suggests that MR may eventually prove more sensitive than CT for the detection of skull base invasion.[13,14] Invasion of NPC into the base of the skull is well demonstrated by a moderately low signal against the high signal of fatty bone marrow on T1-weighted images. However, following administration of contrast, the enhanced tumour may assume a similar signal to the bone marrow and may thus be more difficult to distinguish (4). This has led to the use of MR sequences which combine T1-weighted images after contrast with saturation of the signal from fat. In some centres bone scanning is also used in the detection of bone erosion, but we have abandoned this technique because of its lower spatial resolution.

Advanced disease with extension into the cranium involves the cavernous sinus, middle cranial fossa and less commonly the posterior cranial fossa. Intra-cranial disease is well demonstrated on imaging and, once again, MR imaging is better than CT for delineating the extent of disease.[15]

Invasion of the paranasal sinuses occurs in the sphenoid sinus and posterior ethmoid air cells in 26% and 18% of patients respectively.[6] Extension into the maxillary sinus

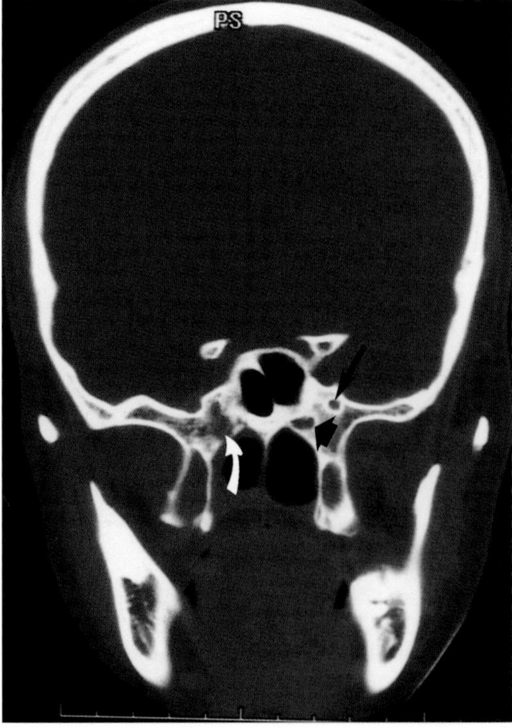

Figure 12. Coronal CT image of the skull base and pterygoid processes demonstrating the normal left foramen rotundum (black arrow) and vidian canal (black arrow head) and early invasion of these foraminae on the right side (curved white arrow).

occurs in 9% of patients and is usually seen in association with sphenoid infiltration and very advanced disease.[14] Patients with NPC often have mucosal disease of the sinuses and contrast enhanced CT or MR imaging is of value in differentiating between inspissated sinus secretions and tumour extension.[11,16]

Nodal Metastases

The clinically important lymph nodes in this disease are the retropharyngeal, submandibular, submental and lateral cervical groups.[17]

In NPC, 75% of the patients have enlarged nodes at presentation which are clinically palpable.[18] Sham *et al.* have suggested that neck node involvement by nasopharyngeal carcinoma is by orderly spread downwards. Node involvement in the lower neck is associated with a poorer prognosis. The detection of lymph node involvement is therefore of great importance. It is well known that clinical palpation of neck nodes is inaccurate, with a false positive rate of about 25% and a false negative rate between 10 and 15%.[19] It is often difficult to differentiate one single large lymph node from multiple matted nodes. Moreover, retropharyngeal lymph nodes and the most superior internal jugular nodes are not detectable by clincial palpation. Accurate assesment of the nodal status therefore relies on imaging.

Imaging modalities available for detection of nodal metastases of the neck include computed tomography, magnetic resonance imaging and ultrasound.

Computed tomography

Diagnostic CT critieria for a metastatic node include:[20]

1. Extracapsular nodal spread or extension of metastatic tumour beyond the lymph node capsule: This is diagnosed when there is enhancement of the nodal capsule and the presence of poorly defined margins around the node (*Figure 13*). However recent surgery, irradiation or active infection may give a similar and therefore false positive result.
2. Size: The widely accepted upper limit of normal for the maximum nodal diameter is 1.5 cm for the jugulodigastric and submandibular nodes and 1 cm for all other cervical lymph nodes. Nodes that exceed these limits have an 80% chance of being metastatic. Recently, it has been suggested that the minimal axial diameter (MAD) is a more accurate criterion for assessment.[21] The accepted upper limit of MAD of lymph nodes in the digastric region is 11 mm and 10 mm for all other cervical nodes except the retropharyngeal groups. Any nodes seen in the median retropharyngeal group should be considered abnormal and 4 mm should be taken as the upper limit of the minimal axial diameter of the lateral retropharyngeal nodes.[5]
3. Nodal shape: Hyperplastic lymph nodes are usually elongated in shape while metastatic nodes are usually more spherical.

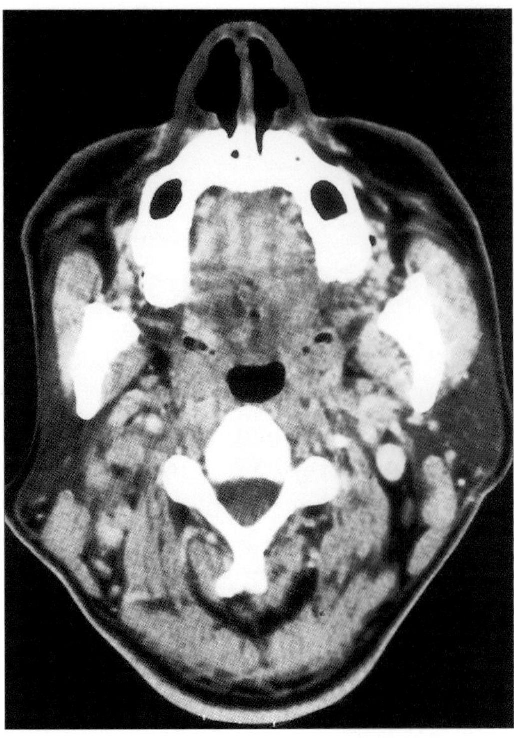

Figure 13. Axial CT image showing the multiple small lymph nodes in the right upper cervical chain. The borders of the lymph nodes are poorly defined, suggestive of extracapsular nodal spread.

4. Nodal grouping: This refers to the presence of three or more contiguous and confluent lymph nodes, each of which should have a maximal diameter of 8–15 mm (or a minimal axial diameter of 8–10 mm) (*Figure 14*).
5. Central necrosis: The most accurate CT criterion for the presence of metastasis is central necrosis. On a non-contrast scan, this appears as an area of low density in the centre of the node. Following administration of intravenous contrast, necrosis appears as an unenhanced area in the centre surrounded by a thin rim of peripheral enhancement (*Figure 15*). Nodal lipid metaplasia or an abscess within the lymph node may sometimes simulate necrosis due to metastasis.

Magnetic resonance imaging

MRI has the advantage of having better soft tissue resolution and multiplanar capability. It might therefore be expected that MRI should demonstrate the presence of nodes and differentiate benign from malignant nodes with a higher sensitivity and accuracy than computed tomography. However, the fat surrounding the nodes decreases their conspicuity on MRI. MRI adopts the same diagnostic criteria as computed tomography. The most accurate diagnostic sign is the presence of central necrosis. Nodes showing central necrosis usually have a heterogeneous MRI appearance on both T1 and T2 weighted images (*Figures 16a, b*). However, blood products may have low, intermediate or high signal intensity and haemorrhage into metastatic nodes may then have a

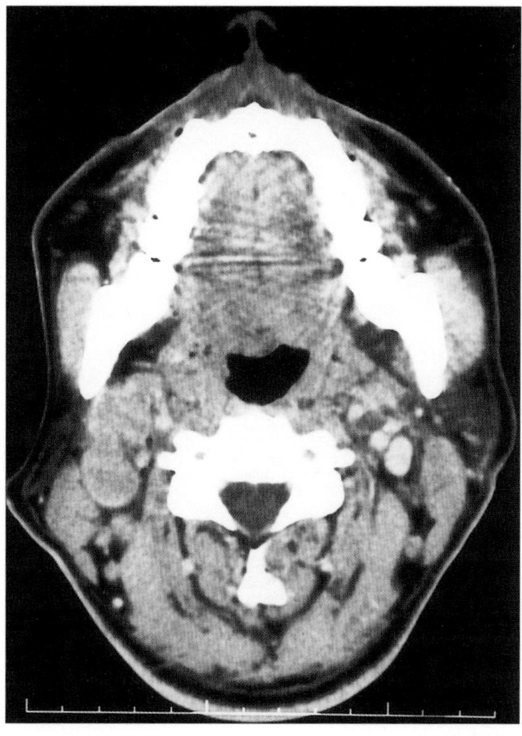

Figure 14. Axial CT images showing multiple enlarged and confluent lymph nodes in right upper cervical chain compatible with nodal grouping.

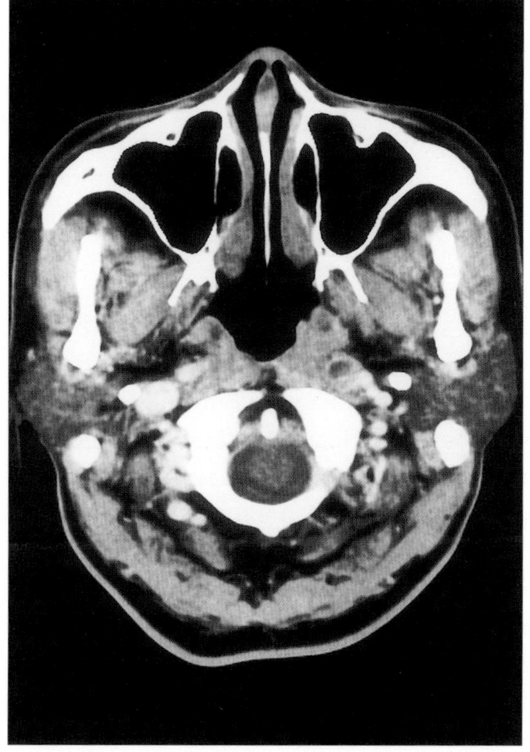

Figure 15. Axial CT post contrast scan showing central necrosis of the lateral group of left retropharyngeal lymph node. Note the hypodense centre and the rim enhancement around the necrotic centre.

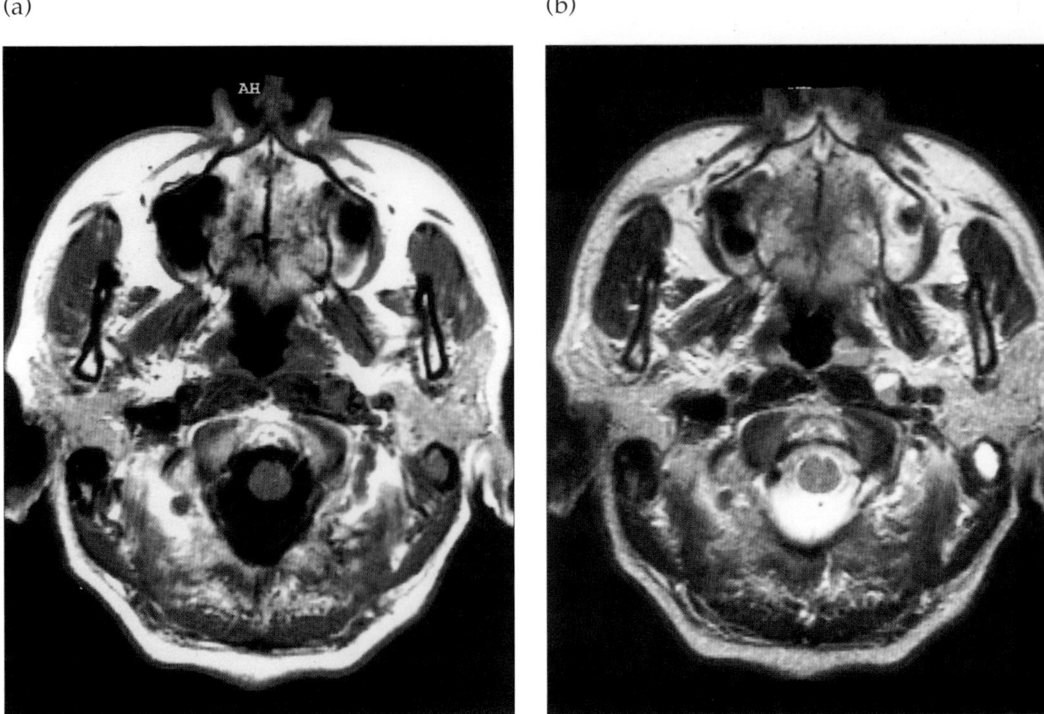

Figure 16 a, b. Axial SE T1 and TSE T2 weighted MR images. Note the enlarged lymph node in lateral chain of left retropharygneal group. There is a necrotic centre which is hypointense on T1 weighted image hyperintense on T2 weighted image.

relatively homogeneous appearance. Enhanced images will increase the sensitivity of detecting central necrosis. However post-gadolinium spin echo T1 weighted images will also decrease the conspicuity of the periphery of the node when viewed against the surrounding high T1 weighted signal intensity of fat. A fat suppressed enhanced sequence is therefore likely to be the optimal MR sequence.[20] Other problems, such as the less than optimal design of the neck coil, motion artefact, artefacts due to non-uniformity of the magnetic field and blood flow, may degrade the image quality. In fact, some authors have shown that CT is more sensitive than MRI in the detection of nodal necrosis and extranodal spread.[22,23] Attempts to characterize lymphadenopathy by magnetic resonance relaxation time shows overlap between nonspecific lymphadenopathy, nodes involved by granulomatous disease and malignant nodes.[24] Anzai *et al.*[25] administered dextran coated iron oxide to 12 patients for imaging of neck nodes. By comparing the signal intensities of the lymph nodes in pre- and post- contrast scans, they showed a substantially lower signal intensity ratio in benign nodes than in metastatic nodes. They achieved a sensitivity of 95% and a specificity of 84% in differentiating benign and malignant nodes in their small series. These preliminary results are promising but this technique is impractical in a routine clinical setting as the pre- and post-contrast studies need to be 10–48 hours apart.[25]

Ultrasound

Ultrasound examination does not involve irradiation or administration of contrast media. It is our chosen technique for the assessment of neck node status of NPC patients. For this reason it is discussed in greater detail in a special section devoted to ultrasound (*vide infra*).

Distant Metastases

Distant metastases from head and neck cancers are considered a rare occurrence. However, nasopharyngeal cancer appears to be a unique entity and has one of the highest rates of distant metastases among head and neck cancers. Whereas lung is the commonest distant metastatic site in other head and neck cancers,[26,27] the most common sites of involvement in NPC are bone, liver and lung, in descending order of incidence. Distant metastases usually develop within a period of three years. There is an association between distant metastases and N stage.[28]

Bone

Skeletal involvement conforms to a general pattern, the spine and pelvis being the commonest sites, followed by femur, ribs, sternum and humerus. Radiologically, the lesions are lytic in 66%, mixed lytic and sclerotic in 12.8% and sclerotic in 21%.[29] The unusually high incidence of mixed and sclerotic bony secondaries is unique is head and neck cancer.The detection rate by scintigraphy of asymptomatic skeletal metastases on presentation is only 1.8%, and the predictive value of an abnormal scan for metastases 30%. Because of the low sensitivity and specificity of bone scanning, bone scintigraphy is not justified as a routine staging investigation for nasopharyngeal carcinoma, but is an option for patients considered to be at risk for distant metastases.[30,31]

Thorax

The incidence of intrathoracic metastases has been reported as 8–13%.[26,28] In patients with lung metastasis, there is a high incidence of thoracic lymphadenopathy (64%). Of all the intrathoracic lymph nodes, hilar nodes are most commonly involved. 12% of the lung deposits are cavitating, these are often associated with squamous cell primary tumours.[32]

Hypertrophic pulmonary osteoarthropathy is reported in 6.6% of NPC patients, out of which 48% have pulmonary metastases.[33,34] The condition can precede lung metastases and should therefore be regarded as a possible early sign of the latter condition.

Liver

In autopsy patients, the liver was the most common site of distant metastases, suggesting that a significant number of patients die with undiagnosed liver metastases.[27] All patients with positive findings in liver scintigraphy and abdominal ultrasound correlate well with clinical findings. Therefore, in the absence of clinical evidence of disease, routine bone and liver scintigraphy are of limited value.[35,36]

Local tumour recurrence

Common symptoms related to local tumour recurrence in nasopharyngeal carcinoma, including nasal bleeding, pain and diplopia usually occur late. Fibre-optic endoscopy is a useful technique in the detection of local recurrence but, due to the propensity of a submucosal pattern in these cases, up to 50% of endoscopically guided or random biopsies may be negative in patients that are subsequently proven to have recurrent tumours.[37] This underlines the importance of cross-sectional imaging techniques such as CT or MRI in the detection of recurrence. Furthermore, these studies provide a comprehensive assessment of the extent of tumour when recurrence is present.

Most cases take the form of a recurrent mass, bone destruction or the appearance of tumour in previously unaffected areas. The diagnosis is straightforward when a mass grows larger than the residual dimension after RT. Almost half of the patients who had no paranasopharyngeal extension before primary RT extended into this region at the time of recurrence.[37] Without an increase in size, diagnosis of recurrence is more difficult. Asymmetry of the NP on either CT or MRI is not a reliable criterion as this can be due to post-RT change. Abnormal signal or density in a soft tissue mass can be attributed to post-RT oedema, inflammation, fibrosis as well as recurrent tumour. Compared with CT, MRI enables a better differentiation and separation between tumour, muscle and fibrosis.[38] Oedema, inflammation, fibrosis and recurrent tumour are isodense and difficult to differentiate on CT. On MRI, mature fibrosis is hypointense on T1W and T2W sequences and can be differentiated from the slightly hyperintense recurrent tumour on T2W.[10,39,40] Hyperintensity , however, is also seen in post-RT oedema, inflammation, and immature fibrosis.[40] Although inflammation and oedema tend to be more hyperintense than recurrent tumour on T2W sequence, there is an overlap in signal intensity which can preclude differentiation.[10] The frequent association of sinonasal inflammation with NPC especially after RT, frequently poses a problem of differentiation between inflammation and tumour recurrence in those regions. In this situation MRI is more accurate than CT with less false positive diagnoses.[10]

Bone erosion occurs frequently with local tumour recurrence, which underlines the importance of skull base assessment. About one third of patients without prior involvement show erosion on recurrence on CT.[37] Persisting or progressive bone erosion on CT is also seen in the majority of patients with recurrence who had bone erosion prior to RT.[37] New bone erosion or infiltration found on post-treatment follow-up scans, or increase in bone erosion in cases with pre-RT involvement, should raise a strong suspicion of tumour recurrence: The converse however may not be true. Bony reconstitution may be identified within four to six months after RT along with reformation of the foramina ovale and spinosum in some cases that had skull base destruction prior to RT.[41] An increase of clival marrow signal intensities on T1W on MRI after RT has also been documented.[37] However, it is not known whether the persistence of static bone erosion or infiltration after RT, seen on CT as a lytic focus or on MR as a hypointense focus on T1W or hyperintense focus on T2W, should be equated with persisting or recurrent tumour. As the natural course of these lesions is not fully understood, and biopsy is hazardous, serial scanning is advised.

Increased uptake of F18-fluoro-2deoxy-D-glucose (FDG) on positron emission tomography (PET) can differentiate hypometabolic post-RT oedema, or scarring from hypermetabolic recurrent head and neck cancer.[42] However, the expense involved and general lack of availability make it less useful than single photon emission computed tomography (SPECT). Thallium 201 SPECT imaging has also been shown to be more effective during follow up imaging than CT in the differentiation of viable neoplastic tissue and RT induced changes.[43] It is therefore useful in NPC for assessing tumour response to irradiation and for detecting local recurrence.[44]

Complications of RT

Radiotherapy for NPC inevitably results in radiation exposure of adjacent normal structures. Late radiation injury is the major, dose-limiting complication of brain irradiation and it occurs in focal and diffuse forms.[45] Focal necrosis demonstrates the CT and MR characteristics of a mass lesion. Diffuse radiation injury is characterised by increased signal on T2-weighted MR images and hypodensities on CT.

In NPC, radiation injury of the brain can involve the temporal lobes, brainstem, cervical cord, basal ganglia and frontal lobes. Temporal lobe radiation changes are by far the most common and most important. It is the most worrying complication accounting for 65% of irradiation-induced mortalities.[46] Aggravating factors include diabetes mellitus, hypertension, and repeat courses of irradiation.[46] A hyperfractionation schedule may also pose more risk than conventional RT.[47] Both CT and MRI are capable of detecting abnormalities in the temporal lobe in clinically asymptomatic cases.[47,48] On the other hand, irradiated patients with normal CTs have been found to perform more poorly in intellectual and memory functions than controls.[49] Early radiation injury to the temporal lobes is represented by white matter encephalopathy seen as finger like hypodensities on CT[48,50] (*Figure 17*), and hyperintense white matter changes on T2W sequences on MRI. MRI is more sensitive than CT in the detection of such changes.[51] Radiation white matter encephalopathy may progress or regress. Progression to more severe injury results in temporal lobe necrosis (*Figure 18*). Haemorrahge and atrophy may also be found. In the delineation of the liquefactive necrotic cavity, MRI is (*Figure 19*) more precise than CT (*Figure 20*). Haemorrhage is an unusual complication of cerebral radiation necrosis but can be fatal.[52] Acute haemorrhage accompanying brain necrosis is better shown on CT but repeated small petechial haemorrahges are better seen on MRI (*Figure 21*). Half of the radiation injuries in the temporal lobes show enhancement on contrast-CT[50] and the enhancement is confined to the target volume.[48] When tumour

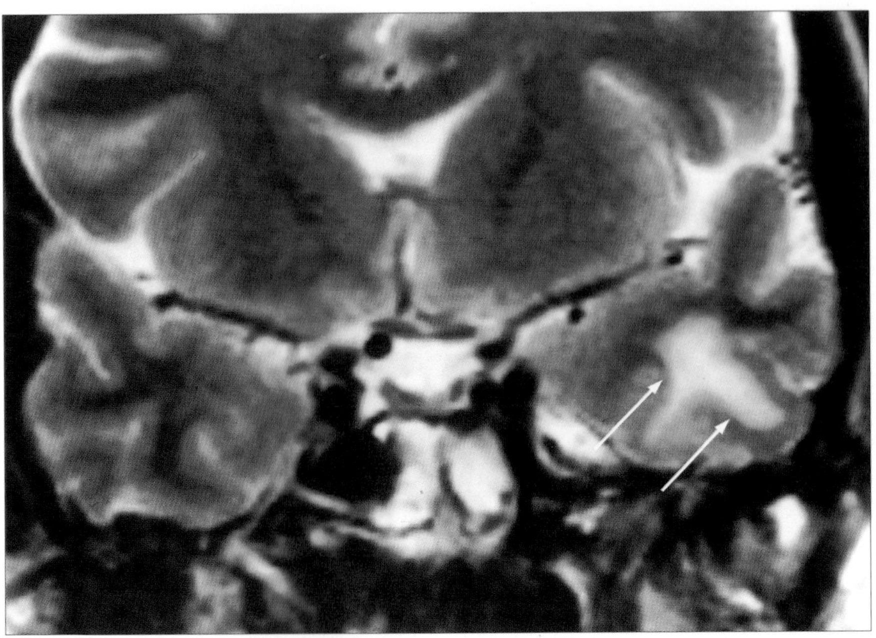

Figure 17. Homogeneous hyperintense change involving the white matter in the inferior two-thirds of the left temporal lobe (arrows) on T2-weighted MRI image. This radiation induced white matter encephalopathy is probably due to oedema or gliosis.

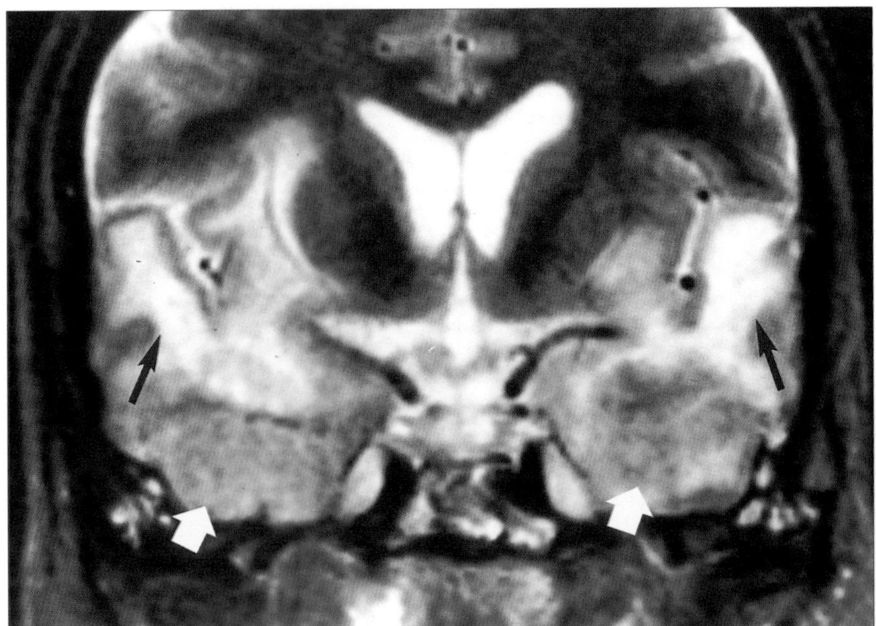

Figure 18. Heterogeneous signal change due to radiation induced injury in both temporal lobes on T2-weighted MRI sequence. Homogeneous component (black arrow) represent vasogenic oedema. The heterogeneous intermediate signal component (white arrow) represents necrosis.

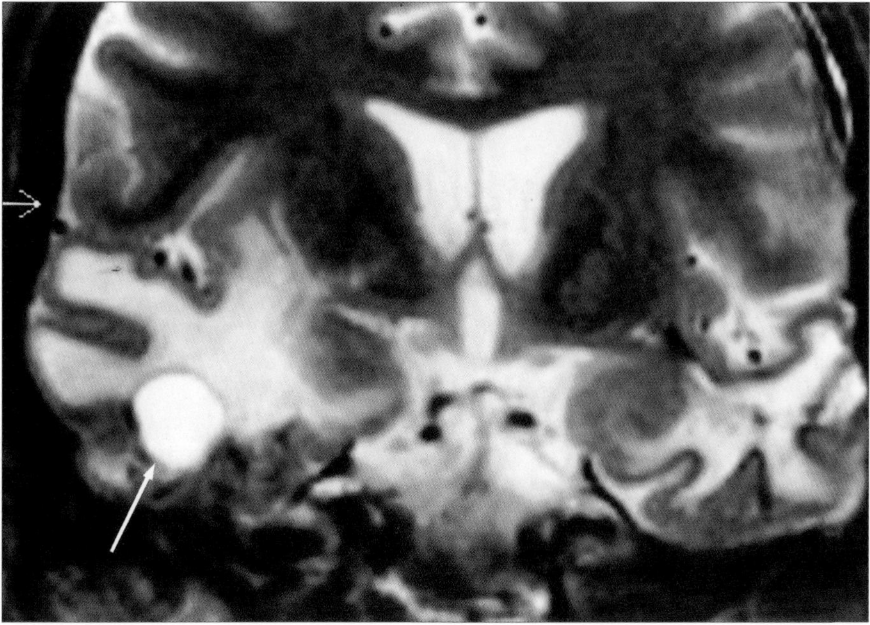

Figure 19. Bilateral radiation induced injury of temporal lobes on T2-weighted sequence. The right temporal lobe is swollen with mass effect and the presence of a well defined cyst (arrow).

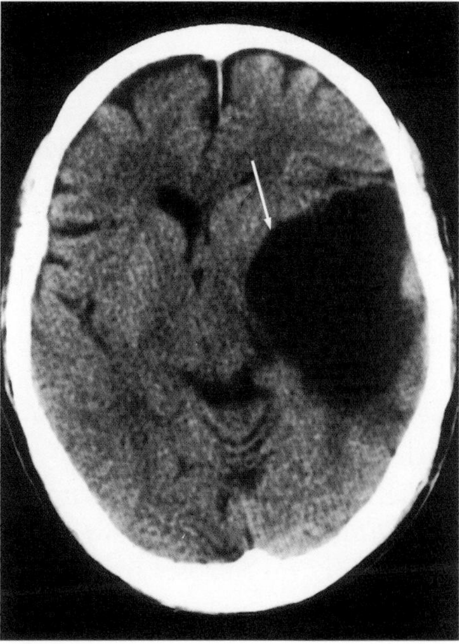

Figure 20. Non-contrast CT shows radiation-induced injury of left temporal lobe with large cystic change (arrow). Severe mass effect with compression of left frontal horn and midline shift is observed.

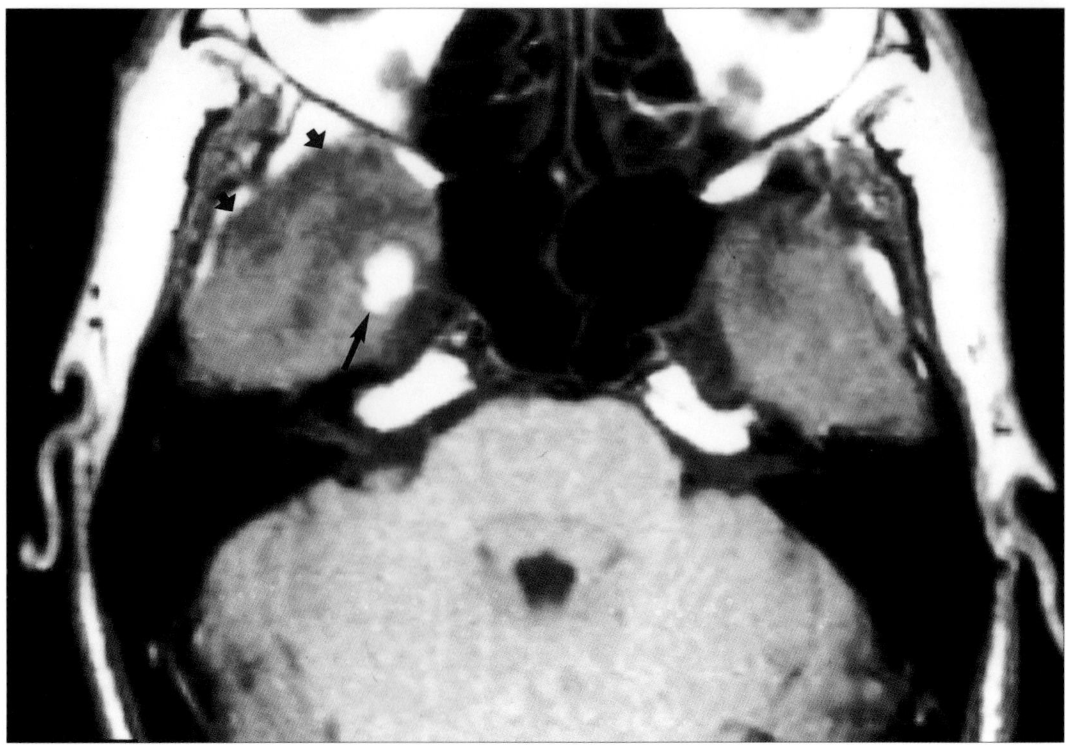

Figure 21. Axial SE T1-weighted MRI image showing hyperintense focus (arrow) consistent with methaemoglobin due to subacute haemorrhage. The low-signal areas (short arrows) represent radiation induced oedema and necrosis.

infiltration in the skull base is contiguous with abnormal changes in the temporal lobe, differentiation between radiation necrosis and tumour infiltration in the temporal lobe is diffficult.[53] One may diagnose tumour if the enhancing part extends outside the radiation field (*Figure 22*). For less extensive tumour, FDG-PET has been successfully applied in differentiating recurrent brain tumour from radiation injury.[54]

Brainstem encephalopathy/cervical cord myelopathy are infrequent but serious sequelae. Both CT and myelograms are diagnostically unhelpful. MRI demonstration of a swollen cord, or hyperintense changes on T2W representing oedema or demyelination would confirm the diagnosis.[55]

Cranial/cervical sympathetic nerve injury can occur without coexisting brainstem and cord involvement. The last four cranial nerves are by far the commonest affected, with an incidence of 4%.[46] Perineural fibrosis in the retropharyngeal space, as a contributing cause to the neuropathy, may be shown on CT/MRI as non-specific soft tissue thickening. The sequela of damage to the hypoglossal nerve can be demonstrated indirectly on MRI as atrophy of tongue (*Figure 23*). Barium swallow can also demonstrate swallowing dysfunction, which may result in fatal aspiration pneumonia.[46] Direct demonstration of nerve damage by CT or MR is not yet possible.

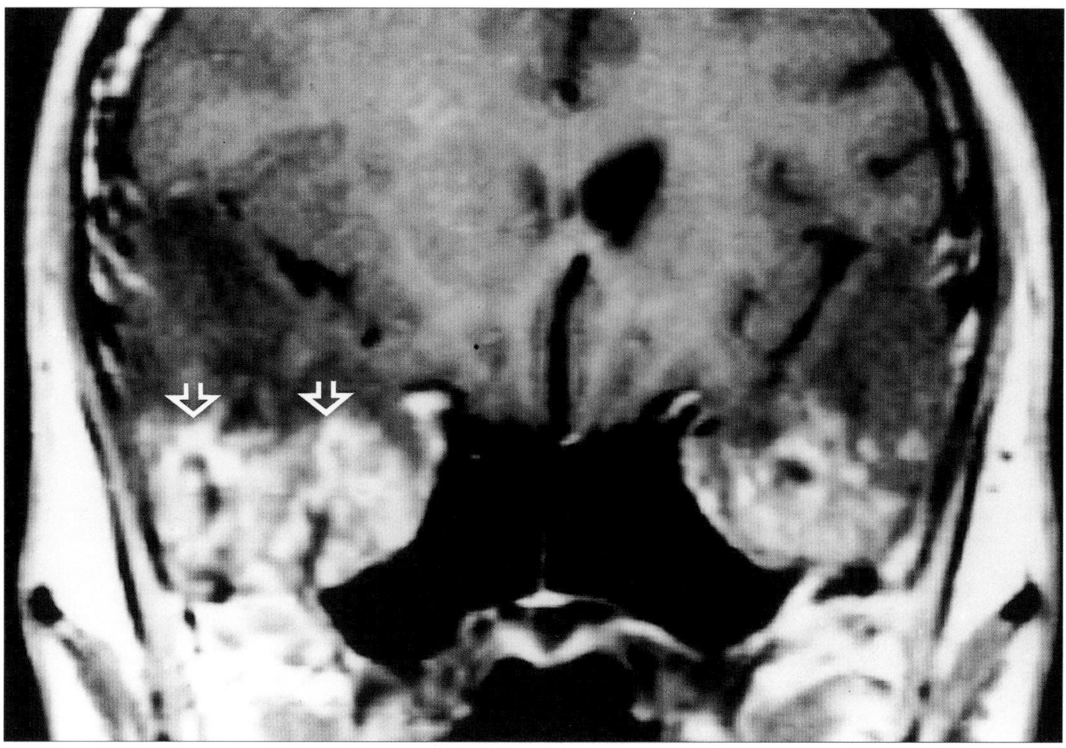

Figure 22. Contrast-enhanced SE T1 weighted coronal MRI image showing marked enhancement in both temporal lobes with radiation necrosis. The enhancement is confined to the radiation field with a straight upper margin corresponding to the field margin (open arrows).

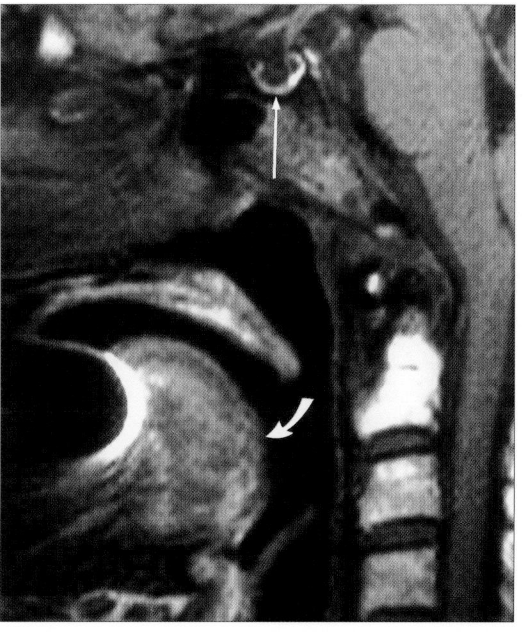

Figure 23. Sagittal T1-weighted MRI image showing an atrophic pituitary gland (arrow) with a relatively empty sella. The tongue (currved arrow) is atrophic and withdrawn from the palate.

As the hypothamlamus and pituitary are included in the radiation field damage to these structures is unavoidable. The cumulative probability of endocrine dysfunction has been estimated to be 62% after 5 years with damage to the hypothalamus being suggested as the major cause of radiation-induced hypopituitarism.[56] Radiation injury of the hypothalamo-pituitary axis is demonstrable as different degrees of pituitary atrophy culminating in a frank empty sella (*Figure 23*), and these changes are much better shown on MRI than on CT.

Mastoid effusion is encountered in 9% of patients after radiotherapy.[57] Post-RT xerostomia is associated with shrinkage and fatty change of the parotid glands. Changes in the mastoid sinuses and parotid glands can be detected with CT or MRI. The decrease in salivary function can also be assessed using Tc-99 m sialography.[58]

ULTRASOUND OF METASTATIC CERVICAL NODES

Anil T. Ahuja and *Constantine Metreweli*

As already detailed, cervical nodal metastases are common as a presenting feature of NPC. This is especially the case in patients under the age of 21 years.[59] However enlarged reactive nodes of inflammatory origin are often found in the adult Chinese population[60] and tuberculous cervical adenitis still remains a diagnostic dilemma. High resolution ultrasound (US) with its greater sensitivity than clinical examination (92% vs 70%)[61] and its high specificity when combined with fine needle aspiration cytology (92.7%) is a useful initial investigation in distinguishing benign from malignant disease.[19]

Although CT and MRI play an important role in the evaluation of NPC, the sonologist presented with a patient who has cervical lymphadenopathy may be the first to make the primary diagnosis by differentiating the swelling from the other causes of neck node enlargement. The sonologist must therefore be aware of the distinguishing features of the primary tumour Ultrasound has a further role in management, by monitoring post therapy changes and confirming the neck is disease free. For this reason the effects of therapy on the ultrasonic appearances must also be known.

Ultrasound features of an abnormal node

Size

Most US studies define metastatic nodes on the basis of size; nodes in the internal jugular group greater than 9 mm in transverse diameter are considered metastatic. The corresponding criterion for nodes in the submental and submandibular areas is 7 mm.[62] In general nodes less than 5 mm are rarely metastatic.[63] Note that these

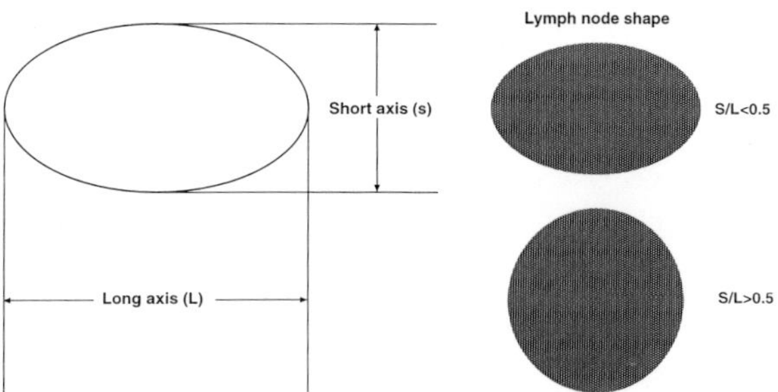

Figure 24. Line drawing showing the short axis to long axis ratio (S/L ratio). An S/L ratio less than 0.5 represents an oval node whereas round nodes have an S/L ratio greater than 0.5.

dimensions differ from and are generally smaller than the limits accepted for CT and MRI.

Shape

Shape is assessed on the basis of the short axis (SA) to long axis (LA) ratio.[64] An SA/LA ratio greater than 0.5 indicates a round node, while less than 0.5 indicates an oval node (*Figure 24*). Based on shape it has been suggested that benign nodes tend to be oval while malignant nodes are round.[65] Employing the combined parameters of shape and size, lymph nodes greater than 10 mm in long axis, with a short to long axis ratio greater than 0.5 show a higher incidence of malignancy.[64]

Internal Architecture

In assessing internal architecture, the features to note are the echogenic hilus, coagulation necrosis and cystic necrosis.

The echogenic hilus (*Figure 25*) in a lymph node is due to the converging sinuses within the medulla of the node providing numerous parallel interfaces.[66] Its presence used to be considered a sign of benignity. However more recent studies suggest that the sign is of limited value in this context.[67]

Coagulation necrosis (*Figure 26*) is portrayed as echogenic foci within abnormal nodes. The affected area is less echogenic than the normal hilus, separate from it and discontinous from surrounding fat.[62] Cystic necrosis (*Figure 27*) is seen as a focal echoluscent area within an abnormal node. Sakai *et al.*[62] in a correlative in vitro study of US with pathological specimens demonstrated coagulation necrosis and cystic necrosis within metastatic nodes. However, even in benign nodes they observed similar alterations in echogenicity.[62,66,68] Thus, based on internal architecture, one is not often able to distinguish a benign from a malignant condition.

Distribution

On US the distribution of nodes in the neck is normally classified into 8 areas,[63] (*Figure 28*): 1. Submental. 2. Submandibular. 3. Inferior angle of parotid. 4. Upper cervical,

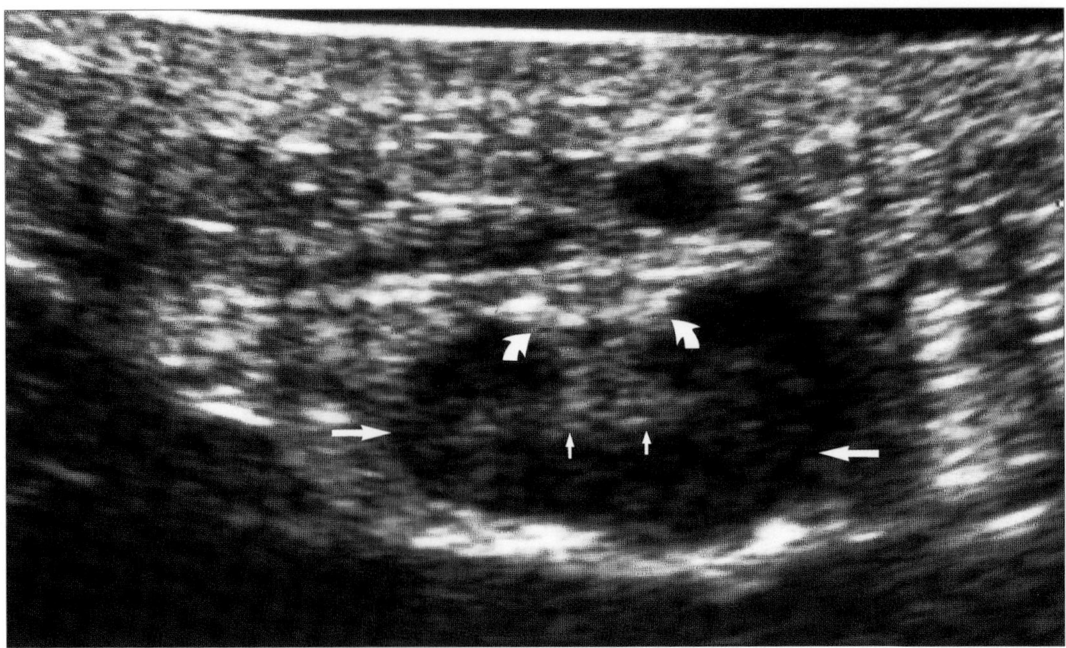

Figure 25. Transverse sonogram of a hypoechoic node (large arrows) with a echogenic hilus (small arrows). Note its continuation with adjacent soft tissues (curved arrows).

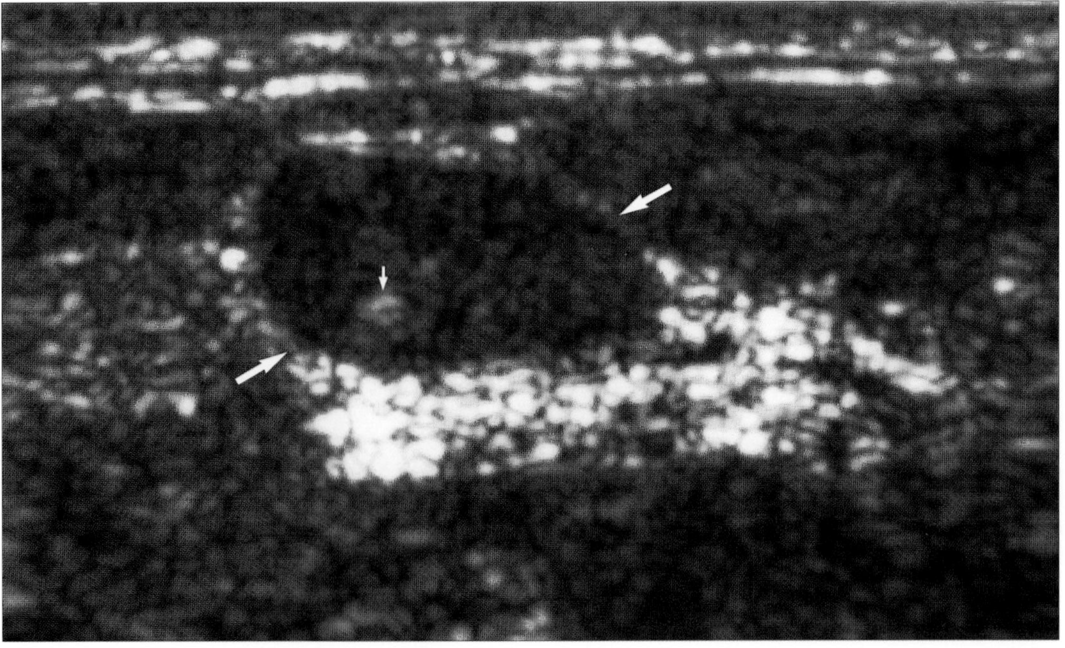

Figure 26. Transverse sonogram of a hypoechoic node (large arrows) showing coagulation necrosis (small arrow). Note that it is not continuous with adjacent soft tissues.

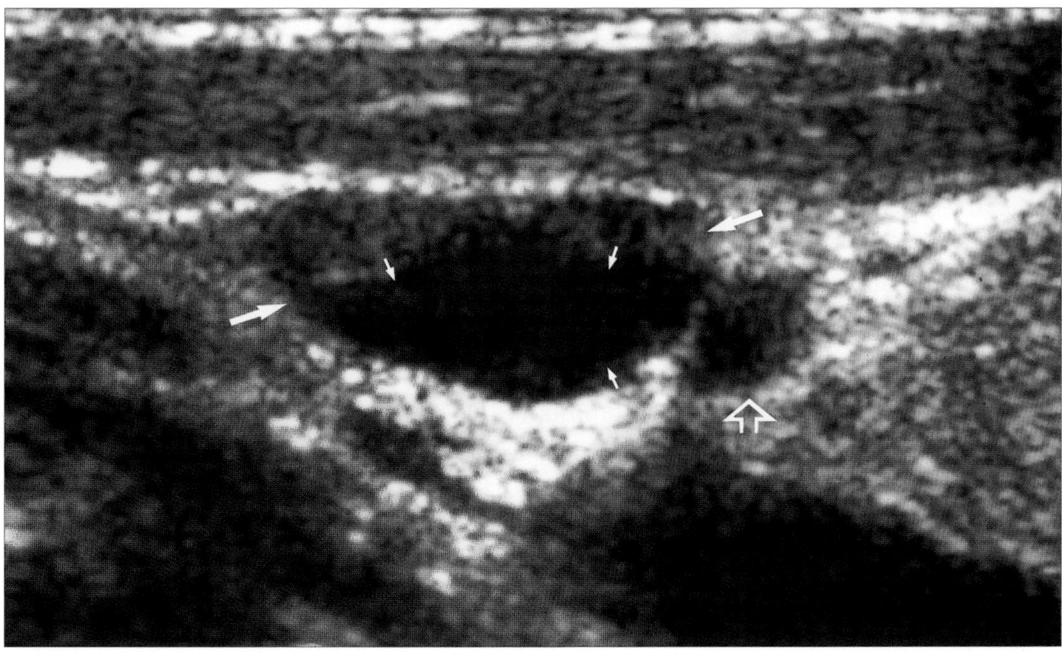

Figure 27. Transverse sonogram of a hypoechoic node (large arrows) with intranodal necrosis (small arrows). The open arrow identifies the common carotid artery.

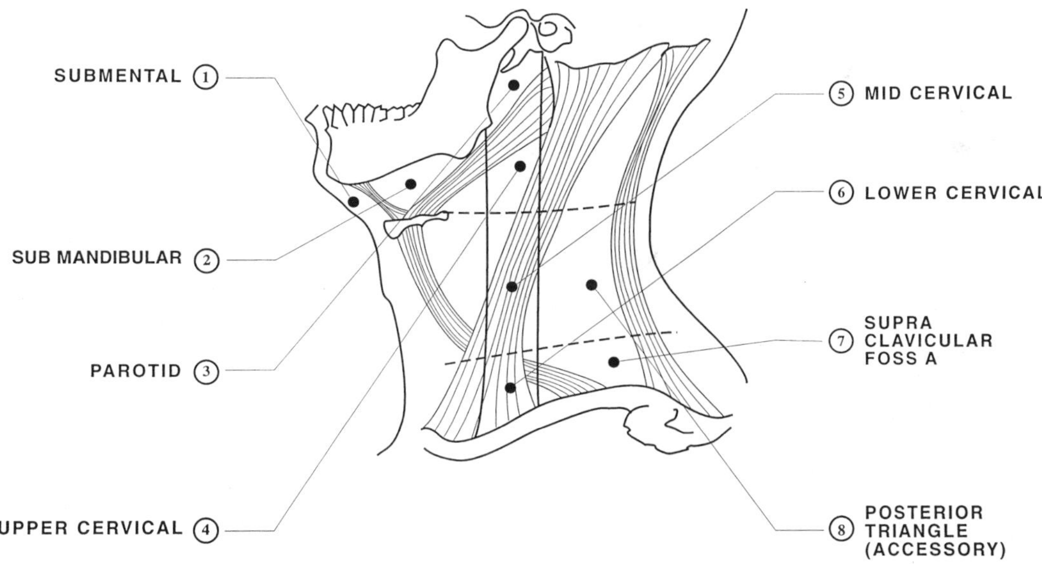

Figure 28. Line diagram showing the subdivision of the neck into eight areas to map lymph node distribution.

above hyoid and along internal jugular vein (IJV) and common carotid artery (CCA). 5. Mid cervical, between hyoid and cricoid cartilage and along the IJV/CCA. 6. Lower cervical, below cricoid cartilage and along the IJV/CCA. 7. Supraclavicular fossa. 8. Posterior triangle.

Metastatic nodes in the neck are site specific. If the primary lesion itself is not visible the pattern of distribution of lymphadenopathy may suggest its location. The distribution of the abnormal nodes is a consistent and reliable feature in distinguishing between the various causes of cervical lymphadenopathy.

Nodal Border

Lymph nodes with a well delineated boundary (*Figure 29*) are more likely to be malignant compared to those with poorly delineated borders.[69]

Ancillary Features

Matting: defined as clumps of nodes adherent to each other with no normal echogenic connective tissues intervening (*Figure 30*).

Soft tissue oedema: indicated by diffuse decrease in echogenicity in adjacent tissues, loss of fascial planes and thickening of skin (*Figure 31*).

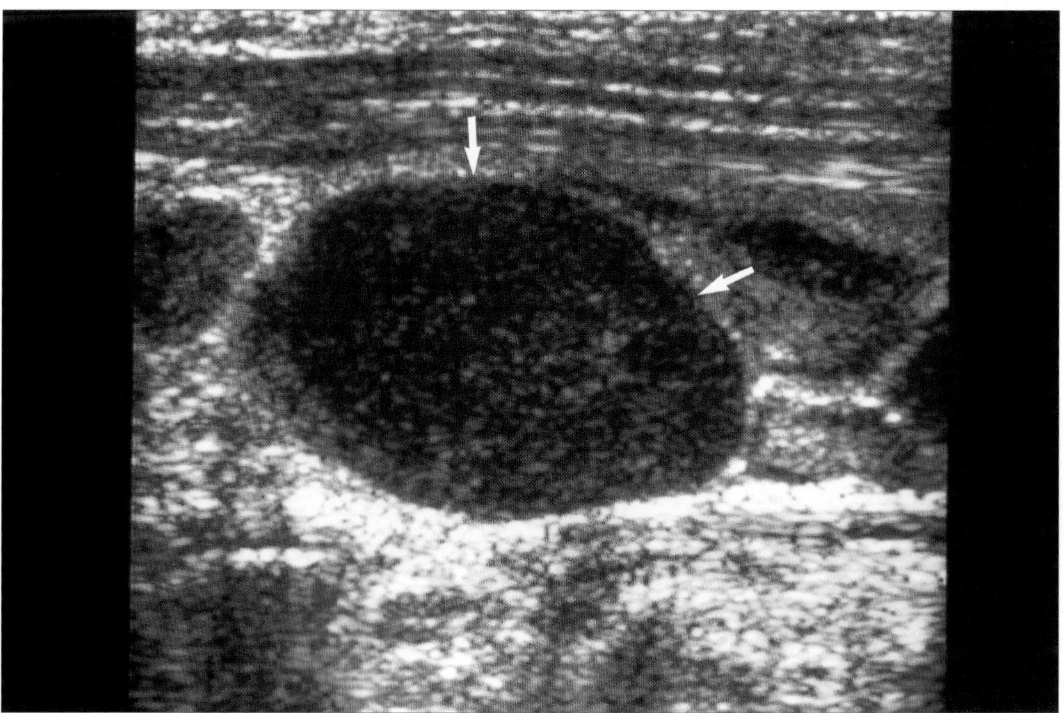

Figure 29. Transverse sonogram of a hypoechoic node with sharply defined borders (arrows).

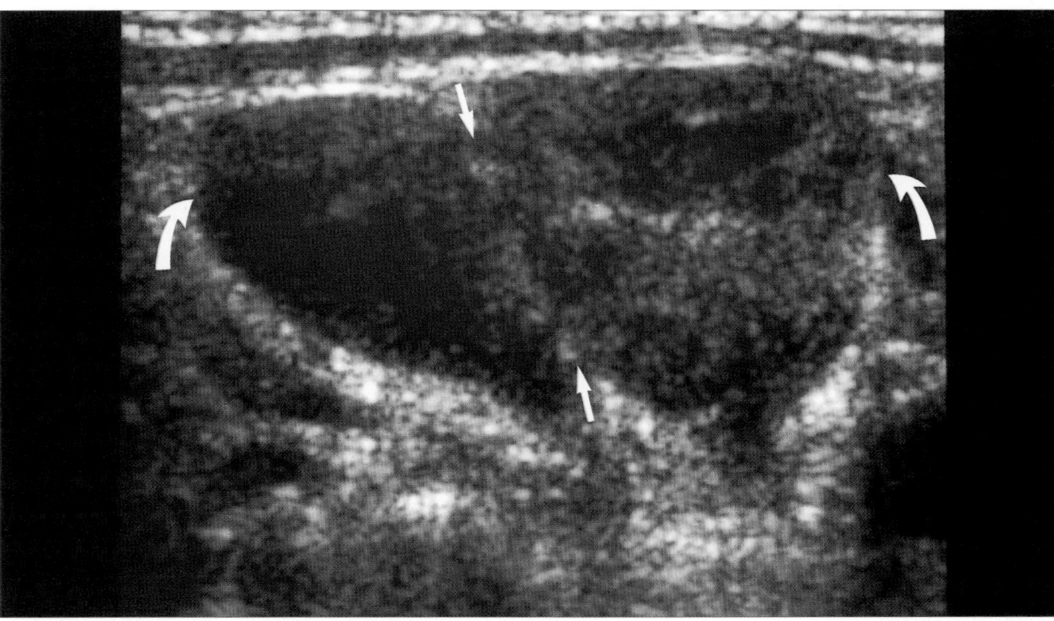

Figure 30. Longitudinal sonogram showing two hypoechoic, heterogeneous nodes (curved arrows). Note the loss of fascial planes between the nodes (straight arrows).

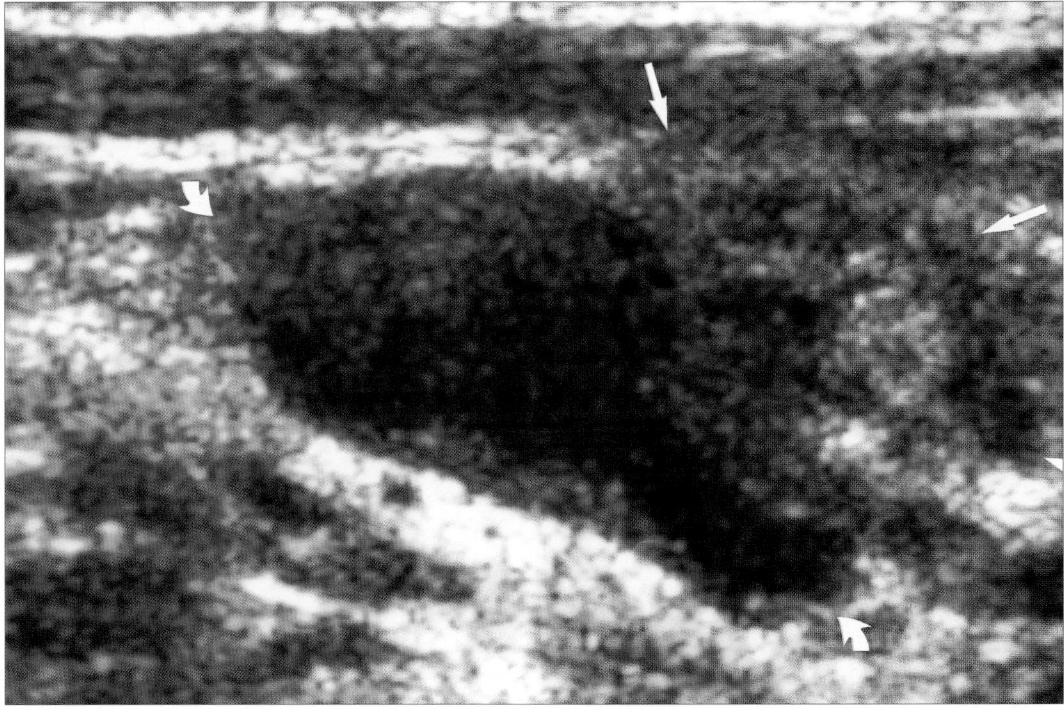

Figure 31. Longitudinal sonogram of a hypoechoic, heterogeneous node (curved arrows) with adjacent soft tissue oedema (straight arrows).

All the foregoing ancillary features are commonly seen in tuberculous adenopathy[70] and following radiotherapy to the neck.[71]

Ultrasound features of metastatic NPC nodes

Metastatic neck nodes from NPC are always hypoechoic relative to surrounding tissues: calcification is absent: 74% are round in shape (SA/LA ratio greater than 0.5) and have sharp nodal borders (91%): 84% show no echogenic hilus: most are homogeneous (94%), and only a few show intranodal necrosis (6%) and distal enhancement (12%). The majority of the nodes are seen in the upper cervical chain (22%) and in the posterior triangle (64%). Although none of the above features are specific for NPC, other pathological conditions having similar appearances,[72] nodes with these features are considered to be diagnostic of malignancy in a patient with known NPC. In particular their predominant distribution in the upper cervical area and the posterior triangle should alert the sonologist to the possibility of NPC, particularly in the southern Chinese. A US guided FNAC at this time may further help to indicate the primary.

Ultrasound helps to map the distribution of these nodes prior to RT. The scans can then be used as a baseline to monitor the nodes following RT to the neck.

Differential diagnosis

In patients who present initially with adenopathy the common differential diagnoses include TB, lymphoma and malignant metastases from other areas such as oral cavity (OC), pharynx, larynx and oesophagus (PLO) and papillary carcinoma of the thyroid. Infraclavicular primary tumours should also be borne in mind.

The following features help in the differential diagnosis:[72]

1) Metastases from oral cavity tumours are commonly seen in the submental/submandibular areas (43%) and the upper cervical chain (43%); 23% of the nodes show intranodal necrosis.
2) Metastases from PLO tumours are commonly seen all along the cervical chain (37%), in the supraclavicular fossa (30%) and in the posterior triangle (22%). Intranodal necrosis is present in 38%.
3) Metastatic nodes from papillary carcinoma of the thyroid are seen along the cervical chain (80%). The nodes are hyperechoic (79%), show punctate intranodal calcification (50%) and 21% demonstrate intranodal necrosis.[73]
4) Metastatic nodes from infraclavicular primaries are frequently seen in the supraclavicular fossa (43%) and lower posterior triangle (51%) and 28% have unsharp borders.
5) Tuberculous nodes are commonly seen in the posterior triangle (70%). The nodes have intranodal necrosis (63%), and unsharp borders (31%). They are frequently matted (46%) and show adjacent soft tissue edema (37%).

6) Lymphomatous nodes are frequently seen in the submental and submandibular areas (39%) and in the posterior triangle (32%): most of them show distal enhancement (84%).[74]

US appearances after RT

Following RT for NPC, the incidence of persistent or recurrent disease in the neck nodes is around 18%.[75] As further treatment is necessary it is important to identify affected abnormal nodes.

Although clinical examination can detect progressive enlargement of nodes during treatment, which is normally indicative of persistent active disease, it is unable to identify for certain whether there is residual tumour within the nodes. Furthermore, due to post radiation induration, nodes are frequently not palpable. However some nodes may still harbour malignant disease which may predispose to distant metastases.

Ultrasound would therefore appear to be an ideal initial investigation to evaluate the nodes after RT. However apart from shrinkage of the nodes and the appearance of oedema, the features of previously abnormal nodes remain unaltered for at least three months following RT.[71] Apart from a reduction in soft tissue oedema, a similar result may occasionally be seen even at one year after RT. However many of the abnormal features of nodes have disappeared after one year and 15–16 months after RT almost all the nodes show normal post radiotherapy features as follows:

1) One year following RT there is a 49.6% reduction in size in the long axis and 66.6% in the short axis of the largest malignant node. All these nodes return to the normal size limits for their respective area and do not show shrinkage below normal values.
2) The shape of the node reverts to normal around 13 months after therapy.
3) The echogenic hilus returns to normal around 15 months after RT and is seen in a minority of patients. In most patients the nodes demonstrate a thin, discontinuous, faint echogenic line separate from surrounding soft tissues. This most probably represents fibrosis (*Figure 32*).
4) Although all the nodes still remain poorly reflective compared to surrounding soft tissues, post RT nodes are slightly more echogenic than normal nodes when compared to the adjacent sternomastoid muscle.
5) Soft tissue induration still persists in a small percentage of patients (12.5%) one year after RT particularly in the posterior triangle.

Based on the above data the best time to perform a baseline scan for neck nodes is close to one year post RT. The US appearances and distribution of nodes at this time should be carefully mapped. Any change in the subsequent scans should alert the sonographer to the possibility of recurrence.

The role of ultrasound guided FNAC, although well documented as significantly increasing the specificity of ultrasound,[19] is not useful after RT. Following therapy to

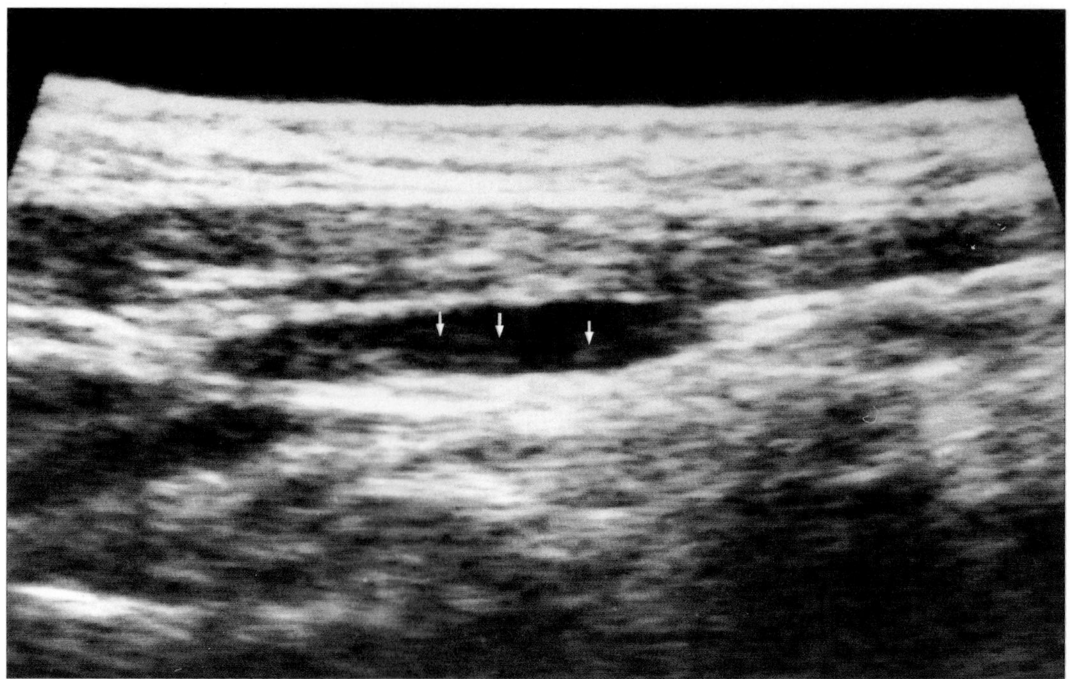

Figure 32. Longitudinal sonogram of an eliptical, hypoechoic post RT node with echogenic lines (arrows) presumably representing fibrosis.

neck nodes it is often difficult to obtain positive samples[76] and the cytological interpretation of the aspirate is difficult. This is particularly true in the early post-treatment period as tumour cells are not uniformly viable.[77]

Concluding Remarks

Computed tomography is the most widely available technique for evaluating patients with new and recurrent NPC. However, MR imaging has several advantages related to the excellent contrast resolution. It is better in evaluating early paranasopharyngeal extension, in distinguishing the primary tumour from enlarged lateral retropharyngeal nodes, and in assessing invasion of the sinuses and cranium. MR may prove also to be as good as, or better than, CT in the evaluation of skull base invasion.

In a Chinese patient who presents with cervical adenopathy, US and guided FNAC of neck nodes may provide the first clue to the presence of an NPC. In a patient with known NPC the role of US is to identify the presence and map the distribution of metastatic nodes in the neck. Following RT, US is useful in evaluating the neck for recurrent disease and may help to identify an enlarging node in the post radiation period, prior to its becoming palpable.

References

1. Parker, G.D., Harnsberger, H.R., Jacobs, J.M. 1990. The pharyngeal mucosal space. *Sem. Ultrasound*; 11:460–475.
2. Dillon, W.P., Mills, C.M., Kjosb, B., DeGroot, J., Brant-Zawadzki, M. 1984. Magnetic resonance imaging of the nasopharynx. *Radiology*; 152:731–738.
3. Teresi, L.M., Lufkin, R.B., Vinuela, F., Dietrich, R.B., Wilson, G.H., Bentson, J.R., Hanafee, W.N. 1987. MR imaging of the nasopharynx and floor of the middle cranial fossa. Part I. Normal anatomy. *Radiology*; 164:811–816.
4. Vogl, T., Dresel, S., Bilaniuk, L.T., Grevers, G., Kang, K., Lissner, J. 1990. Tumors of the nasopharynx and adjacent areas: MR imaging with Gd-DTPA. *Am. J. Radiology*; 154:585–592.
5. Lam, W.W.M., Chan, Y.L., Leung, S.F., Metreweli, C. 1997. Retropharyngeal lymphadenopathy in nasopharyngeal carcinoma. *Head Neck*; 19:176–181.
6. Ichimura, K. 1993. Can Rouviere's Lymph nodes in non-malignant subjects be identified with MRI? *Auris Nasus Larynx*; 20:117–123.
7. Teresi, L.M., Lufkin, R.B., Vinuela, F., Dietrich, R.B., Wilson, G.H., Bentson, J.R., Hanafee, W.N. 1987. MR imaging of the nasopharynx and floor of the middle cranial fossa. Part II. Malignant tumors. *Radiology*; 164:817–821.
8. Sham, J.S.T., Cheung, Y.K., Choy, D., Chan, F.L., Leong, L. 1991. Nasopharyngeal carcinoma: CT evaluation of patterns of tumour spread. *AJNR*; 12:265–270.
9. Sato, H., Kurata K., Yen, Y.H., Honjo, I., Yong, Y.H., Hsieh, T. 1988. Extension of nasopharyngeal carcinoma and otitis media with effusion. *Arch. Otolaryngol. Head Neck Surg.*; 114:866–867.
10. Olmi, P., Fallai, C., Colagrande, S., Giannardi, G. 1995. Staging and follow up of nasopharyngeal carcinoma: magnetic resonance imaging versus computerized tomography. *Int. J. Radiat. Oncol. Biol. Phys.*; 32:795–800.
11. Crawford, S.C., Harnsberger, H.R., Lufkin, R.B., Hanafee, W.N. 1989. The role of Gadolinium — DTPA in the evaluation of extracranial head and neck mass lesions. *Radiol. Clin. North Am.*; 27:219–241.
12. Mineura, K., Kowada, M., Tomura, N. 1991. Perineural extension of nasopharyngeal carcinoma into the posterior cranial fossa detected by magnetic resonance imaging. *Clin. Imaging*; 15:172–175.
13. Poon, P., Tsang, V., Munk, P. 1996. Comparison of MRI and CT in the T-staging of nasopharyngeal carcinoma. *Proceedings of 4th International Conference on Head and Neck Cancer*; 302:134.
14. Wong, J.R. 1996. Radiological studies of the clivus/base of skull invasion by nasopharyngeal cancer using MRI/CT and bone scan. *Proceedings of 4th International Conference on Head and Neck Cancer*; 303:134.
15. Curran, W.S., Hackney, D.B., Blitzer, P.H., Bilaniuk, L., 1986. The value of magnetic resonance imaging in treatment planning of nasopharyngeal carcinoma. *Acta Radiol. Oncol. Radiat. Phys. Biol.*; 12:2189–2196.
16. Chong, V.F., Fan, Y.F., Toh, K.H., Khoo, J.B., Lim, T.A. 1995. Magnetic resonance imaging and computed tomography features of nasopharyngeal carcinoma with maxillary sinus involvement. *Australas Radiol.*; 39:2–9.
17. Som, P.M. 1987. Lymph nodes of the neck. *Radiology*; 165:593–600.
18. Sham, J.S.T., Choy, D., Wei, W.I. 1990. Nasopharyngeal carcinoma: orderly neck node spread. *Int. J. Radiat. Oncol. Biol. Phys.*; 19(4):929–933.
19. de Jong, B., Rongen, R.J., Lameris, J.S., *et al.* 1989. Metastatic neck disease. *Arch. Otolaryngol. Head Neck Surg.*; 115:689–690.
20. Som, P.M. 1992. Detection of metastasis in cervical lymph nodes: CT and MR criteria and differential diagnosis. *Am. J. Radiology*; 158:961–969.
21. Van den Brekel, M.W.M., Stel, H.V., Castelijns, J.A., *et al.* 1990. Cervical lymph node metastases: assessment of radiologic criteria. *Radiology*; 177:379–384.

22. Chong, V.F.H., Fan, Y.F., Khoo, J.B.K. 1996. MRI features of cervical nodal necrosis in metastatic disease. *Clin. Radiol.*; 51;103–109.
23. Yousem, D.M., Som, P.M., Hackney, D.B., Schwaibold, F., Hendrix, R.A. 1992. Central nodal necrosis and extracapsular neoplastic spread in cervical lymph nodes: MR imaging versus CT. *Radiology*; 182:753–759.
24. Dooms, G.C., Hricak, H., Moseley, M.E., Bottles, K., *et al.* 1985. Characterization of lymphadenopathy by magnetic resonance relaxation times: preliminary results. *Radiology*; 155:691–697.
25. Anzai, Y., Blackwell, K.E., Hirschowitz, S., Rogers, J.E., Sato, Y., Yuh, W.T.C., *et al.* 1994. Initial clinical experience with dextran-coated superparamagnetic iron oxide for detection of lymph node metastases in patients with head and neck cancer. *Radiology*; 192;709–715.
26 . Leung, S.F., Teo, P.M.L., Shiu, W.W.T., Tsao, S.Y., Leung, T.W.T. 1991. Clinical features and management of distant metastases of nasopharyngeal carcinoma. *J. Otolaryngol.*; 20:1, 27–29.
27. Ahmad, A., Stefani, S. 1986. Distant metastases of nasopharyngeal carcinoma: a study of 256 male patients. *J. Surg. Oncol.*; 33:194–197.
28. Sham, J.S.T., Choy, D., Choi, P.H.K. 1990. Nasopharyngeal carcinoma: the significance of neck node involvement in relation to the pattern of distant failure. *Brit. J. Radiol.*; 63:108–113.
29. Sham, J.S.T., Cheung, Y.K., Chan, F.L., Choy, D. 1990. Nasopharyngeal carcinoma: pattern of skeletal metastases. *Brit. J. Radiol.*; 63:202–205.
30. Leung, S.F., Stewart, I.E.T., Tsao, S.Y., Metreweli, C. 1991. Staging bone scintigraphy in nasopharyngeal carcinoma. *Clin. Radiol.*; 43:314–315.
31. Sham, J.S.T., Tong, C.M., Choy, D., Yeung, D.W.C. 1991. Role of bone scanning in detection of subclinical bone metastais in nasopharyngeal carcinoma. *Clin. Nucl. Med.*; 16(1):27–29.
32. Daly, B.D., Leung, S.F., Cheung, H., Metreweli, C. 1993. Thoracic metastases from carcinoma of the nasopharynx: high frequency of hilar and mediastinal lymphadenopathy. *Am. J. Radiology*; 160:241–244.
33. Liu, R.S., Chen, Y.K., Yen, S.H., Chu, Y.K., *et al.* 1995. Hypertrophic pulmonary osteoarthropathy in nasopharyngeal carcinoma: an early sign of pulmonary metastasis. *Nucl. Med. Commun.*; 16 (9):785–789.
34. Daly, B.D. 1995. Thoracic metastases from nasopharyngeal carcinoma presenting as hypertrophic pulmonary osteoarthropathy: scintigraphic and CT findings. *Clin. Radiol.*; 50:545–547.
35. Kraiphibul, P., Atichartakarn, V., Clongsusuek, P., Kulapaditharom, B., *et al.* 1991. Nasopharyngeal carcinoma: value of bone and liver scintigraphy in the pretreatment and follow up period. *J. Med. Assoc. Thai*; 74(7):276–279.
36. Leung, S.F., Metreweli, C., Tsao, S.Y., van Hasselt, C.A. 1991. Staging abdominal ultrasonography in nasopharyngeal carcinoma. *Australas Radiol.*; 35(1):31–32.
37. Sham, J.S.T., Choy, D., Wei, W.I., Yau, C.C. 1992. Value of clinical follow-up for local nasopharyngeal carcinoma relapse. *Head Neck*; 14:208–217.
38. Glazer, H.S., Niemeyer, J.H., Balfe, D.M., Hayden, R.E., Emami, B., *et al.* 1986. Neck neoplasms: MR imaging. Part II. Posttreatment evaluation. *Radiology*; 160:349–354.
39. Gong, Q.Y., Zhu, H.Y., Zheng, G.L., Wang, Y., Yuan, C.M., *et al.* 1992. MRI-T2 values in the differentiation of recurrence and fibrosis after radiation of nasopharyngeal carcinoma. *Chin. Med. J. (Engl.)*; 105:135–138.
40. Gong, Q.Y., Zheng, G.L., Zhu, H.Y. 1991. MRI differentiation of recurrent nasopharyngeal carcinoma from postradiation fibrosis. *Comput. Med. Imaging Graph.*; 15:423–429.
41. Unger, J.D., Chiang, L.C., Unger, G.F. 1978. Apparent reformation of the base of the skull following radiotherapy for nasopharyngeal carcinoma. *Radiology*; 126:779–782.
42. Kim, K.H., Sung, M.W., Jang, Y.J., Yun, J.B., Chung, J.K. 1996. F-18 FDG whole body PET in the evaluation of postoperative recurrence of head and neck cancer patients. *Proceedings of the 4th International Conference on Head and Neck Cancer*; Abstract:434.

43. Gapany, M., Grund, F., Faust, R., Fehling, S., Hildebrandt, W. 1996. Thallium-201 SPECT imaging of head and neck tumours. *Proceedings of the 4th International Conference on Head and Neck Cancer;* Abstract:437.
44. Togawa, T., Yui, N., Kinoshita, F., Shimada, F., Omura, K., *et al.* 1993. Visualization of nasopharyngeal carcinoma with Tl-201 chloride and a three-head rotating gamma camera SPECT system. *Ann. Nuc. Medicine;* 7(2):105–113.
45. Valk, P.E., Dillon, W.P. 1991. Radiation injury of the brain. *AJNR;* 12:45–62.
46. Lee, A.W.M., Law, S.C.K., Ng, S.H., Chan, D.K.K., Poon, Y.F., *et al.* 1992. Retrospective analysis of nasopharyngeal carcinoma treated during 1976-1985: late complications following megavoltage irradiation. *Brit. J. Radiol.;* 65:918–928.
47. Leung, S.F., Kreel, L., Tsao, S.Y. 1992. Asymptomatic temporal lobe injury after radiotherapy for nasopharyngeal carcinoma: incidence and determinants. *Brit. J. Radiol.;* 65:710–714.
48. Lee, A.W.M., Ng, S.H., Ho, J.H.C., Tse, V.K.C., Poon, Y.F., *et al.* 1988. Clinical diagnosis of late temporal necrosis following radiation therapy for nasopharyngeal carcinoma. *Cancer;* 61:1535–1542.490.
49. Lee, P.W.H., Hung, B.K.M., Woo, E.K.W., Tai, P.T.H., Choi, D.T.K. 1989. Effects of radiation therapy on neuropsychological functioning in patients with nasopharyngeal carcinoma. *J. Neurol. Neurosurg. Psychiatry;* 52:488–492.
50. Hu, J.Q., Guan, Y.H., Zhao, L.Z., Xie, S.X., Guo, Z., *et al.* 1991. Delayed radiation encephalopathy after radiotherapy for nasopharyngeal cancer: a CT study of 45 cases. *J. Comput. Assist. Tomogr.;* 15:181–187.
51. Lee, A.W.M., Cheng, O.C., Ng, S.H., Tse, V.K.C., O, S.K., *et al.* 1990. Magnetic resonance imaging in the clinical diagnosis of late temporal lobe necrosis following radiotherapy for nasopharyngeal carcinoma. *Clin. Radiol.;* 42:24–31.
52. Woo, E., Chan, Y.F., Lam, K., Lok, A.S., *et al.* 1987. Apoplectic intracerebral hemorrhage: an unusual complication of cerebral radiation necrosis. *Pathology;* 19:95–98.
53. Batnitzky, S., Halleran, W.J. 3rd, McMillan, J.H., Price, H.I., Kalsbeck, J.E. 1986. Radiologic manifestations of delayed radiation necrosis of the brain. *Acta Radiol. Suppl.;* 369:231–234.
54. Ogawa, T., Kanno, I., Shishido, F., Inugami, A., Higano, S., *et al.* 1991. Clinical value of PET with 18F-fluorodeoxyglucose and L-methyl-11C-methionine for diagnosis of recurrent brain tumor and radiation injury. *Acta Radiol.;* 32:197–202.
55. Wang, P.Y., Shen, W.C. 1991. Magnetic resonance imaging in two patients with radiation myelopathy. *J. Formos. Med. Assoc. (Taiwan);* 90:583–585.
56. Lam, K.S.L., Tse, V.K.C., Wang, C., Yeung, R.T.T., Ho, J.H.C. 1991. Effects of cranial irradiation on hypothalamic-pituitary function — a 5-years longitudinal study in patients with nasopharyngeal carcinoma. *Quart. J. Med.;* 286:165–176.
57. Tang, N.L., Choy, A.T., John, D.G., van Hasselt, C.A. 1992. The otological status of patients with nasopharyngeal carcinoma after megavoltage radiotherapy. *J. Laryngol. Otol.;* 106:1055–8.
58. Kuo, W.R., Wu, C.C., Lian, S.L., Ching, F.Y., Lee, K.W., *et al.* 1993. The effects of radiation therapy on salivary function in patients with head and neck cancer. *Kao Hsiung I Hsueh Ko Hsueh Tsa Chih;* 9:401–409.
59. Sham, J.S.T., Poon, Y.F., Wei, W.I., Choy, D. 1990. Nasopharyngeal carcinoma in young patients. *Cancer;* 65:2606–2610.
60. Ying, M., Ahuja, A., Brook, F., Brown, B., Metreweli, C. 1996. The sonographic appearances and distribution of normal cervical lymph nodes in Chinese population. *J. Ultrasound Med.;* 15:431–436.
61. Bruneton, J.N., Roux, P., Caramella, E., Demard, F., Vallicioni, J., Chauvel, P. 1984. Ear, nose, and throat cancer: ultrasound diagnosis of metastasis to cervical nodes. *Radiology;* 152:771–773.
62. Sakai, F., Kiyono, K., Sone, S., *et al.* 1988. Ultrasonic evaluation of cervical metastatic lymphadenopathy. *J. Ultrasound Med.;* 7:305–310.
63. Hajek, P.C., Salomonowitz, E., Turk, R., Tscholakoff, D., Kumpan, W., Czembriek, H. 1986. Lymph nodes of the neck: evaluation with US. *Radiology;* 158:739–742.

64. Tohnosu, N., Onada, S., Isono, K. 1989. Ultrasonographic evaluation of cervical lymph node metastases in esophageal cancer with special reference between the short to long axis ratio (S/L) and the cancer content. *J. Clin. Ultrasound*; 17:101–106.
65. Vassallo, P., Wernecke, K., Roos, N., *et al.* 1992. Differentiation of benign from malignant lymphadenopathy: the role of high resolution US. *Radiology*; 183:215–220.
66. Rubaltelli, L., Proto, E., Salmaso, R., *et al.* 1990. Sonography of abnormal lymph nodes in vitro: correlation of sonographic and histologic findings. *Am. J. Radiology*; 155:1241–1244.
67. Evans, R.M., Ahuja, A., Metreweli, C. 1993. The linear echogenic hilus in cervical lymphadenopathy — a sign of benignity or malignancy? *Clin. Radiol.*; 47:262–264.
68. Bruneton, J.N., Balu-Maestro, C., Marcy, P.Y., *et al.* 1994. Very high frequency (13 MHz) ultrasonographic examination of the normal neck: detection of normal lymph nodes and thyroid nodules. *J. Ultrasound Med.*; 13:87–90.
69. Shozushima, M., Suzuki, M., Nakashima, T., Yanagisawa, Y., Sakamaki, K., Takeda, Y. 1990. Ultrasound diagnosis of lymph node metastasis in head and neck cancer. *Dento. Maxillo. Fac. Radiol.*; 19:165–170.
70. Ahuja, A., Ying, M., Evans, R., King, W., Metreweli, C. 1995. The application of ultrasound criteria for malignancy in differentiating tuberculous cervical adenitis from metastatic nasopharyngeal carcinoma. *Clin. Radiol.*; 50:391–395.
71. Ahuja, A., Ying, M., Leung, S.F., Metreweli, C. 1996. The sonographic appearance and significance of cervical metastatic nodes following radiotherapy for nasopharyngeal carcinoma. *Clin. Radiol.*; 51:698–701.
72. Ahuja, A., Ying, M., King, W., Metreweli, C. 1997. A practical approach to ultrasound of cervical lymph nodes. *J. Laryngol. Otol.*; 111:245–256.
73. Ahuja, A., Chow, L., Mok, C.O., King, W., Metreweli, C. 1995. Metastatic cervical lymph nodes in papillary carcinoma of the thyroid: ultrasound and histological correlation. *Clin. Radiol.*; 50:229–231.
74. Ahuja, A., Ying, M., Yang, W.T., Evans, R., King, W., Metreweli, C. 1996. The use of sonography in differentiating cervical lymphomatous nodes from cervical metastatic nodes. *Clin. Radiol.*; 51:186–190.
75. Bedwinek, J.M., Perez, C.A., Keys, D.J. 1980. Analysis of failures after definitive irradiation for epidermoid carcinoma of the nasopharynx. *Cancer*; 45:2725–9.
76. Wei, W.I., Lam, K.H., Ho, C.M., Sham, J.S.T., Lau, S.K. 1990. Efficacy of radical neck dissection for the control of cervical metastasis after radiotherapy for nasopharyngeal carcinoma. *Am. J. Surg.*; 160:439–442.
77. Woo, J.K.S., Waldron, J. 1991. In: *Nasopharyngeal Carcinoma*, eds. van Hasselt, A., Gibb, A. Hong Kong: The Chinese University Press, 93–104.

CHAPTER 9

Epstein-Barr Virus Serological Markers

John S. Tam

Introduction

Nasopharyngeal carcinoma (NPC) has a well defined geographical distribution. This malignancy occurs relatively infrequently in Europe and North America, but is common among certain ethnic groups such as Cantonese in southern China and south-east Asia,[1] Maghreb Arabs in North Africa[2] and Eskimos in Greenland and Alaska.[3] In endemic areas the disease is most common among males over 30 years of age. In addition to genetic predisposition, dietary and other environmental factors, and chemical carcinogens as possible causes of NPC, extensive data in immunological, biological and molecular biological investigations have shown that NPC is closely associated with the Epstein-Barr virus (EBV). The serological relationship between EBV and NPC was first described by Old *et al.* in 1966[4] using immunodiffusion. This observation was subsequently confirmed by indirect immunofluorescence using EBV transformed cell lines and it was shown that patients with NPC had elevated antibody levels against various EBV-associated antigens.[5,6] The level of antibody in NPC patients correlated with the stage of the disease and the total tumour burden.[7,8] It had been reported that NPC cells, which are of epithelial origin, contain multiple copies of the EBV genome and that several EBV specific antigens are expressed in such cells.[9,10] The demonstration of high levels of IgA type immunoglobulin to EBV specific antigens[11] in NPC patients and subsequent sero-epidemiological studies showed that the detection of such antibodies is useful in the diagnosis of NPC.[12] This chapter addresses the relationship of EBV specific markers in NPC patients and the application of these markers in the diagnosis and monitoring of treatment of the disease.

Epstein-Barr Virus and Virus Induced Antigens

Characterization and epidemiology of Epstein-Barr virus

EBV is a double-stranded DNA virus and is classified as a member of the *Herpesviridae* family. The virus was first described by Epstein *et al.*[13] from electron microscopic examination of cultured Burkitt's lymphoma cells. The morphology of the virus is indistinguishable from that of other members of the herpes family. It has a DNA containing icosahedral viral nucleocapsid enclosed in a lipoprotein envelope with virus specific membrane glycoproteins.

EBV infection is ubiquitous in the human population world-wide as demonstrated in serological surveys and the majority of populations are infected by adulthood.[14] The age of acquisition of EBV infection is determined by socio-economic factors associated with the population. Primary infection acquired early in life is asymptomatic or may present as an upper respiratory infection. Infection usually occurs in the first decade of life in lower socio-economic groups. Infection in older children and young adults occurs commonly in higher socio-economic groups and may present as infectious mononucleosis.[15] Other clinical symptoms include nonspecific febrile illness, pharyngotonsillitis, rash, lymphadenopathy, hepatosplenomegaly and pneumonia. The virus has also been found to be associated with Burkitt's lymphoma (BL), NPC and a wide variety of neoplastic diseases of man such as B cell lymphoma in immunocompromised hosts, Hodgkin's disease, T cell lymphomas and other carcinomas.[16] Transmission of the virus is thought to occur by means of saliva. Infectious virus particles have been isolated in throat washings in 15–20% of normal EBV seropositive individuals indicating that virus excretion may occur periodically even after many years of clinical infection.

Replication of Epstein-Barr virus

The lack of a fully permissive nasopharyngeal epithelial cell culture system for the propagation of EBV rendered initial studies on the replication of the virus in such cells difficult. Human B lymphocytes were found to be the only susceptible cells for EBV infection *in vitro*.[17] EBV infection of B lymphocytes is latent with or without the production of infectious virions.[18] In latent infection, the EBV DNA usually persists in cells as a closed circular episome, but can also be integrated into cellular DNA or exist in both forms.[19] A number of different latent gene products are expressed in such transformed cells. These include six EBV nuclear antigens and three membrane glycoproteins (see below). EBNA2 and LMP1 are important gene products in latent EBV infection especially in the initiation and maintenance of the transformed state of infected cells.[20] Latent infection by EBV can be disrupted and the EBV genome activated. This process of activation can appear spontaneously in a proportion of tumour cells under *in vitro* cultivation (< 10%) or it may be induced by superinfection and chemicals in latently infected lymphoid cultures (see *Figure 1*). Chemicals used for induction include n-butyrate and phorbal ester tumour promoter 12-*o*-tetra decanoyl phorbal-13-acetate (TPA) which are also promoters of cell differentiation.[21]

Initiation of lytic EBV infection is mediated by the expression of the BamH I Z EBV replication activator (ZEBRA) encoded in the BZLF1.[22] A number of different gene products related to the different stages of the lytic replication cycle have been

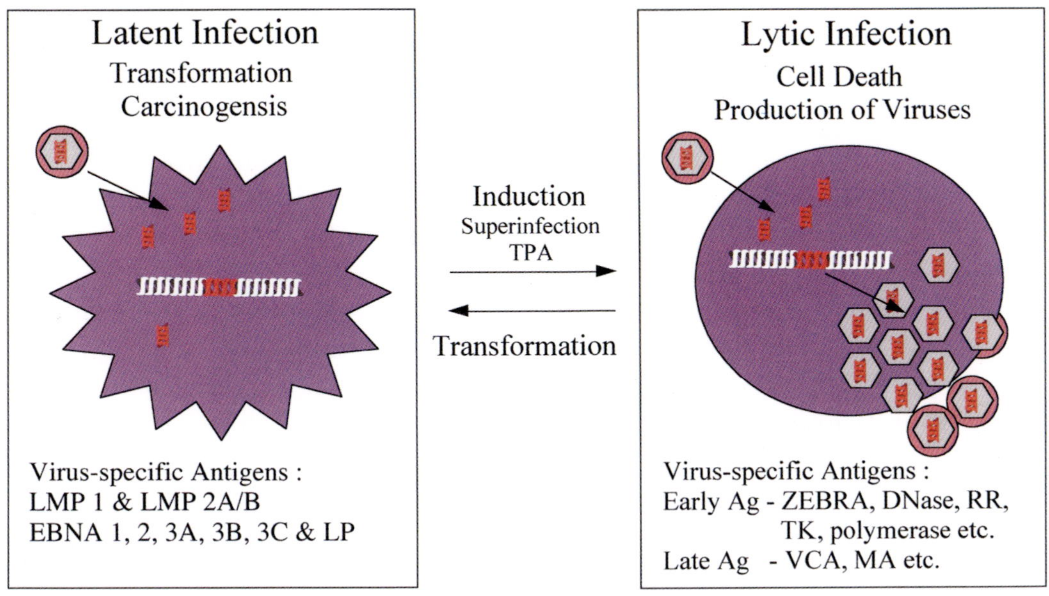

Figure 1. The latent and lytic replication cycle of Epstein-Barr virus in cells.

identified in addition to those associated with latent infection. These can be categorized into immediate early genes and late genes including the viral structural genes.[23]

It has been shown that NPC cells passaged through athymic nude mice contain EBV DNA and EBV specific antigens.[24] In addition, EBV DNA and Epstein-Barr virus associated nuclear antigens (EBNA) have been detected in NPC biopsy material.[9,10] The lytic cycle of EBV is known to take place in differentiated epithelial cells.[25] However EBV replication in epithelial cells is not efficient and little or no virus is produced *in vitro*. How EBV enters nasopharyngeal epithelial cells *in vivo* remains unclear since these cells do not have receptors for EBV.

Epstein-Barr virus specific antigens in infected cells

As discussed above, infection of B cells by EBV may lead to two different outcomes: (1) transformation or immortalization of B cells into lymphoblastoid lines or (2) spontaneous or induced activation of the latent virus into its lytic growth cycle in a proportion of cells of established lymphoblastoid lines, leading to cell death with or without the production of infectious virions. Using these cells and sera from EBV antibody positive patients, a number of different antigens associated with the replication cycle of EBV have been elucidated.

During the latent infection stage, two families of viral specific antigens can be detected in EBV transformed cells. These are designated as Epstein-Barr virus associated nuclear antigens (EBNA) and latent membrane proteins (LMP).[26] EBNA is present in all EBV DNA containing cells and is the first antigen to be expressed in these cells. The EBNA complex consists of at least six proteins (EBNA1, EBNA2, EBNA3A, EBNA3B, EBNA3C and EBNA-LP).[23] All of the known EBNAs are expressed in B cells infected latently by EBV during transformation *in vitro*. However there are considerable differences in the expression of EBNAs in different latent EBV-infected cells *in vivo*.[27] The EBNA proteins are nuclear DNA-binding proteins and are believed to be essential for the maintenance of episomal EBV DNA replication (EBNA1)[20] and to act as *trans*-activators of latent viral genes (EBNA2).[28] EBNA proteins are the only EBV-specific antigen expressed persistently in carcinoma cells in NPC biopsies.[29]

The LMP expressed in latent EBV infection is thought to be an important component of the lymphocyte-detected membrane antigen (LYDMA).[30] Three proteins can be distinguished in EBV-LMP namely LMP1, LMP2A (TP1) and LMP2B (TP2). LMP1 is a dominant transforming oncogene in mouse fibroblast cells[31] which induces B-lymphocyte activation markers, and enhances CD23 (a soluble autocrine B cell growth factor) expression.[32] LMP2A is expressed in most cells latently infected by EBV.[33] LMP2A is phosphorylated by the *src* family of tyrosine kinases leading to the modulation of transmembrane signal transduction and blocking of the switch from latent infection to lytic infection.[34] LMP2B is identical to LMP2A except that the transcription of LMP2B is initiated from the second exon in the LMP2 gene.[35]

The switch between latent and lytic infection of EBV is mediated by the BZLF1 gene which encodes a 40 kDa nuclear protein.[22] When the EBV infected cells enter the lytic cycle, different antigens are produced in sequence. These include: (1) early membrane antigen (EMA);[36] (2) early intracellular antigen (EA);[37] (3) viral capsid antigen (VCA)[38] and (4) late membrane antigen (LMA).[36]

The early antigen (EA) complex consists of a group of non-structural polypeptides divided classically into two components designated as "diffuse" (EA-D) or "restricted" (EA-R) based on the location and appearance of the antigen in the cells as well as their stability after methanol fixation.[37] The EA-R component as detected by immunofluorescence is confined to the cytoplasm. Four EBV-specific antigens associated with the EA-R complex have been described; ribonucleotide reductase (large subunit of 85kDa),[39] protein kinase (17 kDa),[40] alkaline deoxyribonuclease[41] (DNase, 52 kDa) and thymidine kinase[42] (67 kDa). Other viral encoded proteins have also been identified as members of the EA complex. These include the ZEBRA protein[22] and the viral DNA polymerase.[43]

The viral capsid antigen (VCA) and late membrane antigen (LMA) are viral specific late proteins and are integral components of the full virion. VCA is the main building block of the virus nucleocapsid. LMA are associated with the viral envelope and are responsible for the induction of virus neutralizing antibodies. These structural proteins are made prior to the production of virion.

Immunological Responses to Epstein-Barr Virus Antigens in Natural Infections

The immunological response of EBV infected patients to the different virus specific antigenic markers can be characteristic of the type of EBV-associated disease and is therefore of diagnostic and prognostic significance. The immunological response to the different EBV-specific antigens and the associated diseases are listed in *Table 1.*

Table 1. EBV specific antigens and immunological response in patients with EBV associated diseases.

Antigen	Latent infection	Lytic infection	Immune response	Disease association
LYDMA	+	+	cellular	Prognostic of NPC treatment
EBNA	+	+	IgG	Past infection
EA-D	–	+	IgG	IM, NPC
			IgA	NPC
EA-R	–	+	IgG	BL, chronic infection
VCA	–	+	IgG	Recent or past infection
			IgM	Primary infection, IM
			IgA	NPC
LMA	–	+	IgG	Past infection

NPC = nasopharyngeal carcinoma
IM = infectious mononucleosis
BL = Burkitt's lymphoma

EBV Serology in the Diagnosis of Undifferentiated NPC

Patients with NPC regularly exhibit high levels of antibodies directed against EBV-specific antigens. In addition to the IgA responses of NPC patients to VCA and EA-D antigens of EBV-infected cells, several EBV-specific antigenic markers have been studied. These include antibodies against: (1) EBV-specific membrane antigens (LYDMA, LMP and LMA); (2) the individual components of EBNA; (3) EBV-specific DNase; (4) EBV-specific DNA polymerase; (5) EBV-specific thymidine kinase; (6) EBV-specific ribonucleotide reductase and (7) the BamH I Z EBV replication activator protein (ZEBRA).

IgA antibodies against EBV VCA and EA-D in NPC patients

The most striking difference in the immunological response of NPC patients to EBV as compared to healthy populations is their high level of IgA response to VCA and EA-D.[11] Such serological profiles are now used routinely as diagnostic criteria for undifferentiated NPC.[44] *Table 2* summarizes published results on the detection of IgA

Table 2. IgA immune response of NPC patients to EBV specific VCA and EA in different geographical areas.

			% of patients with elevated IgA level					
			NPC		Non-NPC cancer		Healthy individuals	
Ethnic origin	Reference	Country	VCA	EA	VCA	EA	VCA	EA
Chinese Caucasian African	[11]	Hong Kong Europe Kenya	93	73	10	6	8	0
Chinese	[45]	Hong Kong	93	78	9	2	0	0
Chinese	[46]	China	100	65	—	—	0	0
Chinese	[47]	Taiwan	89	60	—	—	3	0
Eskimo	[3]	USA	75	71	—	—	2	0
Eskimo	[48]	Greenland	80	50	—	—	—	—
Caucasian	[50]	USSR & Cuba	91	58	15	0	5	0
Caucasian	[51]	USA	85	—	15	—	9	—
Jews	[52]	Israel	82	—	—	—	6	—

against EBV specific antigens in NPC patients in different geographical locations. However the detection of anti-VCA and EA-D antibodies is traditionally performed by the indirect immunofluorescence test (IFT) using EBV infected producer and nonproducer cell lines.

The method of IFT suffers the major drawback of observer subjectivity. The method must be well controlled and the sensitivity and specificity should be evaluated in each laboratory. In order to evaluate this method in our laboratory, the sensitivity and specificity of IFT for IgA anti-VCA and EA-D for the diagnosis of NPC were calculated using 228 cases of NPC, 143 cases of head and neck tumours other than NPC and 752 non-NPC cases from the Prince of Wales Hospital, Hong Kong. All cases of NPC and head and neck tumours were histologically confirmed. Non-NPC cases were randomly selected from patients with histopathological investigations (other than nasopharyngeal or head and neck specimens) who had also been investigated for IgA anti-VCA and EA-D. As shown in *Table 3*, the geometric mean titres for both IgA anti-VCA and IgA anti-EA-D in NPC patients were respectively 16 and 53 times higher than those of the non-NPC patients indicating the close relationship between NPC and these EBV-specific serological markers. The percentage of NPC patients and non-NPC patients with the various serological endpoints for diagnosis are shown in *Table 4*.

The sensitivity and specificity of IgA anti-VCA alone for the diagnosis of NPC using different serological endpoints are shown in *Table 5* and those for IgA anti-EA-D alone are shown in *Table 6*. These results further demonstrate the high sensitivity (97% at ≥5) of IgA-anti-VCA compared to IgA anti-EA-D (79% at ≥5) and the high specificity (97%

Table 3. Geometric mean titre of IgA anti-EBV VCA and IgA anti-EBV EA in patients with nasopharyngeal carcinoma, other head and neck tumours and non-NPC patients at the Prince of Wales Hospital.

	NPC n = 228	Head & neck n = 143	Non-NPC n = 752
IgA anti-VCA	132.9	20.1	8.4
IgA anti-EA	43.9	1.0	0.8

Table 4. IgA anti-EBV VCA and EA titre in patients with and without NPC at the Prince of Wales Hospital.

	NPC n = 228		Non-NPC n = 752	
Titre	VCA (%)	EA (%)	VCA (%)	EA (%)
< 5	9 (3.9)	45 (19.7)	525 (69.8)	735 (97.7)
≥ 5	219 (96.0)	183 (80.2)	227 (30.1)	17 (2.3)
≥ 10	207 (90.7)	162 (71.1)	137 (18.2)	15 (2.0)
≥ 20	196 (86.0)	138 (60.5)	110 (14.6)	14 (1.9)
≥ 40	156 (68.4)	103 (45.2)	47 (6.3)	3 (0.4)
≥ 80	137 (60.1)	69 (30.2)	26 (3.5)	2 (0.3)
≥ 160	70 (30.7)	26 (11.4)	6 (0.8)	2 (0.3)
320	51 (22.4)	0 (0.0)	4 (0.5)	0 (0.0)

Table 5. Sensitivity and specificity of IgA anti-VCA alone at different serological endpoints for the clinical diagnosis of NPC at the Prince of Wales Hospital.

Serological end-point	Sensitivity (%)	Specificity (%)
≥ 5	97.3	67.2
> 5	90.4	79.0
> 10	85.1	82.3
> 20	68.1	91.3
> 40	59.0	94.3
> 80	28.7	98.0
> 160	22.3	98.9
> 320	4.3	99.8

Table 6. Sensitivity and specificity of IgA anti-EA alone at different serological endpoints for the clinical diagnosis of NPC at the Prince of Wales Hospital.

Serological end-point	Sensitivity (%)	Specificity (%)
≥ 5	78.7	97.3
> 5	69.1	97.6
> 10	58.5	98.0
> 20	41.0	99.2
> 40	27.1	99.6
> 80	8.5	99.9

at ≥5) of IgA anti-EA-D compared to IgA-anti-VCA (67.2% at ≥5) in the diagnosis of NPC. However when these two serological markers are used together, a sensitivity of 80% and a specificity of 98% for the diagnosis of NPC can be reached using a serological endpoint of ≥5 for both markers as shown in *Table 7*.

Table 7. Sensitivity and specificity of IgA anti-VCA and EA combined at different serological endpoints for the clinical diagnosis of NPC at the Prince of Wales Hospital.

Serological end-point IgA anti-VCA	IgA anti-EA	Sensitivity (%)	Specificity (%)
≥ 5 – ≥160	≥ 5	80.3 – 29.0	97.7 – 99.3
≥ 10 – ≥160	≥ 5	70.6 – 29.0	98.0 – 99.5
≥ 20 – ≥160	≥ 5	60.1 – 27.6	98.1 – 99.6
≥ 40 – ≥160	≥ 5	43.9 – 24.6	99.6 – 99.7
≥ 80 – ≥160	≥ 5	28.5 – 18.9	99.7
≥ 160	≥ 5	11.4	99.7

It is apparent from these studies that a serological relationship between EBV and NPC exists in the different geographical areas examined and that IgA anti-VCA and IgA anti-EA-D are both sensitive and specific tests for the diagnosis of NPC. In this regard IgA anti-EA-D appears to be a more specific but less sensitive marker than IgA anti-VCA.

Antibodies against EBV LYDMA, LMP and LMA in NPC patients

Antibodies against the LYDMA, LMP and LMA of EBV transformed lymphoblastoid cells in NPC patients have been examined by different methods such as the antibody-dependent cellular cytotoxicity assay (ADCC),[53] indirect immuno-fluorescence (IF)[12] and immunoblotting.[54] Neel *et al.*,[55] using the ADCC assay which measures antibodies against the LYDMA, demonstrated that NPC patients with a low ADCC titre at the time of diagnosis have a relatively poor prognosis. They showed that 75% of NPC patients with high ADCC titres (>7680) were disease free for three years or longer while only 34% of patients with low ADCC titres (<7680) were disease free at three years and only 20% at five years. The three year survival rates of NPC patients with high and low ADCC titres were 80% and 50% respectively. Thus the result of the ADCC assay appears to reflect the clinical course of patients with NPC and the antibody level may help to identify patients with recurrent disease after therapy.

Using highly purified latent membrane protein (LMP), Rowe *et al.*[54] demonstrated that 64% of NPC patients produced an antibody response to LMP while only 22% of normal patients with serological evidence of EBV infection and without evidence of NPC were positive using an immunoblotting assay. Moreover in NPC patients, the IgA anti-MA level was shown to be elevated as compared to controls (58% vs 0%) by IF.[46]

Antibodies against EBV EBNAs in NPC patients

Although all EBV infected patients have antibodies against EBNA, antibodies against the individual components of EBNA in normal and NPC patients have been compared. Miller *et al.*[56] using transfected EBNA DNA in mouse cells identified two EBNA components M and K. A serological survey of patients with different EBV associated diseases showed that 96% and 14% of seropositive patients had antibodies against the K and M components respectively whereas 90% of NPC patients had antibodies against both components. These results demonstrated that high levels of antibodies against both M and K components of EBNA can be used as a diagnostic marker for NPC. In a separate study,[54] a reduced incidence of anti-EBNA2 and an increased incidence of antibodies to EBNA3 and EBNA 6 were noted in NPC patients as compared to healthy EBV-seropositive patients.

Anti-EBNA 1 antibodies have been detected in almost all patients previously infected with EBV.[54] However Foong *et al.*[57] showed that IgA anti-EBNA1 is detectable in 91% of NPC patients as compared to 13.3% in normal individuals and only 10.5% in patients with cancer other than NPC. This indicates that IgA anti-EBNA1 can be used as a marker for NPC. Further work by Cheng *et al.*[58] using synthetic peptide-based antigenic epitopes of the carboxy-terminal region of EBNA1 demonstrated reactivity with high specificity for sera of patients with NPC. These results suggested that IgA antibody to EBNA1 can be used as an additional serological marker for NPC.

Antibodies against EBV-specific DNase in NPC patients

Cheng *et al.*[41] in 1980 described the presence of EBV-specific alkaline DNase enzyme in superinfected or chemically induced lymphoblastoid cells and they further demonstrated a high prevalence (94%) of neutralizing antibody to this enzyme in NPC patients compared to controls (1%). This was confirmed by other studies which showed that the presence of neutralising antibody to EBV-specific DNase has 90% sensitivity and 95% specificity for detecting NPC patients.[59,60] A further study by Chen *et al.*[61] on 13 NPC patients in Taiwan with elevated antibody levels to EBV-specific DNase showed only low levels or virtual disappearance of antibodies to EBV-DNase when the patients were in remission. A mass survey including 3,368 males done by the same group using the anti-EBV-DNase assay gave promising results for the application of this assay to predict NPC in high risk populations.[62] Using this marker for field surveys for NPC in Taiwan,[63] 14 cases of NPC were detected among 1306 patients who were found to be anti-DNase positive. These results demonstrate that antibodies to the EBV-specific DNase can be used for the detection of NPC and to monitor the success of treatment.

Antibodies against EBV-specific DNA polymerase in NPC patients

In lymphoid cells latently infected with EBV, a salt-dependent, EBV-specific DNA polymerase can be detected after induction by TPA and n-butyrate.[43] IgG antibody against this enzyme was detected in 85% of NPC patients while only 3.8% normal individuals were positive.[43] Further study by Liu *et al.*[64] showed that anti-DNA polymerase antibody is highly specific for NPC patients. In addition, high antibody levels can be detected as early as stage 1 of the disease in NPC patients and the level of antibody increases with disease progression. Furthermore in serial samples obtained from 9 patients, anti-DNA polymerase levels decreased with treatment.

Antibodies against EBV-specific thymidine kinase in NPC patients

In addition to EBV specific DNA polymerase production in induced EBV-carrying lymphoid cells, an EBV-specific thymidine kinase (TK) is also expressed. An attempt has been made to study the antibody level to EBV-TK as a marker for the detection of NPC. In a preliminary study, Tureune-Tessier *et al.*[42] showed an enhanced antibody neutralization of EBV-TK activity in 59% of NPC patients while only 10% of normal individuals had antibodies against EBV-TK. In a further study by Littler *et al.*[65] using recombinant EBV-TK expressed in *Escherichia coli* as antigen, high levels of IgA anti-EBV-TK were demonstrated in 8/9 NPC patients while no antibody was detected in 26 patients with Burkitt's lymphoma, infectious mononucleosis or controls. A recent evaluation of the different EBV-associated antigens including the alkaline DNase, TK and membrane antigen produced in recombinant baculovirus or bovine papillomavirus systems showed that these diagnostic markers are useful for NPC detection. Antibody to the EBV-TK was found to be the most sensitive predictor of NPC.[66]

Antibodies against EBV-specific ribonucleotide reductase in NPC patients

Another EA component, the EBV-encoded ribonucleotide reductase (RR) has also been cloned, expressed and used to screen for antibodies in sera from patients with NPC, Burkitt's lymphoma and control subjects.[67] It was demonstrated that 20/33 NPC sera were positive for antibody against RR while all of the 15 BL sera and 10 controls were negative. In a more recent study,[68] 81% of NPC patients as compared to 1% of normal EBV serologically positive individuals had IgG antibodies against a short fragment of the carboxyl terminal of the RR.

Antibodies against EBV-specific ZEBRA protein in NPC patients

The BAMHI Z EBV replication activator (ZEBRA) protein is involved in the switch from latency to lytic cycle in EBV infected cells.[22] Using a recombinant ZEBRA protein in an enzyme immunoassay, Mathew *et al.*[69] demonstrated that in 100 NPC patients who were IgA anti-VCA and EA positive, 75% had IgG anti-ZEBRA activities while only 4% of patients with cancer other than NPC and 3.6% of control healthy persons were positive. In addition, 25% of IgA anti-VCA and EA-D negative NPC patients were also positive for IgG anti-ZEBRA. In another study, the prognostic role of anti-ZEBRA in NPC patients was evaluated.[70] Results showed that in addition to the elevated antibody level of IgG anti-ZEBRA in NPC patients as compared to controls, the actuarial survival of patients with high anti-ZEBRA IgG after radiotherapy was lower than those with low anti-ZEBRA. Thus the anti-ZEBRA serological marker can be used not only for NPC detection, but also for disease prognosis.

Antibodies against LMP2A/2B in NPC patients

LMP2A and LMP2B are expressed in many EBV latently infected cells (see above). In a study by Frech *et al.*,[71] recombinant latent infection terminal proteins (TP1 and TP2, i.e. LMP2A and LMP2B) were expressed and antibodies against these proteins were assayed in patients with or without NPC. Results showed that only NPC patients' sera had anti-TP proteins (32/83) and that the antibody level decreased during therapy. In a more recent study, antibodies against LPM2A/2B expressed in human keratinocytes were assayed in NPC patients using immunoblotting assays.[72] The study demonstrated that antibody against LMP2A/2B had high specificity towards patients with NPC.

Application of EBV Serological Markers in Predicting the Development of NPC in High Risk Groups and as a Prognostic Marker for Treatment

Using the IgA anti-VCA antibody as a marker, Zeng[2,73] initiated mass surveys in three different counties in southern China involving over 195,000 individuals aged 30 and over, including sub-groups of particular high risk such as chemical factory workers, boat people and ethnic minority groups of Molaos and Hans. The percentage of IgA-VCA positive individuals ranged from 0.6% to 10%. From these, 106 NPC cases were identified with a detection rate ranging from 1.5% to 13.6%. In addition, the majority (56% to 92%) of patients detected were in the early clinical stages of NPC. Subsequent follow-up studies on 3533 individuals with elevated IgA-VCA titre in the Zangwu County showed that 55 NPC cases were initially detected. After 1 to 3 years of follow-up, 32 additional NPC cases were diagnosed with an overall detection rate of 2462.5 per 100,000. These results established the value of IgA anti-VCA antibody screening in the early detection of NPC.

The level of anti-EBV antibody has also been shown to be related to the stage of NPC and the total tumour burden in the patient.[7,8] Subsequent studies on long-term follow-up of NPC patients after therapy showed that IgA-VCA antibody level decreases in groups of patients who are "cured", while high levels of IgA-VCA antibodies are maintained in patients with recurrence.[74,75]

As discussed above, another EBV related serological marker has been evaluated for the prognosis of EBV patients.[49] A low antibody level against MA in NPC patients as demonstrated by the ADCC assay can identify those in whom recurrent disease is likely to develop after conventional therapy.

Concluding Remarks

Serological investigation of NPC patients for EBV-associated antigenic markers in combination with clinical and histological examinations is valuable for the early detection of the disease. The discovery of new EBV-associated markers has further enhanced the specificity and sensitivity of serological detection of NPC. With the advent of newly developed, highly sensitive assays for antiviral antibodies together with the newly discovered virus-associated serological markers, we are approaching the ultimate goal of early detection, treatment and control of this disease.

References

1. Ho, J.H.C. 1972. Nasopharyngeal carcinoma (NPC). *Adv. Cancer Res.*; 15:57–92.
2. de Thé, G., Zeng, Y. 1986. Population screening for Epstein-Barr virus markers: towards improvement of nasopharyngeal carcinoma control. In: *The Epstein-Barr Virus: Recent Advances*, eds. Epstein, M.A. Achong, B.G. 237–249.
3. Lanier, A.P., Bornkamm, G.W., Henle, W., Henle, G., Bender, T.R., Talbot, M.L., Dohan, P.H. 1981. Association of Epstein-Barr virus with nasopharyngeal carcinoma in Alaskan native patients: serum antibodies and tissue EBNA and DNA. *Int. J. Cancer*; 28:301–305.
4. Old, L.J., Boyes, E.A., Oettgen, H.F., De Harven, E., Geering, G., Williamson, B., Clifford, P. 1966. Precipitating antibody in human serum to an antigen present in cultured Burkitt's lymphoma cells. *Proc. Natl. Acad. Sci. USA*; 56:1699–1704.
5. de Schryer, A., Friberg, S., Klein, G., Henle, G., Henle, W., de Thé, G., Clifford, P., Ho, H.C. 1969. Epstein-Barr virus-associated antibody positive in carcinoma of the post-nasal space. *Clin. Exp. Immunol.*; 5:443–459.
6. Henle, W., Henle, G., Ho, H.C., Burtin, P., Cachin, Y., Clifford, P., de Schryer, A., de Thé, G., Diehl, V., Klein, G. 1970. Antibodies to Epstein-Barr virus in nasopharyngeal carcinoma, the head and neck neoplasma and control groups. *J. Natl. Cancer Inst.*; 44:225–231.
7. Henle, W., Ho, J.H.C., Henle, G., Kwan, H.C. 1973. Antibodies to Epstein-Barr virus related antigens in nasopharyngeal carcinoma. Comparison of active cases and long-term survivors. *J. Natl. Cancer Inst.*; 51:361–369.

8. Henle, W., Ho, J.H.C., Henle, G., Chau, J.C.W., Kwan, H.C. 1977. Nasopharyngeal carcinoma: significance of changes in Epstein-Barr virus related antibody positives following therapy. *Int. J. Cancer*; 20:663–672.
9. Huang, D.P., Ho, J.H.C., Henle, W., Henle, G. 1974. Demonstration of Epstein-Barr virus-associated nuclear antigens in nasopharyngeal carcinoma cells from fresh biopsies. *J. Int. Cancer*; 14:580–588.
10. Klein, G., Giovanella, B.C., Lindhal, T., Fiakow, P.J., Singh, S., Stehlin, J.S. 1974. Direct evidence for the presence of Epstein-Barr virus DNA and nuclear antigen in malignant epithelial cell from patients with poorly differentiated carcinoma of the nasopharynx. *Proc. Natl. Acad. Sci. USA*; 71:4737–4741.
11. Henle, G., Henle, W. 1976. Epstein-Barr virus-specific IgA serum antibodies as an out-standing feature of nasopharyngeal carcinoma. *Int. J. Cancer*; 17:1–7.
12. Hader, T., Rahima, M., Kahan, E., *et al.* 1986. Significance of specific Epstein-Barr virus IgA and elevated IgG antibodies to viral capsid antigens in nasopharyngeal carcinoma patients. *J. Med. Virol.*; 20:329–339.
13. Epstein, M.A., Achong, B.G., Barr, Y.M. 1964. Virus particles in cultured lymphoblasts from Burkitt's lymphoma. *Lancet*; i:702–703.
14. Henle, G., Henle, W. 1970. Observations on childhood infections with the Epstein-Barr virus. *J. Infect. Dis.*; 121:303–310.
15. Henle, G., Henle, W., Diehl, V. 1968. Relation of Burkitt's tumor associated herpes-type virus to infectious mononucleosis. *Proc. Natl. Acad. Sci. USA*; 59:94–101.
16. Rickinson, A.B. 1994. EBV infection and EBV-associated tumours. *Symposium of the Society for General Microbiology*; 51:81–100.
17. Jondal, M., Klein, G. 1973. Surface markers on human B and T lymphocytes. II. Presence of Epstein-Barr virus receptors on B lymphocytes. *J. Exp. Med.*; 138:1365–1378.
18. Paganal, J.S., Lemon, S.M. 1981. The herpes viruses. In: *Medical Microbiology and Infectious Diseases*, eds. Bradue, A.I., Davis, C.E., Frierer, J. W.B. Philadelphia: Saunders, 545.
19. Matsuo, T., Heller, M., Petti, L., Oshiro, E., Kieff, E. 1989. Persistence of the entire Epstein-Barr virus genome integrated into human lymphocyte DNA. *Science*; 226:1322–1325.
20. Yates, J.L., Warren, N., Sngden, B. 1985. Stable replication of plasmid derived from Epstein-Barr virus in variou mammalian cells. *Nature*; 313:135–140.
21. Hudewentz, J., Bornkamm, G.W., zur Hausen, H. 1980. Effect of the diterpene ester TPA on Epstein-Barr virus antigen and DNA synthesis in producer and nonproducer cell lines. *Virology*; 100:175–178.
22. Miller, G., Tayler, N., Kolman, J., Baumann, R., Katz, D., Himmelfarb, H., Carrey, M., Ptashne, M. 1990. How ZEBRA, a weak transactivator, exerts strong biological effect. In: *Esptein-Barr Virus and Human Disease*. Llifton, New Jersey: Humana Press, 27.
23. Kieff, E. 1996. Epstein-Barr virus and its replication. In: *Fields Virology*, 3rd edn., eds. Fields, B.N., Knipe, D.M., Howley, P.M., *et al.* Philadelphia: Lippincott — Raven Publisher, 2343.
24. Huang, D.P., Lau, W.H., Lung, M., Saw, D., Liu, M. 1988. Establishment and characterization of undifferentiated nasopharyngeal carcinoma xenografts from southern Chinese. *J. Exp. Clin. Cancer Res.*; 7:48.
25. Niedobitek, G., Young, L.S., Lau, R., *et al.* 1991. Epstein-Barr virus infection in oral hairy leukoplakia: virus replication in the absence of a detectable latent phase. *J. Gen. Virol.*; 72:3035–3046.
26. Rowe, M., Rowe, D.T., Gregory, C.D., Young, L.S., Farrell, P.J., Rupani, H., Rickinson, A.B. 1987. Differences in B cell growth phenotype reflect novel patterns of Epstain-Barr virus latent gene expression in Burkitt's lymphoma cells. *EMBO J.*; 6:2743–2751.
27. Rowe, D.T., Heston, L., Metlay, J., Miller, G. 1985. Identification and expression of a nuclear antigen from the genomic region of the Jijoye strain of Epstein-Barr virus which is missing in its non-immortalizing deletion mutant P3HR-1. *Proc. Natl. Acad. Sci. USA*; 82:7429–7433.
28. Wang, F., Gregory, C.D., Rowe, M., Rickinson, A.B., Wang, D., Birkenbach, M., Klkutanl, H., Kishimoto, T., Kieff, E. 1987. Epstein-Barr virus nuclear antigen 2 specifically induces expression of the B-cell activation antigen CD23. *Proc. Natl. Acad. Sci. USA*; 83:3452–3457.

29. Fahraeus, R., Fu, H.L., Finke, J., Rowe, M., Klein, G., Falk, K., Nilsson, E., Yadav, M., Busson, P. 1988. Expression of Epstein-Barr virus-coded proteins in nasopharyngeal carcinoma. *Int. J. Cancer*; 42:329–338.
30. Murray, R.J., Wang, D., Young, L.S., Wang, F., Rowe, M., Keiff, E., Rickinson, A.B. 1988. Epstein-Barr virus-associated cytotoxic T-cell recognition of transfectants expressing the virus-coded latent membrane protein LMP. *J. Virol.*; 62:3747–3755.
31. Wang, D., Liebowitz, D., Kieff, E. 1988. The truncated form of the Epstein-Barr virus latent-infection membrane protein expressed in virus replication does not transform rodent fibroblasts. *J. Virol.*; 62:2337–2346.
32. Liebowitz, D., Kieff, E. 1989. The Epstein-Barr virus latent membrane protein (LMP) induction of B-cell activation antigens and membrane patch formation does not require vimentin. *J. Virol.*; 63:4051–4054.
33. Rowe, D.T., Hall, L., Joab, I., Laux, G. 1990. Identification of the Epstein-Barr virus terminal protein gene products in latently infected lymphocytes. *J. Virol.*; 64:2866–2875.
34. Miller, C.L., Lee, J.H., Kieff, E., Longnecker, R. 1994. An integral membrane protein (LMP2) blocks reactivation of Epstein-Barr virus from latency following surface immunoglobulin crosslinking. *Proc. Natl. Acad. Sci. USA*; 91:772–776.
35. Laux, G., Perricaudet, M., Farrell, P.J. 1988. A spliced Epstein-Barr virus gene expressed in latently transformed lymphocytes is created by circularisation of the linear genome. *EMBO J.*; 7:769–774.
36. Ernberg, I., Klein, G., Komilsby, F.M., Silvestre, D. 1974. Differentiation between early and late membrane antigen on human lymphoblastoid cell lines infected with Epstein-Barr virus. I Immunofluorescence. *J. Natl. Cancer Inst.*; 53:61–68.
37. Henle, G., Henle, W., Klein, G. 1971. Demonstration of two distinct components in the early antigen complex of Epstein-Barr virus-infected cells. *Int. J. Cancer*; 8:272–282.
38. Hummel, M., Keiff, E. 1982. Mapping of polypeptides encoded by the Epstein-Barr virus genome in productive infection. *Proc. Natl. Acad. Sci. USA*; 79:5698–5702.
39. Goldsmidts, W.L., Luka, J., Pearson, G.R. 1983. A restricted component of the Epstein-Barr virus early antigen complex is structurally related to ribonucleotide reductase. *Virology*; 157:220–226.
40. Pearson, G.R., Luka, J., Petti, L., Sample, J., Birkenbach, M., Braun, D., Kieff, E. 1987. Identification of an Epstein-Barr virus early gene encoding a second component of the restricted early antigen complex. *J. Virol.*; 160:151–161.
41. Cheng, Y.C., Chau, J.Y., Glaser, R., Henle, W. 1980. Frequency and levels of antibodies to Epstein-Barr virus specific DNase are elevated in patients with nasopharyngeal carcinoma. *Proc. Natl. Acad. Sci. USA*; 77:6162–6165.
42. de Turenne-Tessier, M., Ooka, T., Calender, A., de Thé, G., Daillie, J. 1989. Relationship between nasopharyngeal carcinoma and high antibody titre to Epstein-Barr virus-specific thymidine kinase. *Int. J. Cancer*; 43:45–48.
43. Tan, R.S., Li, J.S., Grill, S.P., Nutter, L.M., Cheng, Y.C. 1986. Demonstration of Epstein-Barr virus-specific DNA polymerase in chemically induced Raji cells and its antibody in serum from patients with nasopharyngeal carcinoma. *Cancer Res.*; 46:5124–5028.
44. Ho, J.H.C., Ng, M.H., Kwan, H.C., Chau, J.C.W. 1976. Epstein-Barr virus-specific IgA and IgG serum antibodies in nasopharyngeal carcinoma. *Brit. J. Cancer*; 34:655–659.
45. Ho, J.H.C., Lau, W.H., Kwan, H.C., Chan, C.L., Au, G.H.K., Saw, D. 1982. Immunology and diagnosis of nasopharyngeal carcinoma. In: *Herpesvirus: Clinical, Pharymacological and Basic Aspects*, eds. Shioter, H., Cheung, Y.C., Prusoff, W.H. Exerpta Medica International Congress Series No. 571. Amsterdam-Oxford-Princeton: Excerpta Medica, 389–397.
46. Zhu, X.X., Zeng, Y., Wolt, H. 1986. Detection of IgG and IgA antibodies to Epstein-Barr virus membrane antigen in sera from patients with nasopharyngeal carcinoma and from normal individuals. *Int. J. Cancer*; 37:689–691.
47. Lynn, F.C., Hsich, R.P., Chuang, C.Y., Huang, S.C., Hsieh, T. 1984. Epstein-Barr virus-associated antibodies and serum biochemistry in nasopharyngeal carcinoma. *Laryngoscope*; 94:1485–1488.

48. Saemundsen, A.K., Albeck, H., Hansen, J.P.H., Nielson, N.H., Anvset, M., Henle, W., Henle, G., Thomsen, K.A., Kristensen, H.K., Klein, G. 1982. Epstein-Barr virus in nasopharyngeal carcinoma and salivary gland carcinomas in Greenland Eskimos. *Brit. J. Cancer*; 46:721–728.
49. Neel, H.B., Pearson, G.R., Taylor, W.F. 1984. Antibody-dependent cellular cytotoxicity: relation to stage and disease course in North American patients with nasopharyngeal carcinoma. *Arch. Otolaryngol.*; 110:742–747.
50. Gurtsevitch, V., Ruiz, R., Stepina, V., Blachov, I., Le Riverend, E., Glazkova, T., Lavoue, M.F., Paches, A., Aliev, B., Mazurenko, N. 1986. Epstein-Barr viral serology in nasopharyngeal carcinoma patients in the USSR and Cuba, and its value for differential diagnosis of the disease. *Int. J. Cancer*; 37:375–381.
51. Neel, H.B., Pearson, G.R., Taylor, W.F. 1984. Antibodies to Epstein-Barr virus in patients with nasopharyngeal carcinoma and in comparison groups. *Am. J. Otolaryngol.*; 93:477–482.
52. Hader, T., Rahima, M., Kahan, E., Sidi, J., Rakowsky, E., Sarov, B., Sarov, I. 1986. Significance of specific Epstein-Barr virus IgA and elevated IgG antibodies to oral capsid antigens in nasopharyngeal carcinoma patients. *J. Med. Virol.*; 20:329–339.
53. Pearson, G.R., Johansson, B., Klein, G. 1978. Antibody-dependent cellular cytotoxicity against Epstein-Barr virus-associated antigens in African patients with nasopharyngeal carcinoma. *Int. J. Cancer*; 22:120–125.
54. Rowe, M., Finke, J., Szigeti, R., Klein, G. 1988. Characterization of the serological response in man to the latent membrane protein and the six nuclear antigens encoded by Epstein-Barr virus. *J. Gen. Virol.*; 69:1217–1228.
55. Neel, H.B. 1985. Nasopharyngeal carcinoma: clinical presentation, diagnosis, treatment and prognosis. *Otolaryngol. Clin. North Am.*; 28:479–90.
56. Miller, G., Grogan, E., Fisher, D.K., *et al.* 1985. Antibody responses to two Epstein-Barr virus nuclear antigens defined by gene transfer. *N. Engl. J. Med.*; 312:750–755.
57. Foong, Y.T., Cheng, H.M., Sam, C.K., Dillner, J., Hinderer, W., Prasad, U. 1990. Serum and salivary IgA antibodies against a defined epitope of the Epstein-Barr virus nuclear antigen (EBNA) are elevated in nasopharyngeal carcinoma. *Int. J. Cancer*; 45:1061–1064.
58. Cheng, H.M., Foong, Y.T., Sam, C.K., Prasad, U., Dillner, J. 1991. Epstein-Barr virus nuclear antigen 1 linear epitopes that are reactive with immunoglobulin A (IgA) or IgG in sera from nasopharyngeal carcinoma patients or from healthy donors. *J. Clin. Microbiol.*; 29:2180–2186.
59. Hsu, M.M., Chen, J.Y., Liu, M.Y., Lynn, T.C., Tu, S.M., Yang, C.S. 1974. Antibody to Epstein-Barr virus specific DNase in sera of nasopharyngeal carcinoma and other nine most common cancer patients in Taiwan. *Clin. J. Microbiol. Immunol.*; 17:131–137.
60. Chen, J.Y., Chen, C.J., Liu, M.Y., Cho, S.M., Hsu, M.M., Lynn, T.C., Shieh, T., Tu, S.M., Lee, H.H., Kuo, S.L., Lai, M.Y., Hsieh, C.Y., Hu, C.P., Yang, C.S. 1987. Antibodies to Epstein-Barr virus-specific DNase in patients with nasopharyngeal carcinoma and control groups. *J. Med. Virol.*; 23:11–21.
61. Chen, J.Y., Hwang, L.Y., Beasley, R.P., Chien, C.S., Yang, C.S. 1985. Antibody response to Epstein-Barr virus-specific DNase in 13 patients with nasopharyngeal carcinoma in Taiwan: a retrospective study. *J. Med. Virol.*; 16:99–105.
62. Chen, J.Y., Liu, M.Y., Chen, C.J., Hsu, M.M., Tu, S.M., Lee, H.H., Kuo, S.L., Yang, C.S. 1985. Antibody to Epstein-Barr virus-specific DNase as a marker for the early detection of nasopharyngeal carcinoma. *J. Med. Virol.*; 17:47–49.
63. Chen, J.Y., Chen, C.J., Liu, M.Y., Cho, S.M., Hsu, M.M., Lynn, T.C., Shieh, T., Tu, S.M., Beasley, R.P., Hwang, L.Y. 1989. Antibody to Epstein-Barr virus-specific DNase as a marker for field survey of patients with nasopharyngeal carcinoma in Taiwan. *J. Med. Virol.*; 27:269–273.
64. Liu, M.Y., Chou, W.H., Nutter, L., Hsu, M.M., Chen, J.Y., Hsu, M.M., Chen, J.Y., Yang, C.S. 1989. Antibody against Epstein-Barr virus DNA polymerase activity in sera of patients with nasopharyngeal carcinoma. *J. Med. Virol.*; 28:101–105.

65. Littler, E., Newman, W., Arrand, J.R. 1990. Immunological response of nasopharyngeal carcinoma patients to the Epstein-Barr virus-coded thymidine kinase expressed in Escherichia coli. *Int. J. Cancer*; 45:1028–1032.
66. Littler, E., Baylis, S.A., Yi, Z., Conway, M.J., Mackett, M., Arrand, J. 1991. Diagnosis of nasopharyngeal carcinoma by means of recombinant Epstein-Barr virus proteins. *Lancet*; 337:685–689.
67. Ginsburg, M. 1990. Antibodies against the large subunit of the Epstein-Barr virus encoded ribonucleotide reductase in patients with nasopharyngeal carcinoma. *Int. J. Cancer*; 45:1048–1053.
68. Fones-Tan, A., Chan, S.H., Tsao, S.Y., Li, B., Gan, Y,Y. 1994. Enzyme-linked immunosorbent assay (ELISA) and IgG antibodies to Epstein-Barr virus ribonucleotide reductase in patients with nasopharyngeal carcinoma. *Int. J. Cancer*; 23:542–546.
69. Mathew, A., Cheng, H.M., Sam, C.K., Joab, I., Prasad, U., Cochet, C. 1994. A high incidence of serum IgG antibodies to the Epstein-Barr virus replication activator protein in nasopharyngeal carcinoma. *Cancer Immunol. Immunother.*; 38:68 – 70.
70. Yip, T.T.C., Ngan, R.K.C., Lau, W.H., Poon, Y.F., Joab, I., Cochet, C., Cheng, A.K. 1994. A possible prognostic role of immunoglobulin-G antibody against recombinant Epstein-Barr virua BZLF1 transactivator protein ZEBRA in patients with nasopharyngeal carcinoma. *Cancer*; 74:2414–2423.
71. Frech, B., Zimber-Strobl, U., Yip, T.T.C., Lau, W.H., Mueller-Lantzsch, N. 1993. Characterization of the antibody response to the latent infection terminal peoteins of Epstein-Barr virus in patients with nasopharyngeal carcinoma. *J. Gen. Virol.*; 74:811–818.
72. Lennette, E.T., Winberg, G., Yadav, M., Enblad, G., Klein, G. 1995. Antibodies to LMP2A/2B in EBV-carrying malignancies. *Eur. J. Cancer*; 31A:1875–1878.
73. Zeng, Y. 1985. Seroepidemiological studies on nasopharyngeal carcinoma in China. *Adv. Cancer Res.*; 14:121–138.
74. Lynn, T.C., Tu, S.M., Kawamma, A. 1985. Long-term follow-up of IgG and IgA antibodies against viral capsid antigens of Epstein-Barr virus in nasopharyngeal carcinoma. *J. Laryngol. Otol.*; 99:567–572.
75. de-Vathaire, F., Sancho-Grarnier, H., de Thé, G., Pieddeloup, C., Schwaab, G., Ho, J.H.C., Ellouz, R., Micheau, C., Cammoun, M., Cachui, Y., de Thé, G. 1988. Prognostic value of Epstein-Barr virus markers in the clinical management of nasopharyngeal carcinoma (NPC): a multi center follow-up study. *Int. J. Cancer*; 42:176–181.

CHAPTER 10

Cytological Diagnosis

Alexander R. Chang and *May K.M. Chan*

Introduction

A conclusive diagnosis of nasopharyngeal carcinoma (NPC) requires the examination of tissue or cells from either the primary lesion or a metastatic focus. Usually, this implies a histological diagnosis on biopsy material but in the past two decades there has been greater use of cytology in head and neck tumours, including NPC.[1,2] The use of cytology for the diagnosis of NPC is not new. The first paper was published in 1949 when the authors reported the successful cytodiagnosis in seven out of eight cases of NPC.[3] In 1983, a group of Chinese workers reported on the cytology of more than 1,000 cases of NPC and the detection rate was 89%.[4]

There are two ways in which cytology can be used, exfoliative cytology and fine needle aspiration (FNA) cytology. In exfoliative cytology, cells are scraped from the nasopharyngeal mucosa with a sampling device. Generally this method is atraumatic, quick and cheap. This method is suitable for the diagnosis of primary NPC, as well as recurrent or residual tumour. FNA cytology is invaluable in the diagnosis of metastatic NPC, such as when cervical lymph nodes are involved. FNA can also be employed for evaluating a primary tumour. The needles used for FNA are of small calibre (22–25 gauge) and consequently, discomfort and complications are minimal when compared with a surgical biopsy or excision of a lymph node. When FNA is used it can be performed with or without suction. When the latter technique is employed, the needle is moved to and fro in a similar fashion to acupuncture. The cutting action of the needle, combined with capillary pressure, are sufficient to obtain cells from a lesion. Further benefits with this method are less bleeding and as the operator has greater finger-tip sensitivity, it is possible to palpate the various tissue planes with the needle and accurately guide it into the lesion.

Another potential use for cytology is the screening for NPC in high risk communities, in a similar manner to the widely used cervical smear test, which has been successfully employed for cervical cancer detection and prevention. However, if cytology were to be employed to screen for NPC, it would need to be simple, reliable and of proven benefit to the screened population.

The principle of exfoliative cytology applied to the nasopharynx is similar to cervical smear and respiratory tract cytology. The aim is to collect cells, which have been shed into the nasopharyngeal cavity as well as abrading cells from the surface of the nasopharynx. There are a few studies in the literature which report on this subject and the results have been variable[2–10] (*Table 1*). In most of the studies the number of cases were small, except in the report by Dong *et al.*[4] in China, in which over 1,000 cases of NPC were examined by cytology.

Collection of the Specimen

Various devices have been used for collecting cells from the nasopharynx. The simplest and cheapest is the widely available cotton wool swab, which is easy to use even for non-specialists. However, there are some major disadvantages and these are the rigidity of the swab which makes precise placement difficult, and the low cell yield. The paucity of cells is due firstly to cells being trapped by the cotton wool fibres. Secondly, the soft and smooth surface of the swab results in few cells being scraped from the mucosal surface.[10] Several more sophisticated devices have been designed in China to overcome the problem of low cell yield (*Table 2*). The Chinese researchers reported good results with these instruments.[2,4,11]

Table 1. Review of literature on cytodiagnosis of nasophayngeal carcinoma.

Author	Year	No. of Cases	Positive cytology	Diagnostic rate (%)
Morrison *et al.*[3]	1949	8	7	—
Hopp[5]	1958	12	11	—
Ma & Chen[6]	1958	63	24	38
Djojopranoto[7]	1960	23	6	26
Liang[8]	1964	77	40	52
Ali & Shanmugaratnam[9]	1964	79	35	44
Dong *et al.*[4]	1983	1,138	1,016	89
Chan & Huang[10]	1990	42	32	76
Chang, Chan, Liang[2]	1996	76	53	70

Table 2. Instruments used for collection of cells for cytological examination in China and Hong Kong.[2,10–12]

1. Hollow rubber ball with uneven surface (Zhongshan Medical College),
2. Silk cloth within porous steel ball connected to suction pump (Zhanjiang Medical College),
3. Nylon brush (Sichuan Medical College),
4. Copper scraper (Fujian Medical College),
5. Sponge-ball headed instrument (Hunan Medical College).
6. Flexible nylon brush, Uterobrush (Chinese University of Hong Kong)

In the period 1995–1996, to further investigate the use of cytology for the detection of NPC and precursor lesions, the Uterobrush, a brush sampler, was tested.[2] The Uterobrush was designed principally to obtain endometrial cells for the cytological diagnosis of menstrual abnormalities. The instrument (*Figure 1*) measures 24 centimetres long and has a flexible wire shaft with a fine nylon brush attached at one end. To prevent cell loss and contamination, a sliding guard is slid over the brush before and after sampling. A small plastic knob at the tip prevents trauma and the instrument is supplied sterile and is for single use. Specimens were obtained from new and follow-up patients attending a NPC clinic for nasopharyngoscopy. Brush samples were obtained prior to biopsy. After a topical anaesthetic had been applied, the brush was introduced via the nostril under direct visualization with a nasopharyngoscope. The instrument was well tolerated by patients and was easy to use. Direct smears were made from each sample. To ensure optimal cell preservation, each smear was rapidly fixed in 95% alcohol and later stained with the Papanicolaou stain. In addition, each brush was rinsed in a 25% saline alcohol solution and cell blocks or Millipore filter preparations were made from the material collected.

Table 3 details the results obtained with the Uterobrush when 250 patients were evaluated. Cell trapping by the hairs of the instrument was judged by assessing the

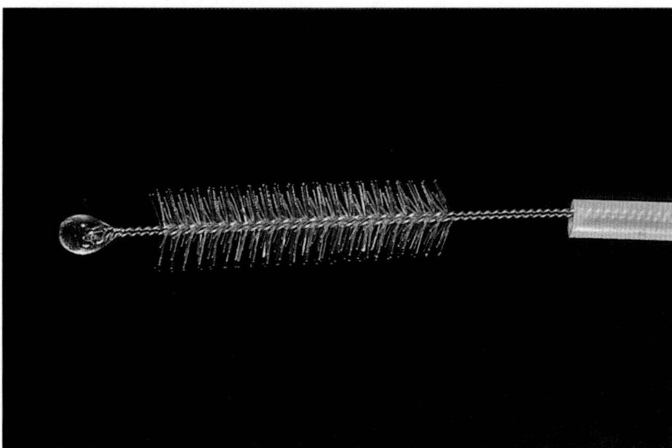

Figure 1. A Uterobrush with soft nylon bristles, plastic knob and retracted protective guard.

Table 3. The cytology result of the clinically positive NPC cases.

Result	Positive	Negative
New cases	47	20
Residual recurrence	6	3
TOTALS	53	23

Diagnostic rate = 69.7%

cellularity of the cell block sections or filter specimens. The results indicated cell trapping was low. However, the detection rate of 69.7% was disappointing and this was due mainly to the shape of the Uterobrush. Whereas in the uterine cervix the cavity is collapsed and the hairs of the Uterobrush are in direct contact with the endometrial surface thus allowing a good sample to be collected, in the more capacious nasopharynx, there is a tendency for the brush to flop around and the smooth plastic tipped knob picks up few cells when it comes into contact with a tumour. This is one explanation why despite an obvious tumour, the smears are negative. If the Uterobrush were modified, the detection rate might be substantially improved. Two changes which might enhance detection would be to replace the plastic tip with hairs, and to have a more ovoid shaped brush. A more radical design would be a brush that is totally round, but small enough to be manoeuvred via the nostril into the nasopharyngeal space. Such modified instruments might improve cell collection and are worthy of further investigation.

All the sampling instruments described can be introduced via the nose or mouth to obtain cells from the nasopharynx. The main disadvantage of the devices used by the Chinese researchers was they were not disposable and had to be carefully cleaned and sterilised before they could be reused. This was a time consuming task.

Irrespective of what device is used for specimen collection, the cells collected are evenly spread onto a clean glass slide. The slide is then either immediately wet-fixed by using a spray fixative or immersed in 95% alcohol. Some pathologists prefer examining air dried smears. Wet-fixed smears are stained with Haematoxylin and Eosin or the Papanicolaou stain. The air dried smears are best stained with Giemsa stain. If extra smears are available, they can be used for additional tests which may substantially enhance diagnostic accuracy. Two useful tests used are for the detection of Epstein-Barr virus (EBV) in NPC cells. One test identifies the EBV associated nuclear antigen (EBNA), and the other detects the EBV-encoded RNAs, known as the EBERs.

Normal Cytology and Non-neoplastic Lesions

Specimens obtained from the normal nasopharyngeal mucosa consist of columnar cells (ciliated or non-ciliated), goblet cells, squamous cells, reserve cells and lymphoid cells (*Figure* 2).

In non-specific infections there is columnar cell hyperplasia along with an increase in goblet cells and reserve cells. The hyperplastic epithelial cells have larger nuclei, coarse chromatin and sometimes perinuclear clearing. There may be an increase in squamous metaplastic cells which may show mild nuclear atypia. Reactive metaplastic squamous cells are also found following radiotherapy treatment (*Figure* 3). Lymphocytes, polymorphonuclear leukocytes, eosinophils, macrophages and plasma cells may also be encountered.

In tuberculosis, which is still prevalent in Asia and may involve the nasopharynx, typical smears show necrosis, Langhan's giant cells and epithelioid cells. However,

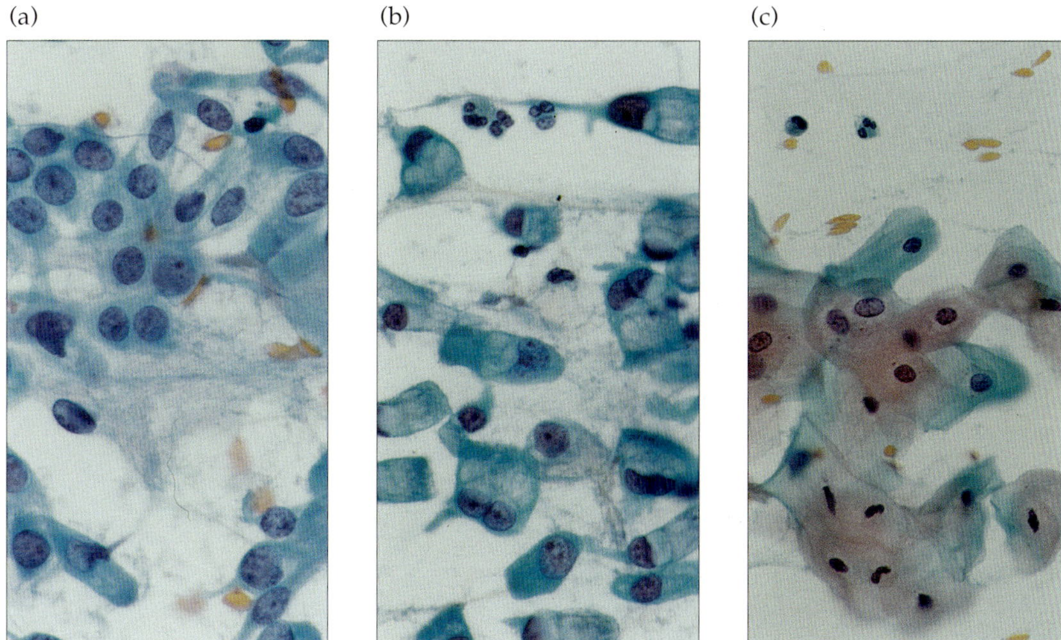

Figure 2. (a) Normal columnar ciliated nasopharyngeal cells with minimal variation in nuclear size. (b) A group of goblet cells with their apical cytoplasm distended with mucus. (c) Normal squamous cells. (All Papanicolaou stain ×600)

specimens consisting of only necrotic material should alert the prudent observer to the possibility of tuberculosis, otherwise a lesion may be overlooked. Staining for acid fast bacilli may provide additional confirmatory evidence and help reach a correct diagnosis.

Neoplastic Lesions

Cytodiagnosis has been applied to various neoplastic lesions including those in the nasopharynx. In the nasopharynx the most commonly encountered neoplasm is the undifferentiated NPC.[13] Well differentiated squamous cell carcinoma, adenocarcinoma, malignant lymphoma and metastatic lesions are uncommon and consequently, experience with the cytological diagnosis of these lesions is limited. In well differentiated squamous cell carcinoma the tumour cells usually have more abundant and dense cytoplasm and intercellular bridges may be seen in cohesive cell clusters. If the tumour is very well differentiated there is evidence of keratinization. In adenocarcinoma, the tumour cells form tight round clusters resembling gland acini and the cytoplasm has secretory vacuoles. An additional diagnostic feature is the presence of eccentrically placed nuclei which may have conspicuous nucleoli (*Figure 4*).

The typical cytological features of undifferentiated NPC are relatively cohesive clumps of large tumour cells with oval to round vesicular nuclei, a high nuclear/

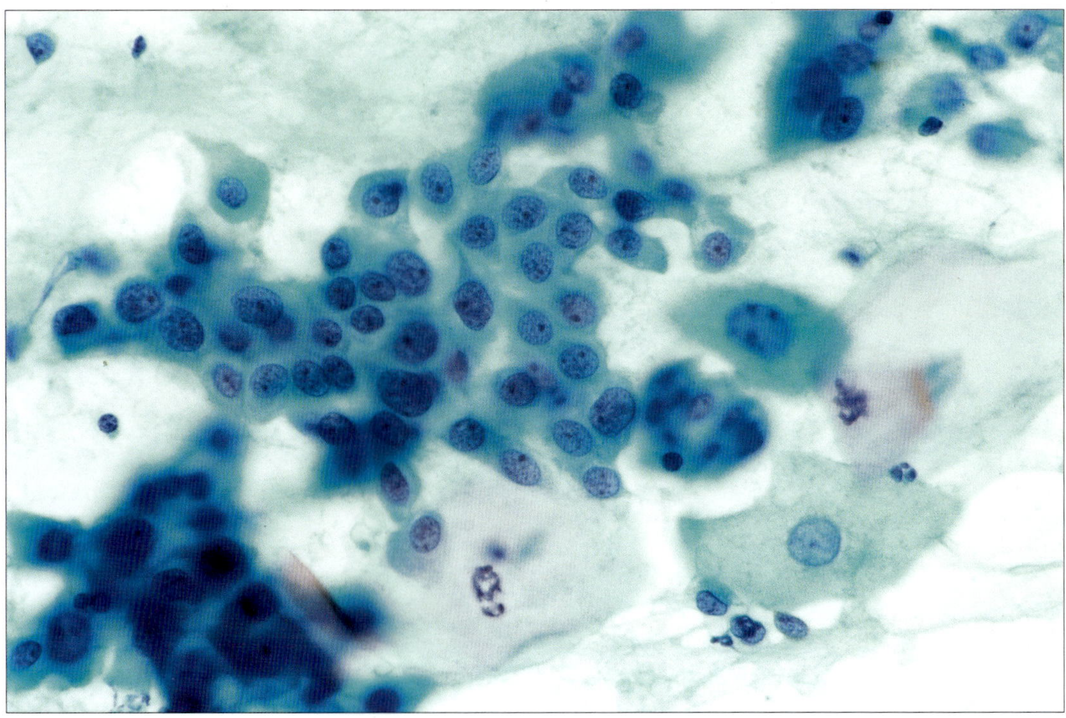

Figure 3. Reactive metaplastic squamous cells with minimally enlarged nuclei. The patient had radiation treatment 12 months previously. Papanicolaou stain ×500.

cytoplasmic ratio and one to two prominent nucleoli.[4,10,14] In some of the specimens collected with the Uterobrush the tumour cells showed more pleomorphism, including nuclei showing notches, indentation, reniform shape and greater variation in size (*Figure* 5). Cytoplasm is usually scanty or poorly preserved. Lymphocytes are usually seen intermingled amongst the tumour cells. Dispersed naked tumour nuclei are also commonly encountered.

Detection of tumour recurrence in post-irradiated cases may be difficult (*Figures 6 and 7*). Care must be taken not to interpret radiation change in benign cells as malignancy. Radiation changes include enlargement of cells, large nuclei with coarse chromatin, multinucleation, prominent nucleoli and cytoplasmic vacuolation (*Figure 8*). Nuclear vacuolation is also seen. An important diagnostic feature is that the nuclear/cytoplasmic ratio is not greatly increased after radiation when compared to cancer cells. In radiation induced cytomegaly, the nuclear membrane remains smooth, without spikes and notches. In some cases obtained with the Uterobrush, squamous metaplasia and increased numbers of goblet cells were seen. These were attributed to the radiation. An additional finding with some Uterobrush cases were elongated columnar ciliated cells. The presence of inflammation and necrosis create further difficulties for the cytopathologist. In general, radiation changes subside after twelve months and by two years there is little residual evidence of the treatment.

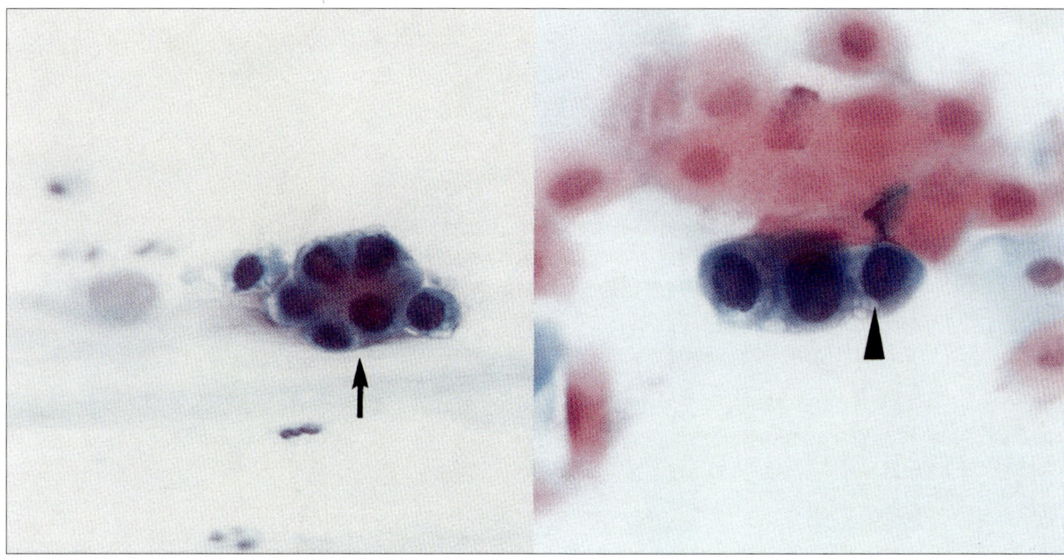

Figure 4. Adenocarcinoma of nasopharynx showing a tight cluster of tumour cells forming acini (arrow), ×440 (original magnification) and vacuolated cytoplasm (arrow head) ×1100 (original magnification): Papanicolaou stain.

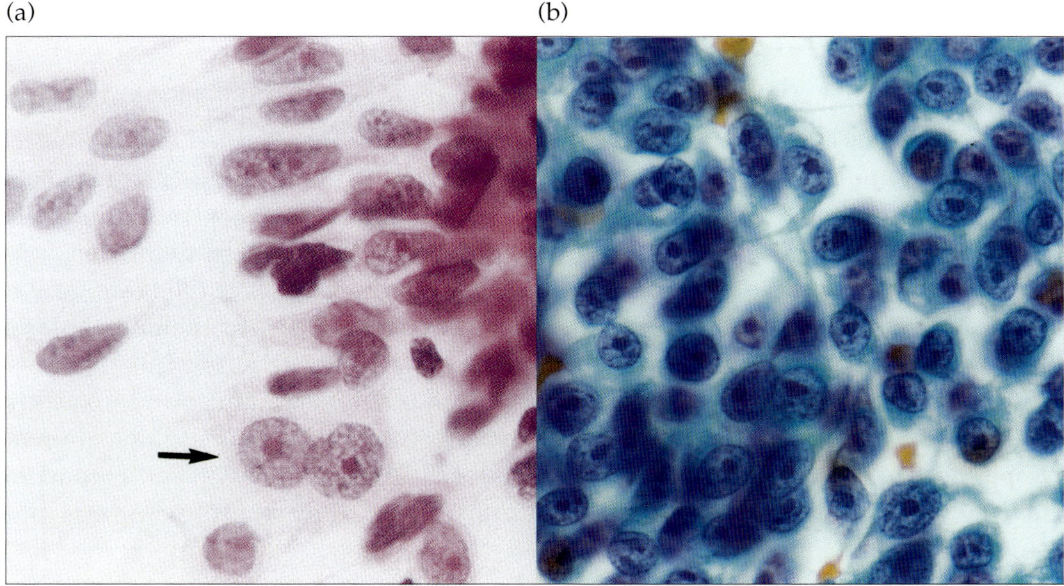

Figure 5. (a) Primary undifferentiated NPC cells (arrow) with vesicular nuclei, prominent nucleoli and mixed with lymphocytes. Papanicolaou stain ×440 (original magnification). (b) A group of well preserved NPC cells obtained with the Uterobrush. The cells exhibit variation in nuclear size and they have distinctive nucleoli. Papanicolaou stain ×800 (original magnification).

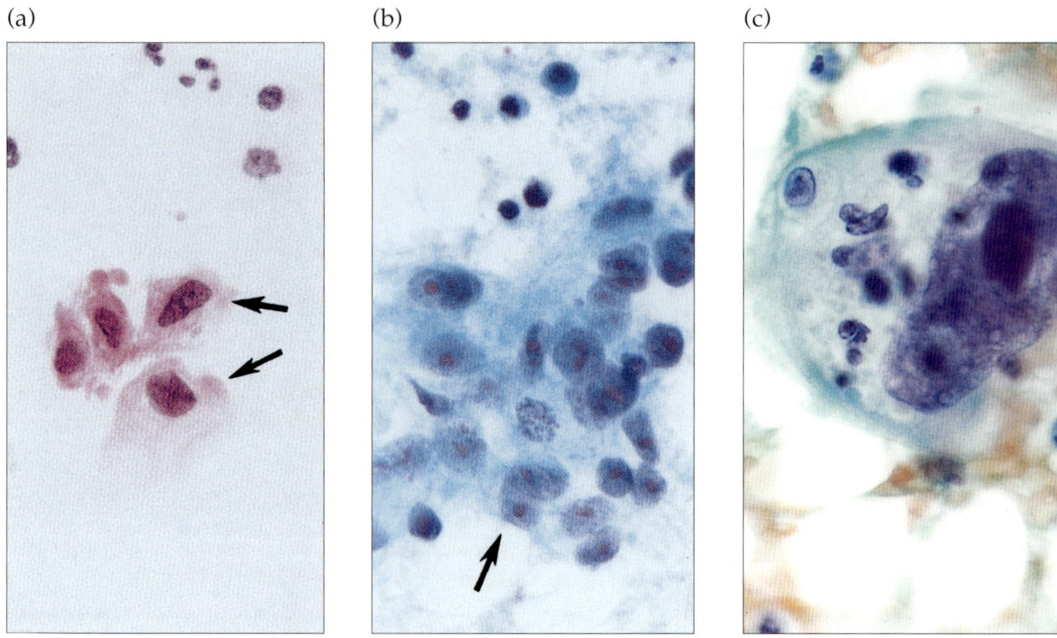

Figure 6. (a and b) Post-irradiated NPC cells (arrows) showing coarse nuclear chromatin, multinucleation and prominent nucleoli. Papanicolaou stain ×440 (c) A bizarre tumour cell showing post-radiation effect. Ingested neutrophils are present. Papanicolaou stain ×500.

Nasopharyngeal Intraepithelial Neoplasia

Preinvasive lesions, termed "nasopharyngeal intraepithelial neoplasia" (NPIN), have been described by authors in China[15] and Hong Kong.[16] NPIN is graded into NPIN I, II and III. These epithelial changes probably precede NPC.[13] A NPIN I lesion corresponds to dysplastic changes confined to the basal part of the epithelium. In NPIN II the abnormal cells occupy the lower 2/3rd of the epithelium. NPIN III denotes full thickness change but there is no evidence of invasion. The abnormal dysplastic cells[17] are similar to those seen in smears of the cervix, when there is cervical intraepithelial neoplasia (CIN). The most important feature that distinguishes dysplastic cells from inflammatory atypia is the chromatin pattern. In dysplasia the chromatin is granular and unevenly distributed whereas in inflammatory conditions it is fine and evenly distributed. Dysplastic cells differ from NPC cells, which have coarse chromatin with peri-chromatin clearing and prominent nucleoli. The literature pertaining to the concept and cytodiagnosis of NPIN is meagre. Nevertheless, the analogy of NPIN preceding NPC and CIN being a precursor of carcinoma of the cervix seems reasonable. At both sites this terminology suggests a disease continuum. Thus, the detection of NPIN in nasopharyngeal smears may aid in the diagnosis of early pre-invasive lesions which precede NPC. If treatment of these early lesions is undertaken, it may prevent the development of future NPC. In theory this should lead to a decrease in the incidence of

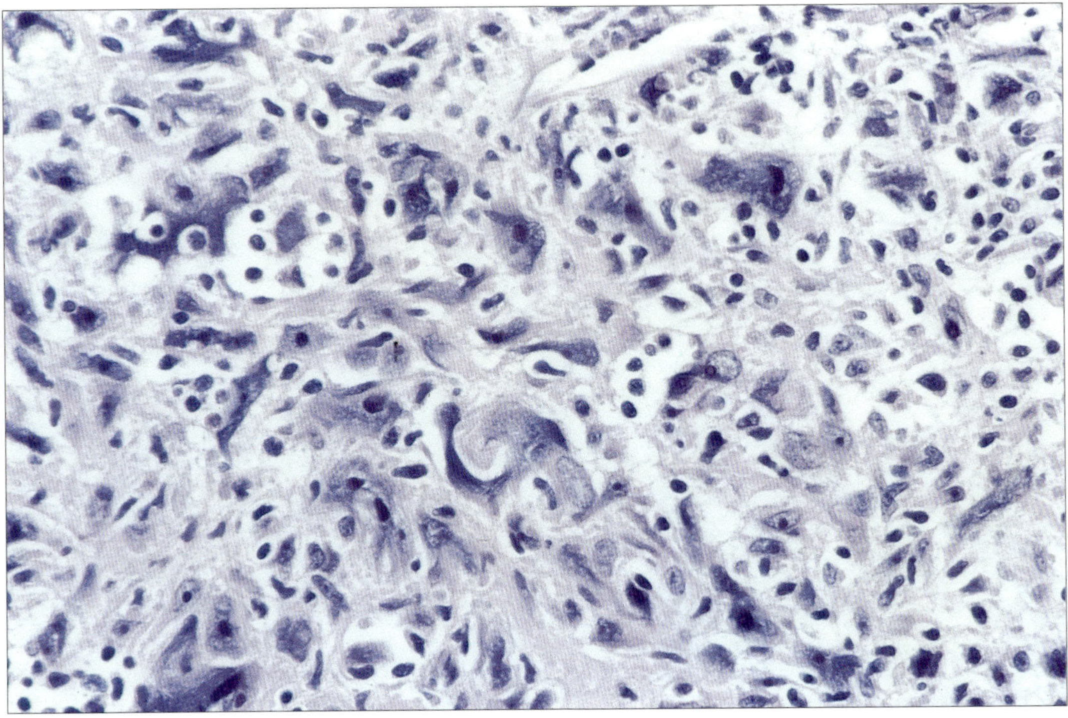

Figure 7. Cell block section of NPC cells retrieved by rinsing the Uterobrush in saline-alcohol after smears had been made. Bizarre tumour cells with radiation induced changes are seen. H&E ×400.

invasive NPC, or improve the prognosis for NPC. In the cervix not all cases of CIN progress to invasive carcinoma and this situation may also be true for NPIN. In the samples collected with the Uterobrush, incontestable cases of NPIN have not been identified. However, more extensive prospective studies are necessary before dogmatic conclusions can be reached.

Fine Needle Aspiration (FNA)

FNA has been proven to be useful in the diagnosis of head and neck tumours. This technique is popular both in Europe and the United States of America. FNA diagnosis of NPC has been carried out in areas where NPC is prevalent.[18] The most common site for FNA diagnosis of metastatic NPC is the cervical lymph node, characterised by painless enlargement of posterior triangle or upper jugulodigastric lymph nodes. Cytodiagnosis of residual or recurrent NPC in metastatic foci is particularly important, as this will spare lymph node excision, which in some cases may affect the long term prognosis.[19] Metastatic NPC has also been diagnosed in bone marrow and lung by using FNA.

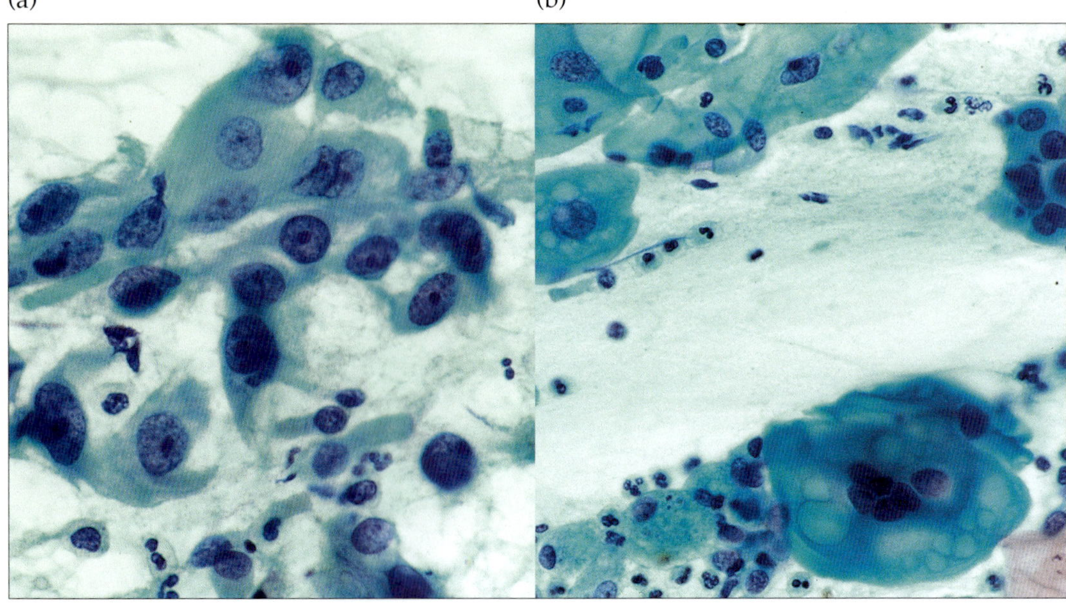

Figure 8. (a) Normal epithelial cells with radiation induced cytomegaly. The nuclear/cytoplasmic ratio is slightly increased and the nucleoli, although prominent, are not as large as those found in NPC cells. Papanicolaou stain ×600. (b) Squamous cells with striking post radiation cytoplasmic vacuolation. In the background are many neutrophils and macrophages with ingested cellular debris. Papanicolaou stain ×400.

Cytological features typical of metastatic undifferentiated NPC include cohesive clumps of large tumour cells with vesicular nuclei, one or two prominent nucleoli and a moderate amount of cytoplasm (*Figure 9*).[18] Among Chinese, most NPCs are the undifferentiated form and a characteristic finding is that the malignant cells are intermingled with lymphocytes. Other carcinomas include well differentiated squamous cell carcinoma, adenocarcinoma, small cell carcinoma and the rare undifferentiated sinonasal carcinoma. In these cancers, the cytological features are less specific and can mimic those of other head and neck tumours.

Granulomatous lesions, especially tuberculosis, are an important consideration in the differential diagnosis of NPC. The epithelioid cells have a low nuclear/cytoplasmic ratio, very fine nuclear chromatin and inconspicuous or small nucleoli (*Figure 10*). Other differential diagnoses include high grade malignant lymphoma, melanoma, and other head and neck carcinoma. High grade malignant lymphoma usually yields loosely scattered tumour cells with prominent nucleoli and scanty cytoplasm (*Figure 11*). In contrast, NPC yields cohesive clumps of tumour cells. However, in some NPCs the tumour cells may be more dispersed, while in some lymphomas cells may be more cohesive. In these instances, immunohistochemical staining for cytokeratin is most useful, as NPC cells are positive and lymphoma cells negative. Metastatic melanoma may also have similar cytological features to NPC. However, other features typical of

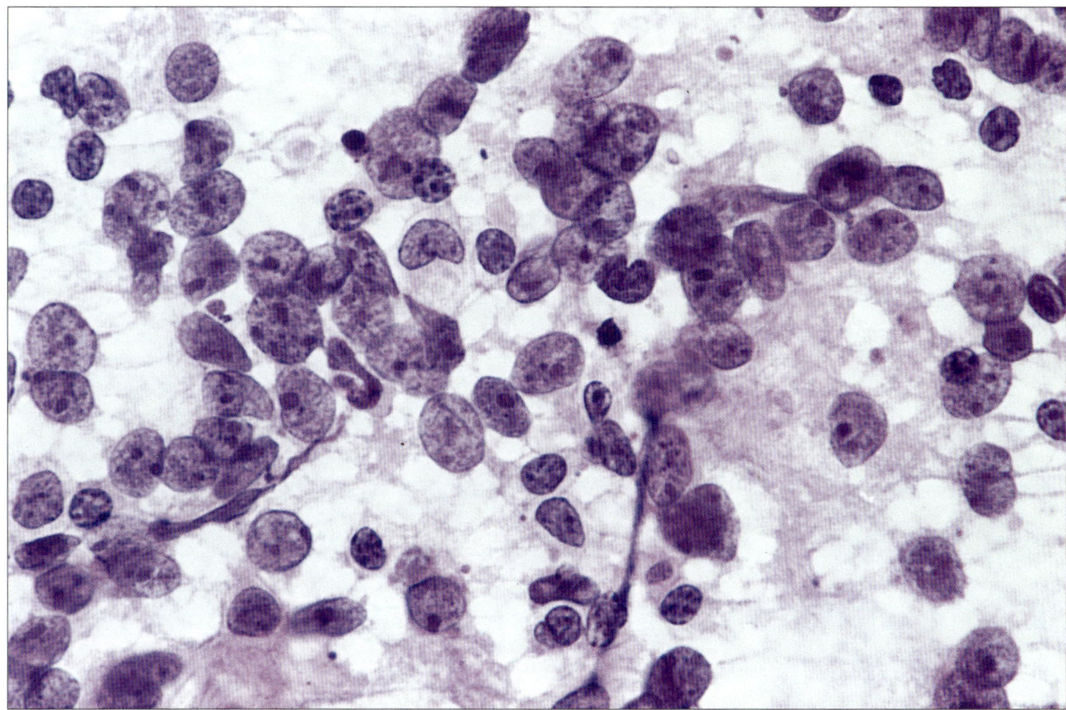

Figure 9. FNA of a cervical lymph node with metastatic NPC. The cancer cells have vesicular nuclei, prominent nucleoli and a few lymphocytes are present. H&E stain ×600.

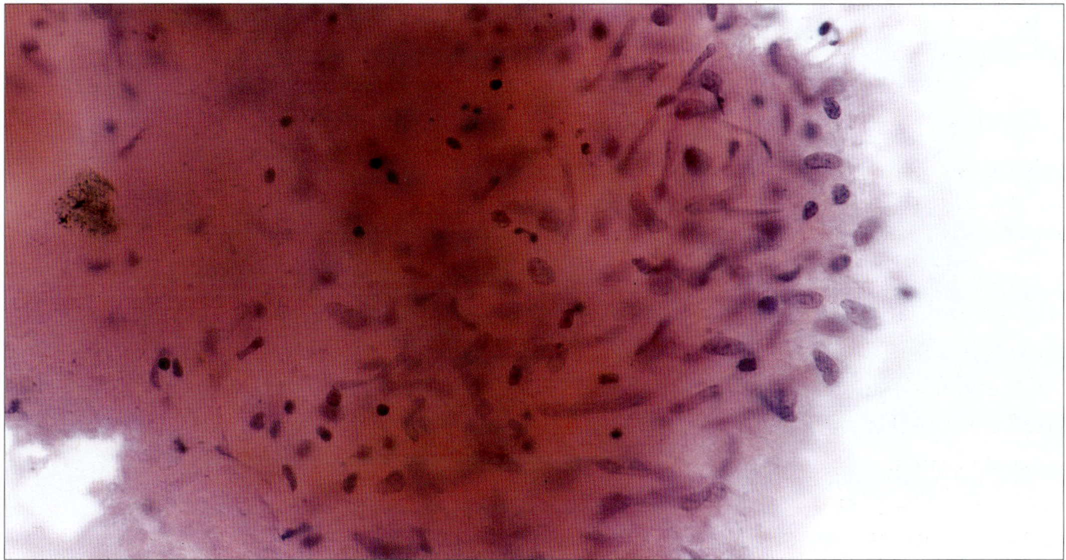

Figure 10. Tuberculous lymphadenitis sampled by FNA. A necrotic focus with epithelioid cells which have low nuclear/cytoplasmic ratio and fine chromatin. H&E ×300.

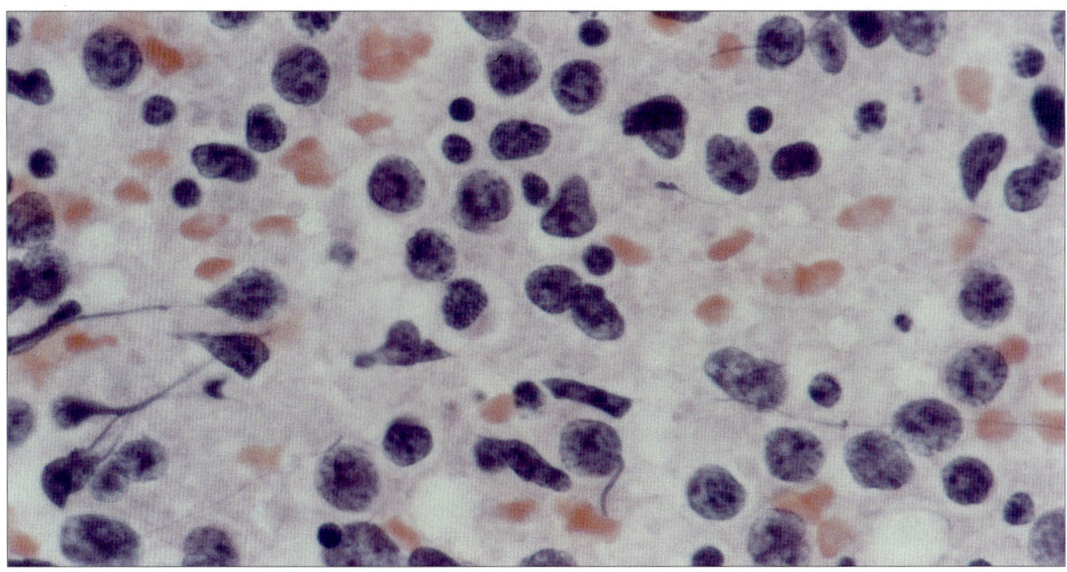

Figure 11. Malignant lymphoma showing pleomorphic tumour cells with prominent nucleoli and scanty cytoplasm. H&E stain ×800.

melanoma, but absent in NPC, should be identified. These include intranuclear cytoplasmic inclusions and intracytoplasmic melanin pigment (*Figure 12*). In difficult cases, immunohistochemical staining for S100 protein is helpful. In melanoma the cells are positive while in NPC the cells are negative.

(a) (b)

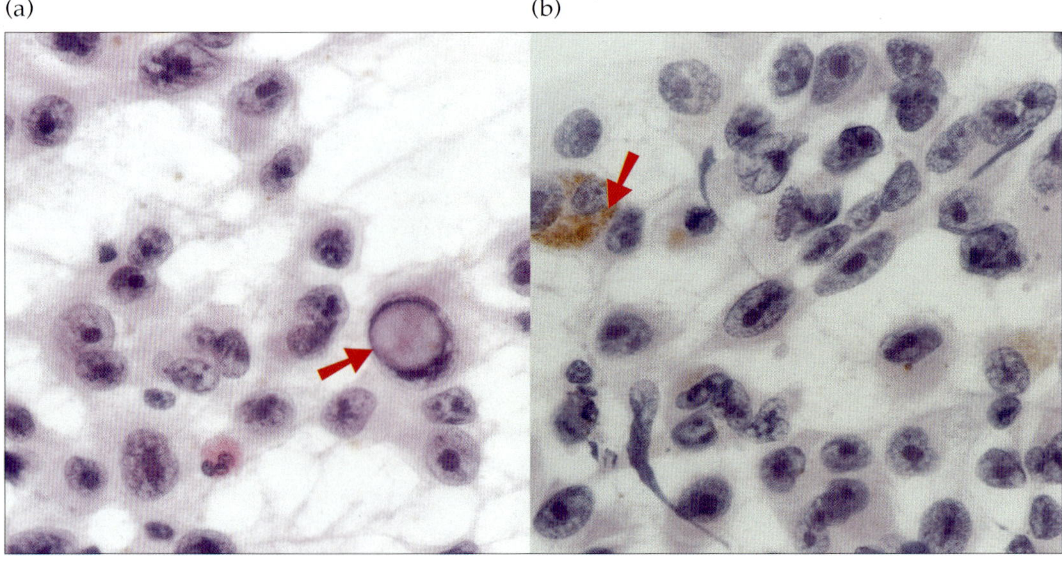

Figure 12. (a) Metastatic melanoma in a lymph node showing an intranuclear vacuole (arrow) and (b) cytoplasmic pigment (arrow). Papanicolaou stain ×600.

FNA can be used to diagnose primary NPC and the results are encouraging, although, only a small number of cases have been studied using this method.[20]

Special Techniques

Immunohistochemical stains can be applied to both exfoliative cytology and FNA specimens in a similar manner to their use in histological sections of surgical specimens. Cytokeratin, a marker for epithelial differentiation, is the single most useful stain used in service laboratories to differentiate carcinoma from non-carcinoma, such as lymphoma (*Figure 13*). Cytokeratin will stain the carcinoma cells, leaving the atypical lymphocytes and lymphoma cells unstained. Staining for S100 protein, a marker for melanocytic differentiation, is useful for distinguishing melanoma from NPC.

More sophisticated antigen detection is undertaken in the research laboratory but service laboratories are increasingly using such panels of antibodies to aid diagnosis. It is well established that NPC is closely linked to the Epstein-Barr virus.[21] A viral antigen which is closely associated with NPC, is the Epstein-Barr virus associated nuclear antigen (EBNA).[22] It has been detected in FNA smears of metastatic NPC, both in China[23] and Hong Kong.[24] EBNA positive cells have nuclei which contain granules which demonstrate strong fluorescence (*Figure 14*). In one Chinese study, the EBNA detection

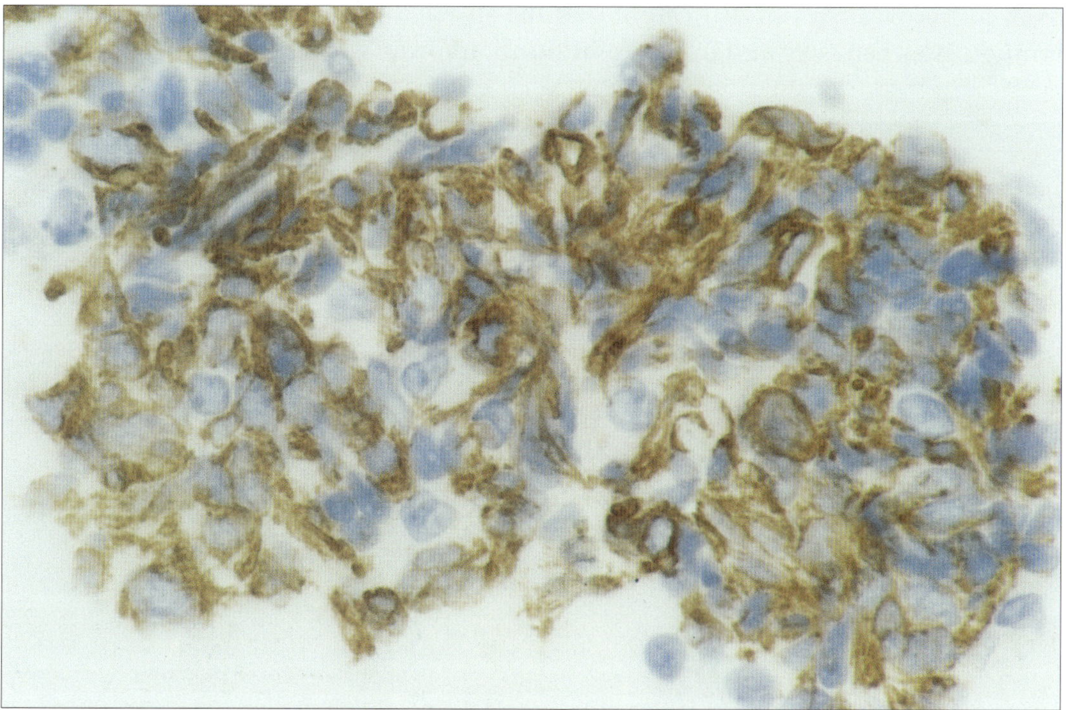

Figure 13. Immunoperoxidase stain for cytokeratin. The brown pigment indicates the NPC cells are of epithelial origin. ×800.

rate was high (82%) in metastatic NPC cervical lymph node aspirates, when compared with 5.1% and 1.2% of other tumours and controls. In a preliminary study of 17 cases of metastatic NPC and other head and neck carcinomas, EBNA was detected in all the NPC cases, while only half of the other head and neck carcinomas were positive. These findings suggest that, whereas a positive result is not specific, a negative result may help to exclude NPC from the diagnosis.[24] More recently the detection of Epstein-Barr virus-encoded RNAs (EBERs) in both histological and cytological material has proved to be very useful in diagnosing NPC. EBV infection of tumour cells can be clearly demonstrated by in situ hybridization with an EBER probe (*Figure 15*).[25,26] This technique permits the detection of EBV when there is highly restricted viral antigen expression and when there is low viral genome copy in infected tissues and conventional immunohistochemistry and in situ hybridization techniques are unhelpful. Thus it is a very useful adjunct in diagnostic pathology. It is applicable to a variety of tissues including old archival material even when "gathered under less than optimal conditions".[26]

Concluding Remarks

Cytological evaluation is simple, cheap, atraumatic and a diagnosis can be made within a very short period of time. In addition, special staining can be performed on smears, as in histological sections. If cell blocks are also available, special stains including immunocytochemistry and in situ hybridisation for EBV can be undertaken and this

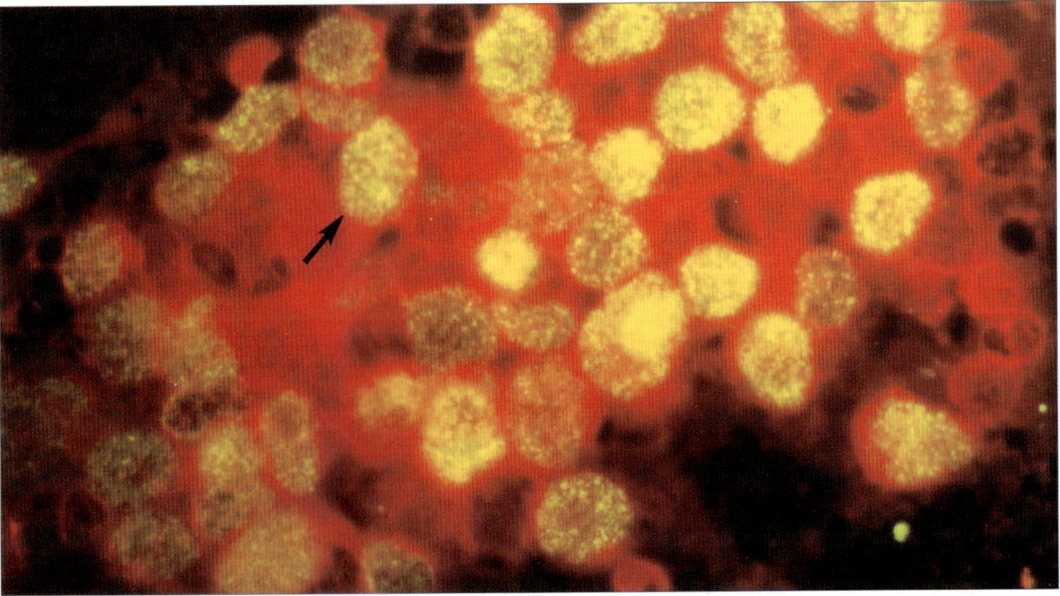

Figure 14. EBNA positive NPC cells showing bright nuclear fluorescence (arrow). Anti-Complement immunohistochemical stain ×1,100.

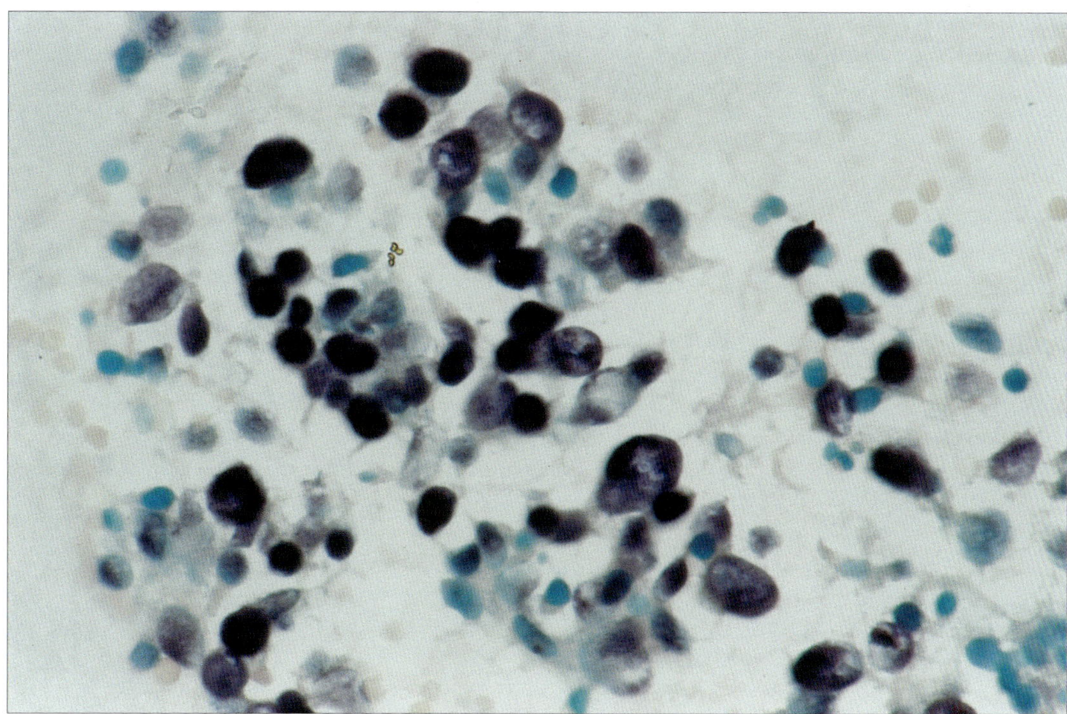

Figure 15. Metastatic NPC in the lung. The pleomorphic cancer cells are EBER positive as denoted by the blue/black colour at the site of hybridisation. Some lymphocytes also show reactivity and this indicates latent infection with the EBV. ×800.

can significantly improve cytodiagnosis. The cytological features of most cases are typical and with an adequate specimen cytodiagnosis is usually straight forward. The limiting factors in diagnosis are an inadequate and non-representative specimen along with poor cellular preservation and an inexperienced cytopathologist. Cellular preservation is directly related to the care and diligence exercised at the time of specimen collection. In the Uterobrush study, technical staff were in attendance to prepare smears to ensure optimal cellular preservation, a prerequisite for cytodiagnosis.

Like its proven role in cervical cancer detection and prevention, cytodiagnosis has the potential to become an effective screening test for NPC in high risk groups. However, before this can become a reality, an easy-to-use and cheap sampling device must be available. The Uterobrush with modification and further experience may be a suitable implement. In the meantime, more widescale prospective studies are required, to assess the diagnostic accuracy of cytological techniques in NPC, before any major initiatives are implemented.

References

1. Frable, W.J., Frable, M.A.S. 1979. Thin needle aspiration biopsy: the diagnosis of head and neck tumours revisited. *Cancer*; 43:1541–1548.

2. Chang, A.R., Chan, M.K.M., Liang, X-M. 1996. The brush cytology of the nasopharynx in a group of Hong Kong subjects. Abstracts of the XXI International Congress of the International Academy of Pathology and 12th World Congress of Academic and Environmental Pathology, Budapest. 46(Suppl. 1):Abstract 167.
3. Morrison, L.E, Hopp, E.S., Wu, R. 1949. Diagnosis of malignancy of the nasopharynx: cytologic study by the smear technique. *Ann. Otolarhngol.*; 58:18–32.
4. Dong, H., Shen, S., Huang, S., *et al.* 1983. The cytologic diagnosis of nasopharyngeal carcinoma from exfoliated cells collected by suction method. *J. Laryngol. Otol.*; 97:727–734.
5. Hopp, E.S.1958. Cytologic diagnosis and prognosis in carcinoma of mouth, pharynx and nasopharynx. *Laryngoscope*; 1,281–1,287.
6. Ma, S.S., Chen, L.H. 1958. Cytology in diagnosis of nasopharyngeal carcinoma. *Taiwan Ta Hsueh I Hsueh Yuan*; 5:1–14.
7. Djojopranoto, M. 1960. Incidence and pathology of nasopharyngeal tumors (translated title). Thesis. Indonesia: Airlangga Di Surabaja University.
8. Liang, P.C. 1964. Studies on nasopharyngeal carcinoma in the Chinese: statistical and laboratory investigation. *Chin. Med. J.*; 83:373–390.
9. Ali, M.Y., Shanmugaratnam, K. 1967. Cytodiagnosis of nasopharyngeal carcinoma. *Acta Cytol.*; 11:54–60.
10. Chan, M.K.M., Huang, D.P. 1990. The value of cytologic examination for nasopharyngeal carcinoma. *Ear Nose Throat J.*; 69:268–271.
11. Chang, A.R., Chan, M.K.M., Liang, X-M., *et al.* Nasopharyngeal carcinoma: obtaining a cytological diagnosis with a Brush sampler (in press).
12. Hunan Medical College. 1980. Atlas of cytology of nasopharyngeal carcinoma (in Chinese).
13. McGuire, L.J., Lee, J.C.K. 1990. The histopathologic diagnosis of nasopharyngeal carcinoma. *Ear Nose Throat J.*; 69:229–233.
14. Chan, M.K.M., McGuire, L.J., Lee, J.C.K. 1988. Cytology of amyloidosis in smears of nasopharyngeal carcinoma. *Acta Cytol.*; 32:429–430.
15. Zong, Y.S., Li, Q.X. 1986. Histopathology of paracancerous nasopharyngeal carcinoma-in-situ. *Chin. Med. J.*; 99:763–771.
16. Suen, M., Lee, J.C.K. 1986. Nasopharyngeal intra-epithelial neoplasia. In: *Abstracts of the XVI International Congress of the International Academy of Pathology, Vienna.*
17. Zong, Y.S. 1985. *Etiology and Pathogenesis of Nasopharyngeal Carcinoma: Cytopathology of Nasopharyngeal Carcinoma.* China: The People's Medical Publishing House.
18. Chan, M.K.M., McGuire, L.J., Lee, J.C.K. 1989. Fine needle aspiration cytodiagnosis of nasopharyngeal carcinoma in cervical lymph nodes. *Acta Cytol.*; 33:344–350.
19. Cai, W.M., Zhang, H.X., Hu, Y.H. *et al.* 1983. Influence of biopsy on the prognosis of nasopharyngeal carcinoma — a critical study of biopsy from the nasopharynx and cervical Iymph nodes of 649 patients. *Int. J. Radiat. Oncol. Biol. Phys.*; 9:1,439–1,444.
20. Scher, R.L., Oostingh, P.E., Levine, P.A. *et al.* 1988. Role of fine needle aspiration in the diagnosis of lesions of the oral cavity, oropharynx and nasopharynx. *Cancer*; 62:2602–2606.
21. Henle, W., Henle, G. 1976. Epstein-Barr virus specific IgA serum antibodies as an outstanding feature of nasopharyngeal carcinoma. *Int. J. Cancer*; 17:1–7.
22. Huang, D.P., Ho, J.H.C., Henle, W., *et al.* 1978. Presence of EBNA in nasopharyngeal carcinoma and control patient tissues related to EBV serology. *Int. J. Cancer*; 22:266–274.
23. Chen, Q.B. 1985. Epstein-Barr virus nuclear antigen (EBNA) assay of the puncture smears from neck masses for the differential diagnosis of nasopharyngeal carcinoma. *Chung Hua Lin Tsa Chih (China)*; 7:29–30.
24. Chan, M.K.M., Huang, D.P., Ho, Y.H., Lee, J.C.K. 1989. Detection of Epstein-Barr virus associated antigen in fine needle aspiration smears from cervical Iymph nodes in diagnosis of nasopharyngeal carcinoma, *Acta Cytol.*; 33:351–354.

25. Khan, G., Coates, P.J., Kangro, H.O., Slavin, G. 1992. Epstein Barr virus (EBV) encoded small RNAs: targets for detection by in situ hybridisation with oligonucleotide probes. *J. Clin. Pathol.*; 45:616–620.
26. Ambinder, R.F., Mann, R.B. 1994. Epstein-Barr-Encoded RNA in situ hybridization: diagnostic applications. *Human Pathol.*; 25:602–605.

CHAPTER 11

Prognostic Factors and Stage-classification

Peter Teo

There are various stage-classifications for NPC[1–9] and yet no concensus has been reached as to which is the most appropriate. The more important classifications are shown in *Table 1*. In these, the differences between the various T-stagings are relatively minor when compared to those relating to the N-stagings. The latter are derived from fundamentally dissimilar concepts related to the independent prognostic significance of the nodal characteristics.[8] Comparison of this feature is therefore of paramount importance. In comparing the different classifications great care must be taken when interpreting historical treatment results and conclusions[1–4,10–12] based on prognostic variables identified prior to the advent of CT and MRI.

It has been shown that Ho's classification[3,13,14] is superior to the UICC/AJC classifications[5,15] because the survival rates of the overall stages differ from one another more significantly and the N-staging is more accurate in predicting the distant metastasis rate.[8] Stages T1 and T2 of UICC/AJC are similar in their free from local failure rate (FLF) and should be grouped together,[8] being equivalent to Ho's T1. Ho's classification has also been compared with the Huang[4] and the Changsha[8] classifications. Again the Ho Classification compared favourably in that it was able to divide patients into the greatest number of distinct prognostic groups with five overall stages and four N-stages. Distribution of patients was also relatively more even among Ho's overall stages. The Huang classification was intermediate in effectiveness between those of Ho and Changsha in predicting prognosis. The overall stages of the Changsha Classification correlated least well with survival, there being no significant difference in actuarial survival rate (ASR) between Stage I and Stages II and III. The Changsha T-staging was also considered inferior in predicting local failure. Other than that of Qin *et al.*,[16] there was no report showing a poorer local control for tumours involving more than one organ beyond the nasopharynx; therefore, the classifying of this as Changsha's T4 was not based on solid scientific grounds. However, even Ho's Classification is now considered outdated as modification is required to incorporate significant prognosticators identified by CT, such as parapharyngeal tumour involvement.[9,12,17–19] Indeed any stage-classification for NPC needs constant updating to take account of advancing imaging technology. Not only is tumour localization becoming more accurate, but the radiotherapeutic methodology continues to improve with the passage of time. These

Table 1. Stage-classifications for NPC.

Stage-H classification	Ho (1978)[13]	Huang (1985)[4]	Changsha (1983)[11]	UICC (1987)[48]
T-stage	T1 NP only T2 T2n Nasal fossa T20 Oropharynx T2p Parapharyngeal region T3 T3a Bone involvement below the base of the skull including floor of the sphenoid sinus T3b Base of the skull T3c Cranial nerve(s) palsy T3d Orbits, laryngopharynx (Hypopharynx) or infratemporal fossa	T Ts Primary soft tissue tumour only Tb Basal skull destruction evident on radiographs Tn Cranial nerve involvement Direct invasion to the adjacent Tc brain evident on CT scan (newly added item)	T0 Subclinical T1 One wall or corner between 2 walls T2 ≥2 walls T3 Nasal fossa, oropharynx (including parapharyngeal region) T4 ≥2 features of T3	T1 One wall NP T2 ≥2 walls NP T3 Nasal cavity, oropharynx (including parapharyngeal region T4 Skull base and/or cranial nerve
N-stage	N0 No nodes N1 Node(s) above skin crease at laryngeal cartilage N2 Node(s) below skin crease but above supraclavicular fossa N3 Supraclavicular node(s)	N Cervical lymph node N0 No palpable nodes N1 Unilateral (ipsilateral) small lymph nodes with total diameter ≤5 cm N2 Bilateral (contralateral) larger lymph nodes with total diameter >5 cm	N0 No node N1 Mobile and/or <3 cm above supraclavicular fossa N2 Fixed and/or 3–8 cm and above supraclavicular fossa N3 Supraclavicular and/or >8 cm	N0 No node N1 Single homolateral node ≤3 cm N2 N2a Single homolateral node >3–≤6 cm N2b Multiple nodes; homolateral, ≤6 cm N3 N2c Bilateral or contralateral nodes ≤6 cm >6 cm node(s)

M-stage M1	M0 No distant metastases M1 Distant metastases	M Distant metastasis evident clinically M M0 No distant metastasis M1 Clinically evident distant metastasis beyond cervical lymph node involvement	M0 No metastases M1 Distant metastases	M0 No metastases
Stage grouping	I T1N0 II T2 and/or N1 III T3 and/or N2 IV N3 (any T) V M1	I TsN0M0 (primary soft tissue only) II T2N1M0 or TbN0-1M0 (any condition with N1 and/or Tb) III TsN2M0 or TbN2M0 or TnN0-2M0 or TcN0-2M0 or involving N2 or Tn or Tc or more combinations) IV M1 (any of the above conditions with distant metastasis evident clinically)	I T1N0 II T2N0; T0-2N1 III T3N0-1; T0-3N2 IV T4N0-2; T0-4N3; M1	I T1N0 II T2N0 III T3N0; T1-3N1 IV T4N0-1 N2-3 (any T); M1 (any T, any N)

Table 1. (Cont'd)

Stage-classification	Kyoto conference (1978)[1]	Proposed modification of Ho (1991)[9]	UICC (1996)[7]
T-stage	T1 Tumour confined to the nasopharynx T2 Extension to nasal fossa, oropharynx or adjacent muscles or nerves below the base of the skull T3 Beyong T2 limits T3a Bone involvement below the base of the skull T3b Involvement of skull base T3c Involvement of cranial nerve(s) T3d Involvement of orbit, laryngopharynx or infratemporal fossa	T1 NP only T2 T2n Nasal fossa T20 Oropharynx T2p Parapharyngeal region T3 T3a Bone involvement below the base of the skull including floor of the sphenoid sinus T3b Base of the skull T3c Cranial nerve(s) palsy T3d Orbits, laryngopharynx (hypopharynx) or infratemporal fossa T3p parapharyngeal region	T1 Confined to nasopharynx T2 T2a Oropharynx and/or nasal fossa T2b Parapharynx extension Bone invasion T3 Intracranial extesion/cranial nerves T4 Infratemporal fossa, hypopharynx, orbit involvement
N-stage	N0 No cervical lymph nodes palpable N1 Node(s) wholly in the upper cervical level bounded below by a line joining the upper margin of the sternal end of the clavicle on the opposite side to the apex of an angle between the lateral surface of the neck and the superior margin of the trapezius on the same side N2 Node(s) extending below the lower boundary line of N1	N0 No nodes N1 Node(s) above skin crease at laryngeal cartilage N2 Node(s) below skin crease but above supraclavicular fossa N3 Supraclavicular node(s)	N1 Unilateral ≤6 cm above supraclavicular N2 Bilateral ≤6cm above supraclavicular N3 N3a Above supraclavicular >6 cm N3b Supraclavicular fossa nodes
M-stage	M0 No distant metastases M1 With distant metastases, or nodal or skin involvement below the clavicle	M0 No haematogenous metastases M1 Haematogenous metastases present, and/or lymph nodal metastases below the clavicle	
Stage grouping	A T1N0 B T1N1; T2N0; T2N1 C T3 (any N); N2 (any T) D M1	I (T1,T2n,T20) N0M0 IIa (T1,T2n,T20)(N1N2)M0 IIb (T2p,T3,T3p)N0M0 IIIa (T2p,T3,T3p)(N1N2)M0 IIIb (T1,T2n,T20)N3M0 IVa (T2p,T3,T3p)N3M0 IVb M1(any T, any N)	Ia T1N0M0 Ib T2aN0M0 II T2bN0M0;T1N1M0;T2N1M0 III T1N2M0;T2N2M0;T3N0-N2M0 IV T4N0-N2M0;Any T N3M0; Any T Any NM1

factors are certain to bring an improvement in prognosis and a change in significant prognosticators.

Significant Prognostic Factors

An analysis of 903 patients at the Prince of Wales Hospital with NPC presenting without distant metastasis between 1984 and 1989 was carried out to determine significant factors influencing prognosis and guiding treatment strategy.[20] We reached the following conclusions by both mono- and multivariate analyses:-

Major prognosticators:

(a) sex and age
(b) Ho's N-stage
(c) The presence of the following:
  i) contralateral cervical nodal metastasis (including bilateral nodes)
  ii) fixed or partially fixed cervical nodal metastasis
  iii) skull base tumour infiltration
  iv) cranial nerve(s) palsy

Cervical nodal parameters:

(i) Among the cervical nodal prognosticators, Ho's N-stage is of paramount importance, because it governs the greatest number of clinical endpoints, apart from local failure rate, with the smallest p-values in comparison to nodal fixation and nodal bilaterality or contralaterality. This has been substantiated by both monovariate and multivariate analyses. Nodal fixation and bilaterality or contralaterality are of secondary prognostic significance only.
(ii) The maximal nodal size (<3 cm vs 3–6 cm vs >6 cm, or, ≤6 cm vs >6 cm, or, as a continuous variable) has not been found to be of independent prognostic significance, even though monovariate analysis has shown that the larger size nodal metastases fare worse.

Local factors:

Local tumour control is not affected by any nodal parameters; among all the tumour parameters, only the presence of skull base tumour infiltration and cranial nerve(s) palsy are significant in worsening local tumour control.

(i) The cranial nerve(s) palsy with or without skull base infiltration has a worse prognosis than skull base infiltration alone, *Figures 1 and 2*.
(ii) Orbital and infratemporal fossa disease carry a significantly poor prognosis even in the absence of skull base infiltration and/or cranial nerve palsy.
(iii) Oropharyngeal and parapharyngeal involvement are less advanced than skull base infiltration and cranial nerve(s) palsy and they are prognostically significant only in the absence of the latter two prognosticators.

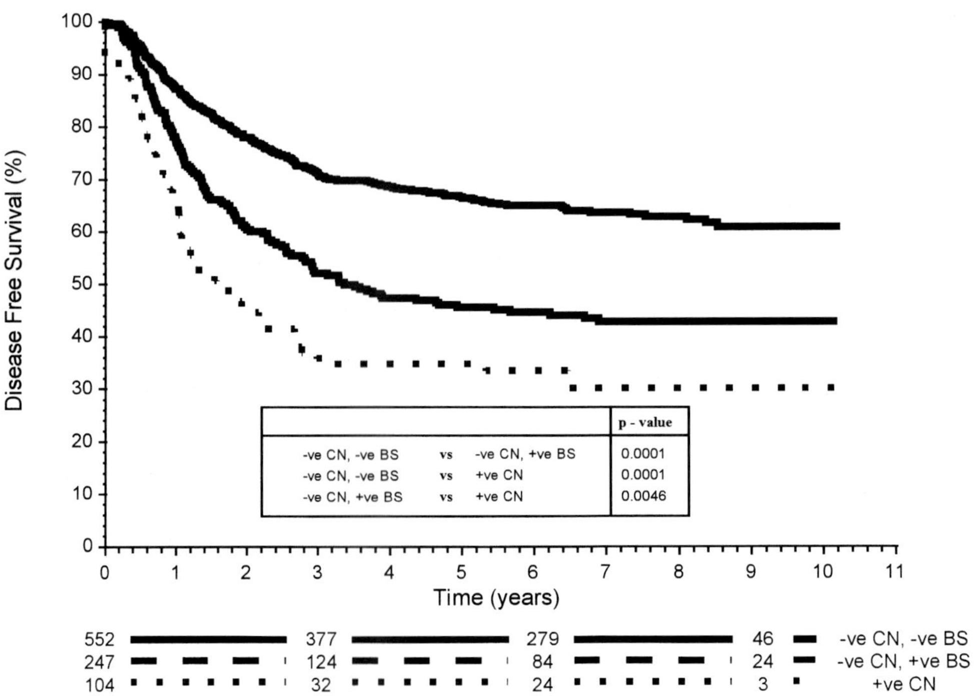

Figure 1. The significance of skull base and/or cranial nerve(s) involvement on DFS.

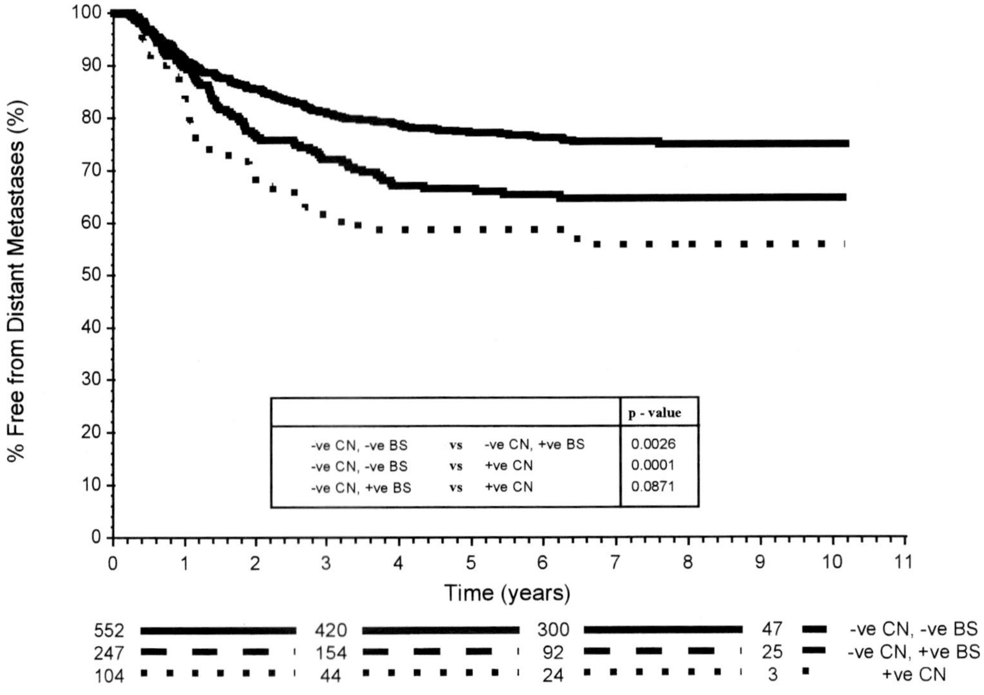

Figure 2. The significance of skull base and/or cranial nerve(s) involvement on FDM.

Minor prognosticators:

The following features were found significant in determining one or more clinical endpoints in the sub-group analyses but not in the overall analysis:-

(a) parapharyngeal, infratemporal fossa or orbital involvement in node-negative patients.

(b) infratemporal fossa involvement and multiple nodal metastasis and the absence of contralateral or bilateral nodal metastasis (as a good prongosticator) in Ho's N1-stage.

(c) laryngopharyngeal or infratemporal fossa involvement in Ho's N2-stage;

(d) oropharyngeal involvement in Ho's N3-stage.

(e) multiple nodal metastasis and orbital tumour infiltration in patients with skull base involvement and/or cranial nerve(s) palsy.

(f) oropharyngeal involvement and multiple nodal metastases in patients without skull base infiltration and/or cranial nerve(s) palsy.

(g) infratemporal fossa involvement in the node-negative patients with skull base involvement and/or cranial nerve(s) palsy.

(h) oropharyngeal involvement or parapharyngeal involvement in the node-negative patients without skull base involvement and/or cranial nerve(s) palsy.

These findings concur with the concept that the further the primary tumour extends or the cervical nodal metastasis occurs from the site of origin in the nasopharynx, the more advanced is the stage of the NPC.

A Comparison of Studies on Significant Prognosticators in NPC

Cervical nodal parameters

In our series, the three nodal parameters significant in determining survival and distant metastasis rates were Ho's N levels, fixed nodes and contralateral neck nodes.

Ho's N stage (or N level)

Ho originally proposed the classification of cervical nodal metastases by their level of occurrence in the neck and demonstrated highly significant survival differences between the individual N stages.

However, in Sham's analysis of 759 Mo-NPC in 1990,[12] the survival rates of Ho's No and N1 stages were comparable. Sham suggested that this could be due to a significant proportion of No-NPC harbouring occult retropharyngeal nodal metastases the prognosis of which was similar to that of Ho's N1.

In an analysis of 4730 Mo-NPC, Lee *et al.*[21] showed that within each of Ho's N levels, the addition of nodal size, multiplicity, and bilaterality could further improve prognostic accuracy. In this series, those with a low Ho level involvement within each

AJC/UICC[5,15] N stage, had significantly more failures but the difference between upper and mid Ho levels did not reach statistical significance.

In a previous study, we found Ho's N-stage to be of paramount significance in determining survival and distant metastasis rates for non-disseminated (Mo) NPC;[19] however, we found a lack of survival difference between Ho's No and N1, which was in agreement with the finding of Sham *et al.*[12] In a more recent study however, we did not classify the retropharyngeal nodal metastasis as N1 but regarded it as parapharyngeal disease and we could then demonstrate a significant survival difference between Ho's No and N1 (*Table 2* and *Figure 3*). Ho's N stage was found to be prognostically significant even among patient sub-groups stratified for maximal nodal size and for fixation. Moreover, the multivariate analysis confirmed that Ho's N stage was a significant prognosticator governing survival, distant metastasis, and regional failure rates (*Table 2*). The minor disagreement between our studies and those of Sham *et al.*[12,22] and Lee *et al.*,[21] regarding the significance of the individual Ho N stages and their relative importance could be explained in several ways. These could include the introduction of the CT parameters, the increasing use of the posterolateral parapharyngeal boosting technique,[23] and the use of the neoadjuvant chemotherapy.[19,23] Even though it has remained controversial whether radiation dose escalation and

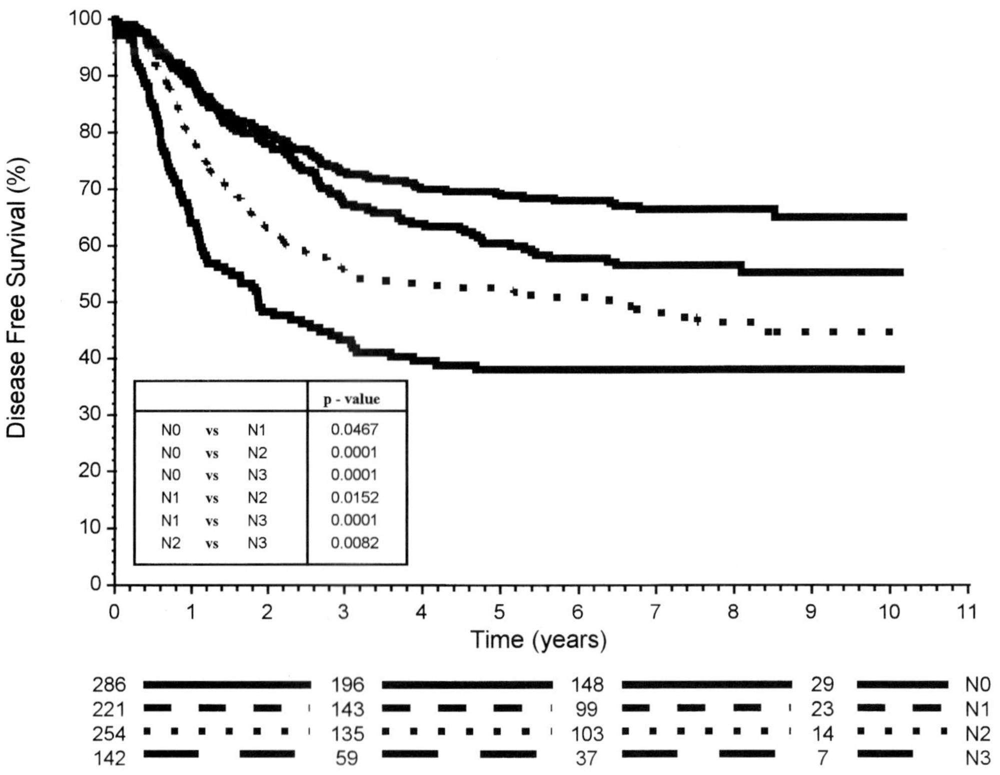

Figure 3. Comparison of Ho's N-stages for DFS.

Table 2. The significant prognosticators for the 903 non-disseminated NPC.[20]

Clinical endpoint	Prognosticator by regression	Cox	Cox regression p-value	Risk ratio	95% confidence interval (CI)	5-year actuarial rates ± 2 standard error (SE)	10-year actuarial rates ± 2 standard error (SE)
ASR	Ho's N-stage	No	0.0001	1.421	1.087,1.858	75.9±0.05	71.3±0.06
		N1				73.3±0.06	63.9±0.07
		N2				59.7±0.06	42.9±0.16
		N3				47.1±0.08	40.8±0.10
	Cranial nerve(s) palsy	Yes	0.0001	2.046	1.529,2.736	36.1±0.10	31.5±0.10
		No				69.7±0.03	61.2±0.05
	Skull base infiltration	Yes	0.0001	1.905	1.520,2.378	51.5±0.06	45.8±0.06
		No				74.4±0.04	65.7±0.06
	Age	<40 years	0.0002	1.016	1.007,1.025	74.1±0.05	67.8±0.06
		≥40 years				61.6±0.04	53.0±0.05
	Fixed cervical node(s)	fixed	0.0093	1.486	1.068,2.068	43.0±0.11	40.1±0.11
		mobile				68.4±0.03	59.8±0.04
	Sex	male	0.0125	1.421	1.087,1.858	62.7±0.04	53.7±0.05
		female				75.5±0.06	69.6±0.06
	Contralateral cervical node(s)		0.0309	1.323	1.026,1.707		
	contralateral/bilateral					52.5±0.06	46.6±0.07
	ipsilateral					72.1±0.04	63.1±0.05

Table 2. (Cont'd)

Clinical endpoint	Prognosticator by regression	Cox	Cox regression p-value	Risk ratio	95% confidence interval (CI)	5-year actuarial rates ± 2 standard error (SE)	10-year actuarial rates ± 2 standard error (SE)
DFS	Ho's N-stage	No	0.0001	1.403	1.273,1.547	69.2±0.05	65.0±0.06
		N1				60.5±0.07	55.4±0.07
		N2				52.2±0.06	44.7±0.07
		N3				37.0±0.08	37.0±0.08
	Cranial nerve(s) palsy	Yes	0.0001	1.813	1.367,2.377	34.9±0.09	30.3±0.10
		No				60.3±0.03	55.5±0.04
	Skull base infiltration	Yes	0.0001	1.788	1.453,2.200	43.0±0.05	38.6±0.06
		No				65.5±0.04	60.1±0.05
	Sex	male	0.0044	1.408	1.108,1.791	53.9±0.04	48.7±0.04
		female				66.9±0.06	63.7±0.06
	Age	<40 years	0.0050	1.010	1.002,1.018	63.3±0.05	60.2±0.06
		≥40 years				54.1±0.04	48.6±0.05
	Fixed cervical node(s)	fixed	0.0235	1.428	1.048,1.947	34.4±0.11	34.4±0.11
		mobile				59.6±0.03	54.5±0.04
FDM	Ho's N-stage	No	0.0001	1.448	1.256,1.699	84.9±0.04	82.2±0.05
		N1				75.9±0.06	73.4±0.06
		N2				67.3±0.06	65.5±0.06
		N3				50.3±0.09	49.4±0.09
	Skull base infiltration	Yes	0.0001	1.607	1.235,2.090	64.3±0.05	62.1±0.06
		No				76.7±0.04	74.5±0.04

	Cranial nerve(s) palsy	Yes	0.0021	1.654	1.150,2.368	58.7±0.10	55.7±0.11
		No				74.0±0.03	71.9±0.03
	Fixed cervical node(s)	fixed	0.0032	1.654	1.158,2.364	47.6±0.11	45.9±0.12
		mobile				74.7±0.03	72.6±0.03
	Contralateral cervical node(s)		0.0098	1.472	1.103,1.964		
	contralateral/bilateral					58.4±0.06	56.3±0.06
	ipsilateral					78.4±0.03	76.2±0.04
	Sex	male	0.0401	1.367	1.013,1.872	69.6±0.04	68.0±0.04
		female				79.8±0.05	76.2±0.06
FLF	Skull base infiltration	Yes	0.0001	1.887	1.355,2.629	66.3±0.06	63.1±0.06
		No				85.6±0.03	79.6±0.04
	Cranial nerve(s) palsy	Yes	0.0001	1.747	1.164,2.623	58.6±0.11	53.7±0.12
		No				81.2±0.03	76.8±0.04
	Age	<40 years	0.0087	1.014	1.003,1.026	82.5±0.04	80.2±0.05
		≥40 years				76.2±0.04	70.0±0.05
FRF	Ho's N-stage	No	0.0001	1.988	1.643,2.406	95.6±0.02	95.0±0.02
		N1				89.0±0.04	87.2±0.05
		N2				84.6±0.05	81.8±0.06
		N3				70.6±0.09	70.6±0.09
	Cranial nerve(s) palsy	Yes	0.0030	1.623	1.084,2.432	83.1±0.05	83.1±0.05
		No				89.5±0.03	87.5±0.04
	Skull base infiltration	Yes	0.0372	1.789	1.025,3.125	78.2±0.10	78.2±0.10
		No				88.2±0.02	86.7±0.03

neoadjuvant chemotherapy are beneficial for NPC, these modifications in treatment, in conjunction with the avoidance of radiotherapy "geographical misses" by CT, might have improved the prognosis of NPC and led to an alteration in composition of the significant prognosticators, including Ho's N stages, and changed their order of statistical significance. Indeed our ratios of 5-year and 10-year local control (79.0% and 73.9% respectively) were superior to those (73% and 67%) in the Lee series.[24] On the other hand, subtle differences in the methodology of analysis for the various parameters could also result in differences in the findings. For example, the nodal size could be analyzed either as a continuous variable or as a categorical variable, and, in the latter case, it could be classified differently by using different maximal nodal sizes.

Nodal Fixation

Sham *et al.*[12,22] classified nodal metastasis into three types: Type 1, mobile nodes less than 4 cm. Type 2, nodes between 4 and 6 cm or partially fixed nodes. Type 3, nodes 6 cm or more, or fixed nodes. In this manner, the nodal characteristic (fixation coupled to size) was found to be an independent prognostic variable in addition to the Ho N stage. However, since nodal fixation was not analyzed separately from the nodal size, Sham *et al.* were unable to reach a conclusion regarding their independent significance. In a recent study by Lee and her group(unpublished), nodal fixation was shown to be an independent nodal prognosticator. Fixation of nodes was classified as N2 or N3 in some studies in the pre-CT era.[10,25–27]

In our studies, nodal fixation was analyzed separately from nodal size, and we were able to demonstrate the prognostic significance of fixed and partially fixed nodes (*Table* 2). For non-disseminated NPC in general, the distant metastasis rate was adversely affected by fixed nodes and contralateral nodes (*Table* 2 and *Figure* 4). The Ho N3 nodes that were fixed or partially fixed had a significantly higher risk of developing distant metastases than freely mobile N3 nodes. However, while there is usually no discrepancy between clinicians in labelling a node as fixed, the differentiation between a partially fixed node and a "freely mobile" node may be problematic. In this respect, there is a higher degree of inter-observer variability. This is the main drawback of using nodal fixation as an N staging criterion because it is less objective than the other nodal characteristics which are based on measurements or locations. From the patho-physiological point of view however, nodal fixation may actually represent the presence of significant extranodal tumour extension or infiltration of soft tissue or bone or surrounding organs. This could explain its adverse impact on the rate of distant metastasis or regional failure.

Contralateral Nodes

Controversies exist concerning the significance of cervical nodal laterality (unilateral/ contralateral/bilateral). In both Sham's[12] and Lee's[24] series, the evaluation of the primary lesion was incomplete and sub-optimal by modern standards. None of Sham's cases had CT or fibreoptic nasopharyngoscopic examinations and only 14% of patients in

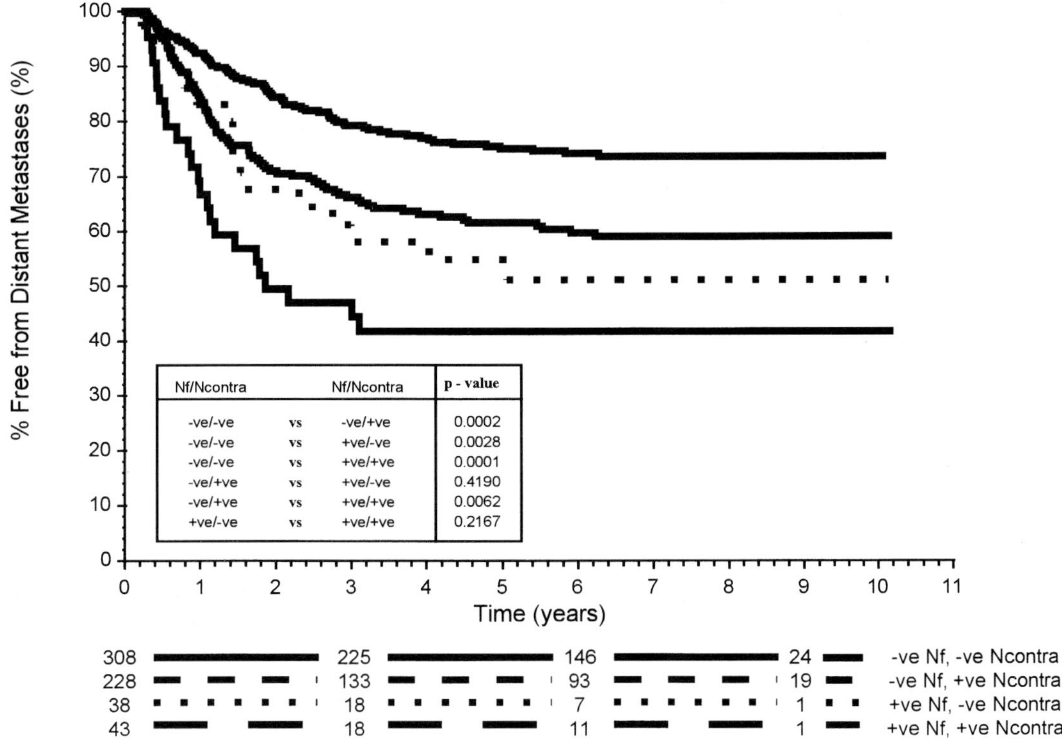

Figure 4. The significance of fixed and contralateral nodal metastasis on FDM.

Lee's series[24] had CT. Therefore, in both series a cervical node could not be labelled as homolateral or contralateral to the bulkiest tumour side in a large proportion of patients in whom the primary tumour was evaluated by no more than a mirror examination and a plain radiograph. Mirror and plain radiographic examinations were sub-optimal for determining the side of the bulkiest primary lesion, and certainly inferior to the combined use of CT and the fibreoptic nasopharyngoscope. Conceptually, Sham (personal communication) regarded the nasopharynx as a midline organ so that all NPCís should be considered as arising from the midline implying that nodal metastases should not be classified as homolateral or contralateral. Furthermore he only classified nodes as unilateral or bilateral in his analysis.[12]

However, we have clearly demonstrated that the presence of contralateral nodes significantly worsens distant metastasis and survival rates (*Table* 2 and *Figure* 4). After stratification by Ho's N stages, the presence of contralateral nodes significantly increased distant metastasis rate in Ho's N2, and, the contralateral N1 nodes were also marginally significant in having a higher risk of distant metastases than the homolateral N1 nodes, $p = 0.06$. In fact, our conclusion on the prognostic significance of nodal laterality is in concordance with that of Wang and Meyer,[25,27] Moench *et al.*,[26] and Hoppe *et al.*,[10] but contrary to that of Ho[1–3,28–31] and Neel *et al.*[32] In view of the accurate delineation of the side of the bulkiest primary lesion by CT and nasopharyngoscopic visualization, which enabled the accurate designation of contralateral cervical nodes, our conclusion on the prognostic significance of contralateral nodes should be valid.

Nodal Size

Discrepancies between the different series[4,12,13,19–22,33] on the prognostic significance of maximal nodal dimension are difficult to explain. It is possible that the maximal cervical nodal size was associated with the occurrence of certain CT-evident primary tumour parameters that were also prognostically significant. Those series in which patients were not routinely investigated by CT-scan suffered from the exclusion of the significant CT-evident prognostic variables associated with maximal nodal size which could have led to erroneous conclusions on the prognostic significance of maximal nodal size. Alternatively, there is a possibility of improvement in NPC prognosis following the administration of the neoadjuvant chemotherapy with cisplatinum and 5-fluorouracil for bulky nodes (≥4 cm) according to the Prince of Wales Hospital protocol (*Table 3*). This could have subtracted from the poor prognostic impact of bulky nodes. However neoadjuvant chemotherapy also strongly correlated with advanced Ho's levels in addition to its significant correlation with large nodal size ($p < 0.0001$ in both cases). Therefore the administration of neoadjuvant chemotherapy by itself could not completely account for the lack of prognostic significance of nodal size, while Ho N levels remained highly significant as a prognosticator (*Table 2*).

On the other hand, according to our investigation and treatment protocol (*Table 3*), the administration of posterolateral booster radiotherapy (PPB)[19,23] of 20 Gy after the conventional radiation treatment[3,13,14,19,23,29–31,34] to NPC's with parapharyngeal tumour extension, resulted in dose escalation not only to the nasopharynx and parapharynx but also to the ipsilateral upper neck which usually contained the bulkiest nodal metastasis. The booster dose could have enhanced the locoregional tumour control directly, and the systemic tumour control indirectly and diluted the possible prognostic impact of nodal size. According to our analysis, the maximal nodal dimension was not significant in predicting any one of the clinical outcomes (*Table 2*).

It is noteworthy that no cervical nodal parameters affected the local failure rate and only Ho's N-level (in addition to cranial nerve(s) palsy and skull base involvement) governed the regional failure rate (*Table 2*). The presence of multiple nodal metastases in contradistinction to a single node was only found to be of prognostic significance in certain subgroup analyses.

Advanced T-parameters

In our series, for each patient, after CT of the nasopharynx and skull base, a chart was filled to record tumour infiltration of the anatomical structures at or below the skull base, including intracranial and parapharyngeal tumour extension. Instead of using Ho's T stages, we used primary tumour characteristics such as nasal, parapharyngeal, and oropharyngeal extension, which characterize Ho's T2 stage, and skull base (BS),

Table 3. Investigative and treatment protocol (1984–1989).

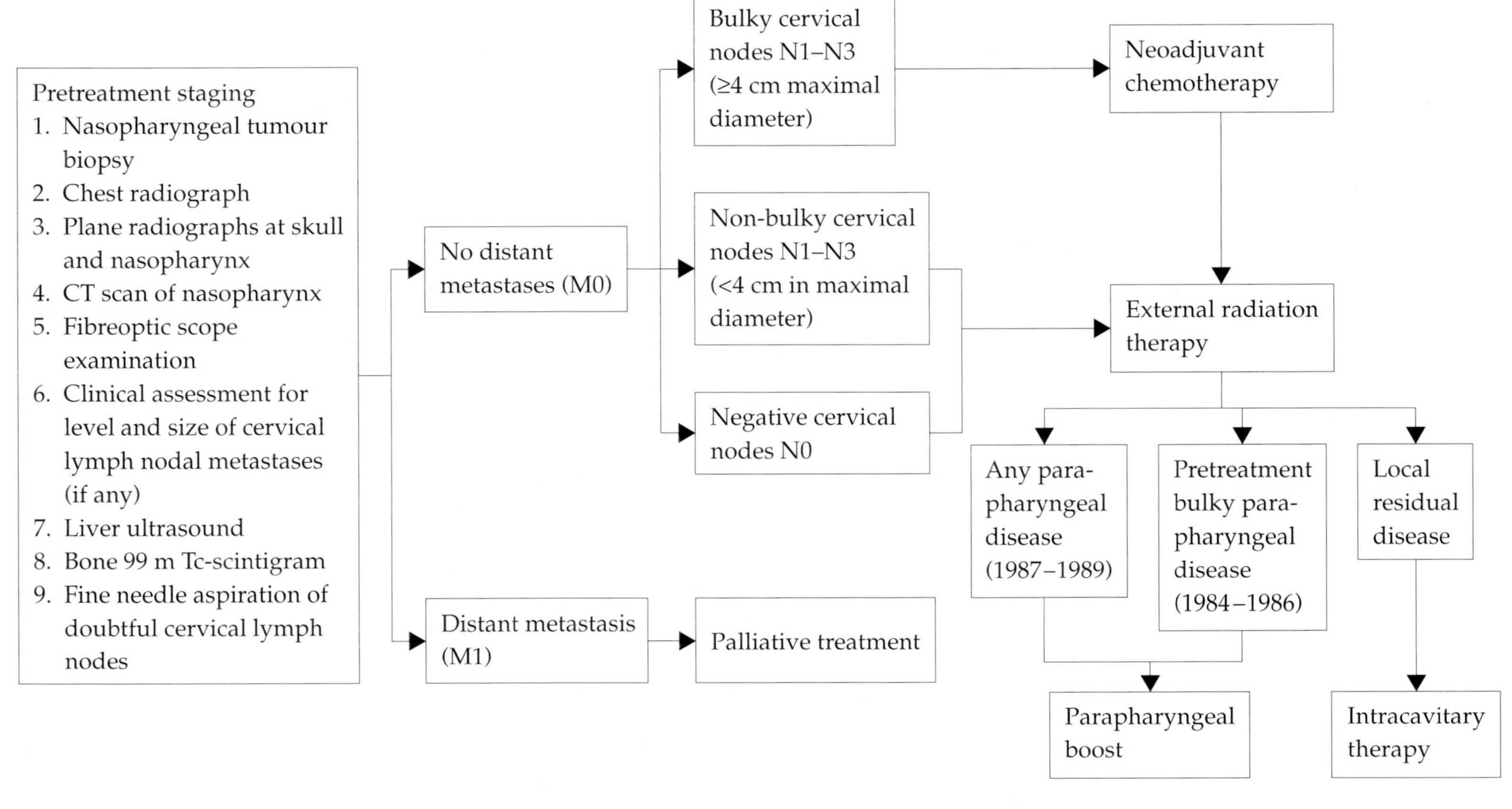

cranial nerve (CN), laryngopharyngeal, orbital, and infratemporal fossa tumour extension, which characterize Ho's T3 (a–d), for the multivariate analysis. In this manner, we could assess the value of each individual tumour characteristic without introducing errors due to artificial grouping of different tumour characteristics into predetermined T stages.

The CT-evident skull base erosion and clinically-evident cranial nerve palsies were found to be independently significant in determining all the clinical endpoints (*Table* 2), thus confirming our former report[19] on their prognostic significance. Skull base erosion was found to worsen survival and systemic and local tumour control significantly (*Table* 2 and *Figures 1 and* 2). Since regional failures were very often associated with, or preceded by, local failures[3,24,35] suggesting that local failures metastasized to the cervical nodes, skull base erosion and cranial nerve(s) palsy, which predicted local failures, also predicted regional failures (*Table* 2).

When cranial nerve(s) palsy was analysed as a single entity, it carried the same order of prognostic significance as skull base erosion (*Table* 2). However, when analyzed separately, the anterior cranial nerve palsies (I–VIII) carried the same prognostic significance as the posterior cranial nerve palsies (IX–XII), which is much less than that of skull base erosion or of cranial nerve palsy (I–XII). Orbital, infratemporal fossa and laryngopharyngeal involvement were individually found to be of independent prognostic significance in determining some clinical endpoints in certain patient subgroups. When grouped together as a single entity, they had a local failure rate comparable to that of cranial nerve palsy which was significantly worse than that of skull base erosion alone. Therefore, it is justifiable to classify tumours involving the orbit(s), intratemporal fossa, and laryngopharynx together with tumours causing cranial nerve(s) palsy in the same T- stage. They should be distinguished from tumours infiltrating the skull base only in view of the significant difference in local control after primary radiotherapy.

Indeed most series in the world literature that report on radiotherapy results and prognosticators of NPC observe that skull base tumour infiltration and cranial nerve(s) palsy significantly reduce rates of survival and local tumour control.[1–4,6,9–11,13,14,19,20,23–33,36–38] However, few report on the significance of these two primary tumour parameters in determining distant metastasis rate. Moreover, only a few recognize the need to classify skull base tumour involvement and cranial nerve(s) palsy separately. While Ho and Huang classify the two separately in their T-stage classifications, Teo *et al.* Sham *et al.* Lee *et al.* and Neel *et al.* all demonstrated that the cranial nerve(s) palsy carry a worse prognosis than the skull base tumour involvement alone. However only Ho catered for the separate classification of laryngopharyngeal, infratemporal fossa, and orbital tumour involvement, within his T-Stage Classification as T3d. Even so, Ho has never proven their distinct prognostic significance. However in Lee's series of more than four thousand patients with NPC, some of whom had a CT-scan for the primary tumour evaluation,[24] the patients with cranial nerve(s) palsy (Ho's T3c) and the patients with orbital, infratemporal fossal, and laryngopharyngeal tumour infiltration (Ho's

T3d) constituted the worst prognostic groups. Despite boosting with additional radiation dose whenever possible, 23% and 12% of the above groups respectively suffered from gross persistent local disease, whereas less than 3% of the others failed to attain an initial local complete response status after radical radiotherapy. The incidence of subsequent recurrence of patients with the Ho T3c and T3d groups was also highest among all patients in Lee's series. Unfortunately, the independent prognostic significance of Ho's T3d features was not proven by multivariate analyses in Lee's study. In our own study, orbital, infratemporal fossa and laryngopharyngeal infiltration (Ho's T3d) were shown to carry independent poor prognosis by both monovariate and multivariate analyses.

Parapharyngeal tumour involvement

Although there is no controversy over the anatomical definition of the parapharyngeal (or paranasopharyngeal) space, the radiological definition of NPC infiltration of the parapharyngeal region lacks concensus.[19,23,24,39–41] We have followed Silver's definition[39] of CT-evident distortion of the fibrofatty tissue plane sandwiched between the pterygoids and lateral pharyngeal wall at C1 vertebral level. In our studies, lateral soft tissue extension from the lateral wall of the nasopharynx with deformity of this fibrofatty tissue plane, effacement of the retroflexion of the pharyngobasilar fascia in the region of the neurovascular bundle, loss of demarcation between the lateral pharyngeal wall and the pterygoid muscles, and presence of tumorous soft tissue posterolateral to the styloid process or inferior to the C1/C2 vertebrae within the paraoropharyngeal region were collectively labelled as parapharyngeal tumour involvement. The lateral limit of the parapharyngeal tumour extension was measured from the midline and recorded for each patient.

From 1984–1986, prior to our first study,[23] bulky parapharyngeal T2 tumour extending ≥4 cm laterally from the midline was given booster radiotherapy of 20 Gy/10 fraction/2 weeks by a posterolateral oblique 6 MV photon beam in addition to the conventional radiotherapy dose of 60–62.5 Gy/6 weeks. Non-bulky tumour was not given the additional booster dose. Surprisingly, the former enjoyed better local tumour control and disease-free survival than the latter.[23] Therefore, after 1986, all parapharyngeal tumours were given booster radiotherapy to minimise local relapses.

In a subsequent study[20] of 659 NPCs, which included 628 non-disseminated cases, routine boosting with escalation of the overall nasopharyngeal radiation dose had been practised for the parapharyngeal tumour without skull base and/or cranial nerve involvement (Tp). Monovariate analysis showed that paranasopharyngeal tumours had significantly more distant metastases than the tumours confined to the nasopharynx or the tumours with nasal and/or oropharyngeal extension only. By multivariate analysis, the parapharyngeal disease was marginally significant in predicting for more distant metastases. The local tumour control was still significantly worse, despite the commencement of the practice of routine boosting.[19] In the more recent study,[20] parapharyngeal disease, perhaps not unexpectedly, was no longer significant in determining local recurrence after a longer practice of the booster radiotherapy which could have nullified the influence of the parapharyngeal tumour on local tumour control. Interestingly, in another study by Sham and Choy on 262 Mo-NPC staged by CT scan,[17] the paranasopharyngeal tumour not subjected to routine radiation boosting was found to be a significantly poor prognosticator for local failures. Unfortunately, they did not report on its impact on the overall survival and the distant metastasis rates.

In our own study,[20] if one eliminated the overriding prognosticators (skull base erosion, cranial nerve palsy and nodal metastasis), the prognostic significance of the radiation-boosted parapharyngeal tumour was unveiled (*Figure 5*), rendering it an important predictor of the distant metastasis rate, actuarial survival rate, and disease-free survival rate. In addition, in the multivariate analysis, it has been proven that parapharyngeal tumour extension significantly predisposes to distant metastasis and worsens survival in the absence of skull base, cranial nerve, and cervical nodal involvement. If booster radiotherapy had not been given, the parapharyngeal disease could have worsened local tumour control as well. In fact, a significant proportion of parapharyngeal tumour involvement actually represents metastasis to the retropharyngeal or retrostyloid lymph node which is not clinically palpable but which may reveal itself by showing a rim of contrast-enhancement in the CT.[23] Conceptually

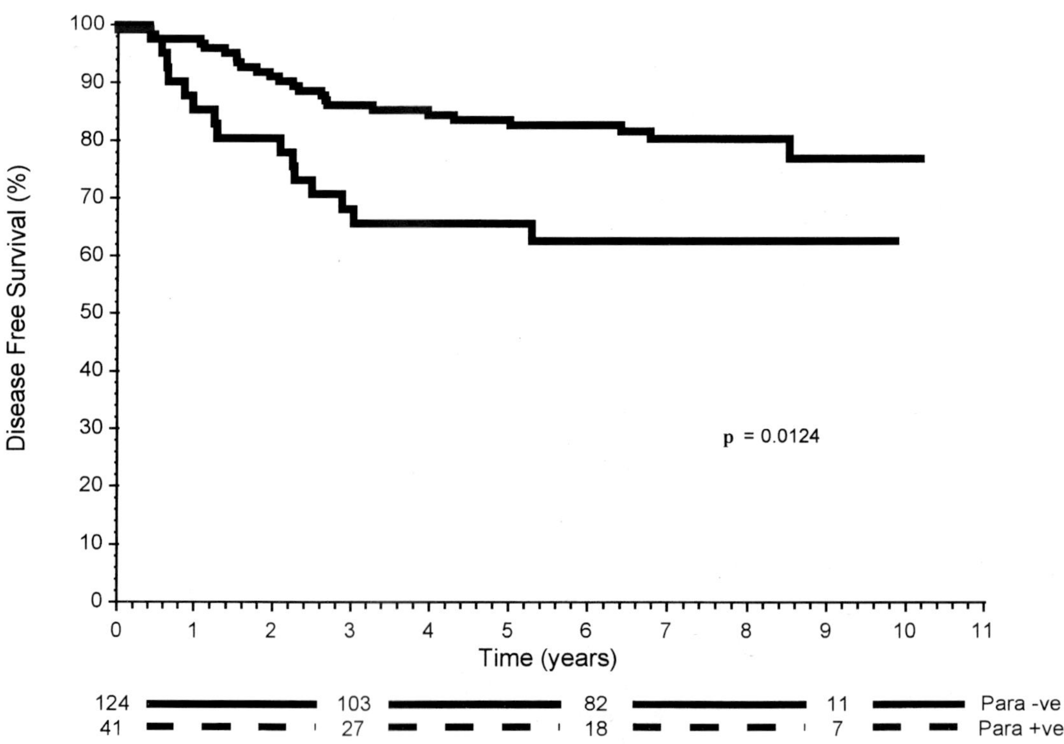

Figure 5. The significance of parapharyngeal involvement on DFS in node-negative patients without skull base infiltration or cranial nerve(s) palsy.

this kind of parapharyngeal disease could be regarded as an intermediate N stage between No and N1. Indeed the first station node of NPC lies in the retropharyngeal space and clinically palpable nodes in the upper neck should be regarded as the second station.[32]

In the presence of more advanced disease with palpable cervical nodal metastasis or skull base or cranial nerve(s) involvement, the parapharyngeal tumour is overshadowed for its prognostic significance. The routine addition of booster radiotherapy since 1986 could have enhanced tumour control by avoiding the "geographical miss" and by achieving a greater log of tumour cell kill with dose escalation (assuming that a dose-response gradient still exists above 60–62.5 Gy). However, improved local tumour control could only have an indirect, perhaps meagre, effect on the distant metastasis rate because the majority of distant metastases occurred without local failures,[35] and only a minor proportion of distant metastases was attributable to local failures.[42] Therefore, while the parapharyngeal tumour lost its predisposition to local failures after the use of booster radiotherapy, it retained its impact on distant metastasis and survival.

It is also significant that booster radiotherapy, used to treat parapharyngeal tumours,[23] also affected the homolateral upper cervical lymphatics. It is therefore not surprising that parapharyngeal tumour involvement has significantly less regional failures in the sub-group without skull base involvement or cranial nerve(s) palsy. Such paucity of regional failures in patients with parapharyngeal tumour involvement is most likely a direct consequence of radiation dose escalation due to the booster radiotherapy to the parapharyngeal region and upper neck, the side of which corresponds, in the vast majority of cases, to the side where clinically evident nodal metastases are located.

Histology

NPC has been classified as undifferentiated carcinoma, poorly differentiated squamous cell carcinoma, and moderate to well differentiated squamous cell carcinoma.[43] There has been much controversy concerning the significance of this histological classification, the presence or absence of a difference in radiosensitivity of the various histological sub-types, and the existence or not of a dose-tumour-response relationship above 60–65 Gy in at least some histological sub-types.[44,46] However, most reports on the prognostic significance and radiosensitivity of different histological subtypes came from Western countries where the undifferentiated carcinoma only constituted 50–80% of all NPC's. However in Southern China, the proportion of the undifferentiated histology is much higher, and various series from Hong Kong reported that over 90% of NPC belonged to this histology. None of the Hong Kong clinical series could show any prognostic significance in the histological sub-typing.[43,47] Our experience in the Prince of Wales Hospital is no exception. In our study, the histology of 903 NPC's has been subject to a uniform review by a single experienced pathologist to exclude the possibility of a wide variation in pathologists' opinion regarding the degree of squamous differentiation of the tumour.[29,45,46] Nonetheless, even by so doing, we could not demonstrate a significant difference in prognosis between the three WHO histological subtypes,[46] *Table 2*. With the exception of the study by Saw *et al.*[45] and some of the studies by Ho, uniform pathological review to confirm the original diagnosis of the histological sub-type[43] was prominent by its absence in all the Hong Kong series. Like all other Hong Kong series, undifferentiated and poorly differentiated squamous cell carcinoma (i.e. WHO Types 2 and 3) accounted for over 98% of our 903 NPC. However, monovariate comparison between well differentiated or keratinizing squamous cell carcinomas (WHO Type 1), poorly differentiated (WHO Type 2) and undifferentiated carcinoma (WHO Type 3)[43,46] with stratification according to the other factors such as the primary tumour extent and the cervical nodal levels was hampered by the small number of patients with WHO Type 1 histology. The small number of well differentiated or keratinizing squamous cell carcinoma (WHO type I) could have also contributed to its lack of prognostic significance in the overall multivariate analysis of the whole NPC population. In contrast, Cox Regression analysis of the North American Prospective Collaborate Study has shown that the WHO Type 1 histology is an independent poor prognosticator among other factors.[32] Therefore, the lack of prognostic significance of WHO Type 1 histology with respect to WHO Types 2 and 3 in our study[19] is the likely result of an overwhelming preponderance of the latter two histologies (98% WHO Types 2 and 3; 2% WHO Type 1). The same can be said about the other Hong Kong series that showed no difference in prognosis between the histological subtypes. As a consequence, our conclusions on significant prognosticators and stage-classifications should be applicable largely to NPC of the WHO Types 2 and 3.[43,46] Their application to the WHO Type 1 is subject to verification in populations in whom this histological sub-type constitutes a greater proportion of NPC histologies.

Thus, after comparing the results of our present series of 903 non-disseminated NPC patients and those of other recently published series in the last decade the following conclusions can be drawn about significant prognosticators affecting NPC in the modern CT era:

1) The independent significant prognosticators that are of primary importance include the age and sex of the patient, presence of cranial nerve(s) palsy, presence of skull base erosion, presence of cervical nodal metastasis and in the case of cervical nodal metastases, their level (Ho's level) in the neck.
2) The independent significant prognosticators that are of secondary importance include the presence of oropharyngeal infiltration, parapharyngeal infiltration, involvement of infratemporal fossa(e), orbit(s) and laryngopharynx (hypopharynx) as a whole group, and nodal fixation and nodal contralaterality/bilaterality in the case of presence of nodal metastasis.

These should form the scientific foundation in the formulation of the modern stage-classification for NPC.

Derivation of a New Stage-classification for NPC

Based on significant prognosticators and using multiple steps of monovariate comparisons for local control, distant metastasis and survival rates, a new stage-classification, which accurately depicts prognosis is proposed (*Table 4*).

The ability to separate the proposed T- and N-stage groupings is demonstrated in *Figures 6, 7 and 8*. A large number of T-N combinations become possible with the newly derived T- and N-stages which facilitate a step-by-step grouping, comparison and regrouping of the various combinations. Those which resemble each other most closely in clinical outcome and DFS (*Figure 9*) are grouped together into overall stages or sub-stages to form the proposed stage-classification for NPC.

This stage-classification is scientifically based on significant prognostic factors in the present era when CT-scan is routinely used for evaluation of tumour extent. It is thus more accurate and useful than the current classifications detailed in Table 1 in depicting NPC prognosis and guiding treatment strategy.

Table 4. New stage-classification for NPC.

T1		Tumours confined to the nasopharynx
T2	T2a	Tumours with nasal cavity involvement only
	T2b	Tumours with oropharyngeal and/or parapharyngeal involvement with or without nasal cavity involvement
T3		Tumours with skull base involvement with or without nasal, oropharyngeal, and parapharyngeal involvement
T4		Tumours causing cranial nerve(s) palsy and/or infiltrating the orbit(s), the laryngopharynx and the infratemporal fossa(e)
No	No cervical nodal metastasis	
N1a	Ho's N1 with either single node or homolateral node(s)	
N1b	Ho's N1 with multiple nodes and contralateral/bilateral nodes	
N2a	Ho's N2 with mobile node(s)	
N2b	Ho's N2 with fixed/partially fixed node(s)	
N3a	Ho's N3 with mobile node(s)	
N3b	Ho's N3 with fixed/partially fixed node(s)	
Stage I	T1NoMo	
Stage II	T2aNoMo	
	T2bNoMo, T1N1Mo (including T1N1a and T1N1b)	
	T2N1Mo (including T2aN1a, T2aN1b and T2bN1b)	
Stage IIIa	T1/T2N2a, T3No, T3N1a	
b	T1/T2N2b, T4No, T4N1a, T3/T4N1b, T3/T4N2	
Stage IVa	T1/T2N3	
b	T3/T4N3	
c	M1 (any T, any N)	

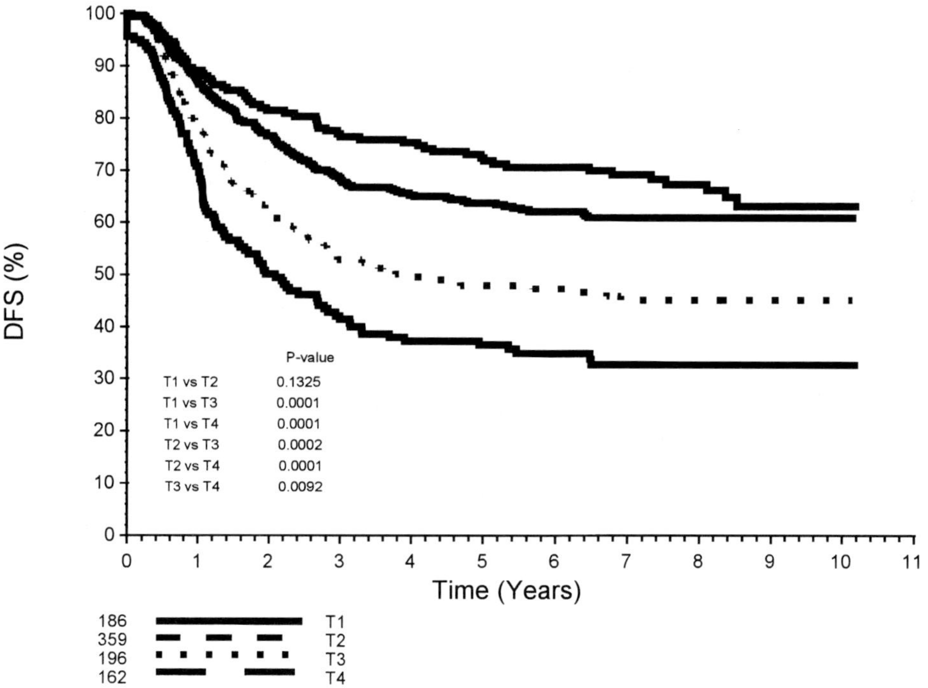

Figure 6. Comparison of DFS between T-stages of the proposed classification.

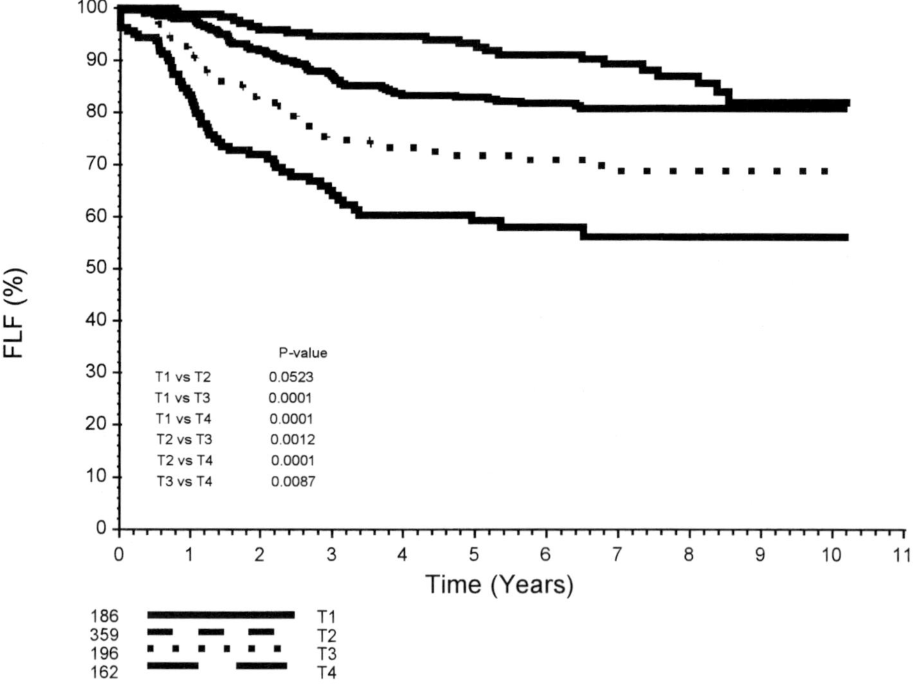

Figure 7. Comparison of FLF between the T-stages of the proposed classification.

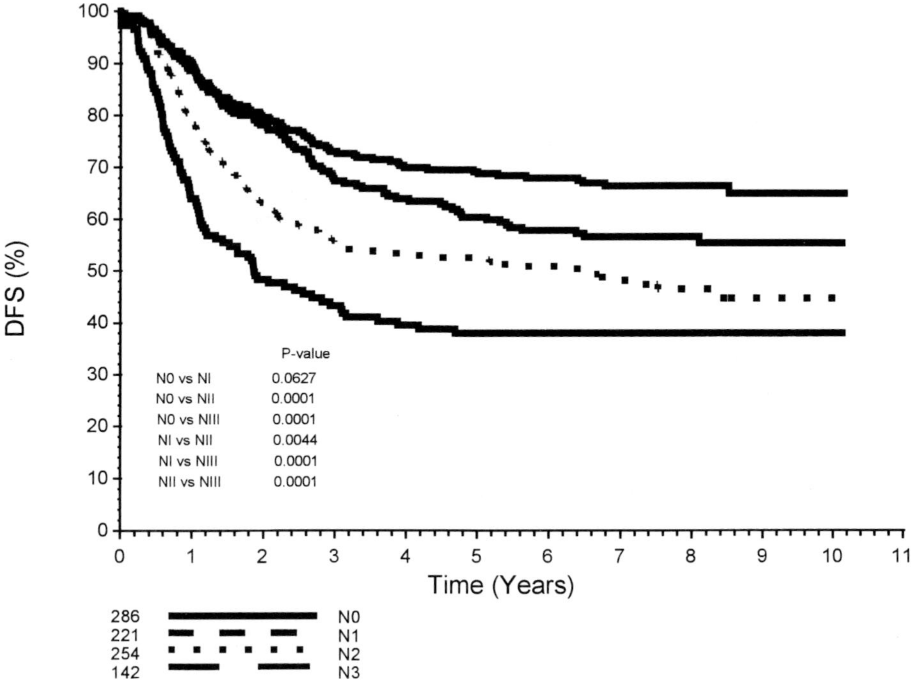

Figure 8. Comparison of DFS between the N-stages of the proposed classification.

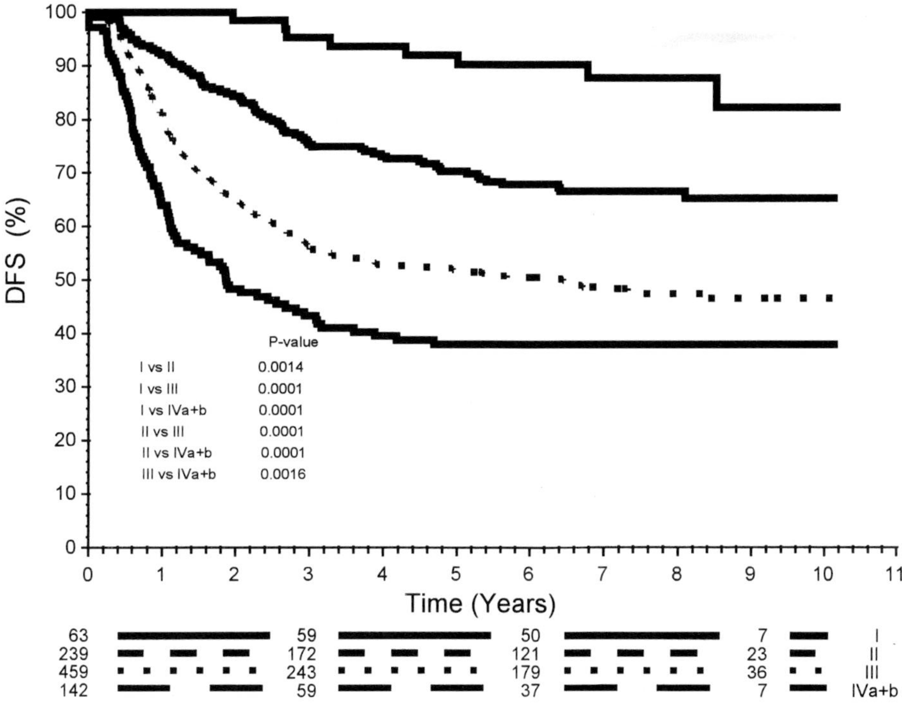

Figure 9. Comparison of DFS between the overall stages of the proposed stage-classification.

References

1. de Thé, G., Ito, Y. (eds.) 1978. *Clinical Staging Recommendation. Nasopharyngeal Carcinoma: Etiology and Control.* Scientific Publications No. 20. Lyon: International Agency for Research on Cancer, 594–595.
2. Fu, K.K. 1980. Prognostic factors of carcinoma of the nasopharynx. *Int. J. Radiat. Oncol. Biol. Phys.*; 6:523–526.
3. Ho, J.H.C. 1978. Stage classification of nasopharyngeal carcinoma: a review. In: *Nasopharyngeal Carcinoma: Etiology and Control*, eds. G. de Thé, G., Ito, Y. Scientific Publications No. 20. Lyon: International Agency for Research on Cancer, 99–113.
4. Huang, S.C. 1980. Nasopharyngeal cacner: a review of 1605 patients treated radically with cobalt 60. *Int. J. Radiat. Oncol. Biol. Phys.*; 6:401–407.
5. International Union Against Cancer. 1987. *TNM Classification of Malignant Tumors.* Berlin: Springer-Verlag.
6. Neel, H.B., Taylor, W.F. 1990. Epstein-Barr virus-related antibody; changes in titers after therapy for nasopharyngeal carcinoma. *Arch. Otolaryngol. Head Neck Surg.*; 116:1287–1290.
7. O'Sullivan, B., Strong, E., Ho, J., Teo, P., Lee, A., Chua, J., Cai, W. 1996. *The AJC/UICC Nasopharyngeal Carcinoma Staging Classification for the 5th Revision of the TNM.* Abstract of 4th International Head and Neck Cancer Conference in Toronto.
8. Teo, P., Leung, S.F., Yu, P., Lee, W.Y., Shiu, W. 1991. A retrospective comparison between different stage classification for nasopharyngeal carcinoma. *Brit. J. Radiol.*; 64:901–908.
9. Teo, P., Tsao, S.Y., Ho, J.H.C., Yu, P. 1991. A proposed modification of the Ho stage-classification for nasopharyngeal carcinoma. *Radiother. Oncol.*; 21:11–23.
10. Hoppe, R.T., Goffinet, D.R., Bagshaw, M.A. 1976. Carcinoma of the nasopharynx. Eighteen year's experience with megavoltage radiation therapy. *Cancer*; 36:2605–2612.
11. Li, C.C., Pan, Q.C., Chen, J.J. 1983. Clinical and experimental research on carcinoma of the nasopharynx. *Science Technol. Guangdong Prov.*; 199–252. (in Chinese).
12. Sham, J.S.T., Choy, D. 1990. Prognostic factors of nasopharyngeal carcinoma: a review of 759 patients. *Brit. J. Radiol.*; 63:51–58.
13. Ho, J.H.C. 1978. An epidemiologic and clinical study of nasopharyngeal carcinoma. *Int. J. Radiat. Oncol. Biol. Phys.*; 4:183–198.
14. Ho, J.H.C. 1982. Nasopharynx. In: *Treatment of Cancer*, eds. Halnan, K.E., Boak, J.L., Crowther, D., von Essen, C.F., Orr, J.S., Peckham, M.J. New York: Igaku-shoin, 249–267.
15. American Joint Committee on Cancer. 1988. *Manual for Staging of Cancer.* Philadelphia: J.B. Lippincott.
16. Qin, D., Hu, Y., Yan, J., Xu, G., Cai, W., Wu, X., Cao, D., Gu, X. 1988. Analysis of 1369 patients with nasopharyngeal carcinoma treated by radiation. *Cancer*; 61:1117–1124.
17. Sham, J.S.T., Choy, D. 1991. Prognostic value of paranasopharyngeal extension of nasopharyngeal carcinoma on local control and short-term survival. *Head Neck*; 13:298–310.
18. Teo, P., Lee, W.Y., Yu, P. 1996. The prognostic significance of parapharyngeal tumour involvement in nasopharyngeal carcinoma. *Radiother. Oncol.*; 38:209–221.
19. Teo, P., Shiu, W., Leung, S.F., Lee, W.Y. 1992. Prognostic factors in nasopharyngeal carcinoma investigated by computer tomography. An analysis of 659 patients. *Radiother. Oncol. I*; 23:79–93.
20. Teo, P., Yu, P., Lee, W.Y., Leung, S.F., Kwan, W.H., Yu, K.H., Choi, P., Johnson, P.J. 1996. Significant prognosticators after primary radiotherapy in 903 nondisseminated nasopharyngeal carcinoma evaluated by computer tomography. *Int. J. Radiat. Oncol. Biol. Phys.*; 36(2):291–304.
21. Lee, A.W.M., Foo, W., Chan, D.K.K. 1994. Nasopharyngeal carcinoma: evaluation of N-staging by Ho and AJCC/UICC System. ASTRO Abstracts No. 86. Proceedings of the American Society for Therapeutic Radiology and Oncology 36th Annual Meeting. *Int. J. Radiat. Oncol. Biol. Phys.*; 30(1):202.
22. Sham, J.S., Choy, D., Choi, P. 1990. Nasopharyngeal carcinoma: the significance of neck node involvement in relation to the pattern of distant failure. *Brit. J. Radiol.*; 63(746):108–113.

23. Teo, P., Tsao, S.Y., Shiu, W., Leung, W.T., Tsang, V., Yu, P., Lui, C. 1989. A clinical study of 407 cases of nasopharyngeal carcinoma in Hong Kong. *Int. J. Radiat. Oncol. Biol. Phys.*; 17:515–530.
24. Lee, A.W.M., Law, S.C.K., Foo, W., Poon, Y.F., Chan, D.K.K., O, S.K., Tung, S.Y., Cheung, F.K., Thaw, M., Ho, J.H.C. 1993. Nasopharyngeal carcinoma: local control by megavoltage irradiation. *Brit. J. Radiol.*; 66:528–536.
25. Meyer, J.E., Wang C.C. 1971. Carcinoma of the nasopharynx, factors influencing results of therapy. *Radiology*; 100:375–378.
26. Moench, H.C., Phillips, T.L. 1972. Carcinoma of the nasopharynx, review of 146 patients with emphasis on radiation dose and time factor. *Am. J. Surg.*; 124:515–518.
27. Wang, C.C., Meyer, J.E. 1971. Radiotherapeutic management of carcinoma of the nasopharynx, an analysis of 170 patients. *Cancer*; 28:566–570.
28. Fletcher, G.H., Million, R.R. 1980. Nasopharynx. In: *Textbook of Radiotherapy*, 3rd edn., ed. Fletcher, G.H. Philadelphia: Lea & Febiger, 364–373.
29. Ho, J.H.C. 1967. *Nasopharyngeal Cancer,* eds. Muir, C.S., Shanmugaratnam, K. UICC Monograph Series, Vol. 1, No, 35. New York: Medical Examination Publ. Co. Inc., 235–246.
30. Ho, J.H.C. 1967. Radiological diagnosis of nasopharyngeal carcinoma with special reference to its spread through the base of skull. In: *Cancer of the Nasopharynx*, eds. Muir, C.S., Shanmugaratnam, K. UICC Monograph Series, No. 1. Copenhagen: Munksgaard, 237–246.
31. Ho, J.H.C. 1970. The natural history and treatment of nasopharyngeal carcinoma (NPC). In: *Proceedings of the 10th International Cancer Congress, Oncology*, Vol. 4, eds. Clark, R.L., Cumley, R.W., McCay, J.E., Copeland, M.M. Yearbook Medical Publishers, 1–14.
32. Neel, H.B., Taylor, W.F. 1989. New staging system for nasopharyngeal carcinoma: long-term outcome. *Arch. Otolaryngol. Head Neck Surg.*; 115:1293–1303.
33. Zhang, E.P., Lian, P.G., Lai, K.L., Chen, Y.F., Cai, M.D., Zheng, X.F., Guang, X.X. 1989. Radiation therapy of nasopharyngeal carcinoma: prognostic factors based on a 10-year follow up of 1302 patients. *Int. J. Radiat. Oncol. Biol. Phys.*; 16:301–305.
34. Ho, J.H.C., Lau, W.H., Fong, M., Chan, C.L. 1983. Treatment of nasopharyngeal carcinoma: current status. In: *Nasopharyngeal Carcinoma: Current Concepts*, eds. Prasad, U., Ablashi, D.V., Levine, P.H., Pearson, G.R. Kuala Lumpur: University of Malaya, 358–385.
35. Yu, K.H., Teo, P., Lee, W.Y., Leung, S.F., Choi, P., Johnson, P.J. 1994. Patterns of early treatment failure in non-metastatic nasopharyngeal carcinoma: a study based on CT scanning. *Clin. Oncol. R. Coll. Radiol.*; 6(3):167–171.
36. Chen, K.Y., Fletcher, G.H. 1971. Malignant tumors of the nasopharynx. *Radiology*; 99:165–171.
37. Vikram, B., Mishra, U.B., Strong, E.W., Manolatos, S. 1985. Patterns of failure in carcinoma of the nasopharynx. I. Failure at the primary site. *Int. J. Radiat. Oncol. Biol. Phys.*; 11:1455–1459.
38. Vikram, B., Strong, E.W., Manolatos, S., Mishra, U.B. 1984. Improved survival in carcinoma of the nasopharynx. *Head Neck Surg.*; 7:123–128.
39. Silver, A.J., Mawad, M.E., Hilal, S.K., Sane, P., Ganti, S.R. 1983. Computed tomography of the nasopharynx and related spaces. *Radiology*; 147:725–731.
40. Yamashita, S., Kondo, M., Hashimoto, S. 1985. Conversion of T-stages of nasopharyngeal carcinoma by computed tomography. *Int. J. Radiat. Oncol. Biol. Phys.*; 11:1017–1024.
41. Yu, Z.H., Xu, G.Z., Huang, Y.R., Hu, Y.H., Su, X.G., Gu, X.Z. 1985. Value of computed tomorgraphy in staging the primary lesion (T staging) of nasopharyngeal carcinoma (NPC): an analysis of 54 patients with special reference to the parapharyngeal space. *Int. J. Radiat. Oncol. Biol. Phys.*; 11:2143–2147.
42. Kwong, D., Sham, J., Choy, D. 1994. The effect of loco-regional control on distant metastatic dissemination in carcinoma of the nasopharynx: an analysis of 1301 patients. *Int. J. Radiat. Oncol. Biol. Phys.*; 30(5):1029–1036.
43. World Health Organization. 1978. *International Histological Classification of Tumours, No. 19. Histological Typing of Upper Respiratory Tract Tumours*. Geneva: World Health Organization, 32–33.

44. Perez, C.A., Ackerman, L.V., Mill, W.B., Ogllra, J.H., Powers, W.E. 1969. Cancer of the nasopharynx: factors influencing prognosis. *Cancer*; 24:1–17.
45. Saw, D., Ho, J.H.C., Fong, M., Chan, C.L., Tse, C.H, Lau, W.H. 1985. Prognosis and histology in stage I nasopharyngeal carcinoma (NPC). *Int. J. Radiat. Oncol. Biol. Phys.*; 11:893–898.
46. Yeh, S.A. 1962. Histological classification of carcinomas of the nasopharynx with a critical review as to the existence of lymphoepitheliomas. *Cancer*; 15:895–920.
47. Shanmugaratnam, K. 1978. Histological typing of nasopharyngeal carcinoma. In: *Nasopharyngeal Carcinoma: Etiology and Control*, eds. de Thé, G., Ito, Y. Scientific Publications No. 20. Lyon: International Agency for Research on Cancer, 3–12.
48. World Health Organization. 1987. *Handbook for Reporting Results of Cancer Treatment*. Geneva: World Health Organization.

CHAPTER 12

Radiotherapy

Peter Teo

In patients without metastatic disease, radiotherapy forms the mainstay of curative treatment.[1–32] There are two main types of delivery, namely external beam radiotherapy, and brachytherapy. External beam radiotherapy is employed as the primary treatment, where the intent is to cure, a radical tumoricidal dose being administered to the primary tumour and, if involved, cervical nodal metastases. The role of brachytherapy is limited to supplementing the nasopharyngeal dose in cases where the tumour persists and to irradiating the cervical tumour bed after radical neck dissection has been performed to eliminate persisting regional tumour. In cases of recurrent tumour, a repeat course of external beam radiotherapy can be given. However, in view of the high radiation dose already given in the primary therapy to the nasopharynx, neck and other organs such as the temporal lobe of brain, it carries a high morbidity.

External Beam Radiotherapy in the Primary Radical Treatment of NPC

Target Volume

The target volume should include the gross tumour, as defined by appropriate clinical and radiological means, together with a "safety margin" where no gross tumour is detected but where microscopic disease is likely to be present. As the sensitivity and accuracy of modern imaging technologies increases, the need to include a large safety margin of normal-looking organs to avoid recurrence due to "geographical miss" diminishes. However, there is still a general lack of consensus on the minimal amount of radiological and clinically normal tissue that should be included in the target volume after MR and CT imaging. In some areas, more than 1 cm of apparently normal tissue beyond the gross tumour volume can be safely included without much added morbidity from radiation. However in other areas, such as the clivus and the ethmoid, such a generous safety margin cannot be included in the target volume without irradiating critical organs to high dose.

In general, the organs at high risk of tumour recurrence include all the structures adjacent to the lesion namely the posterior nasal cavity, the nasopharynx, part of the oropharynx, the parapharyngeal region, the soft palate, the posterior part of the hard palate, the pterygoid plates, the posterior part of the maxillary antra, the posterior ethmoid sinuses, the floor of the sphenoid sinus (or the whole of the sphenoid sinus when its floor is infiltrated by tumour), the foramina lacerum, ovale, spinosum and rotundum, the petrous bones, the basi-sphenoid and basi-occiput, the petro-occipital fissures, the posterior quarter of the bony orbits and the upper neck. However with improved accuracy of modern imaging technology in differentiating between tumour tissue and normal tissue and with increasing availability of 3D-conformal and stereotactic radiotherapy, some of these "normal" organs may, in carefully selected cases, be excluded without jeopardizing local tumour control. However much work is required in this direction before the optimal target volume can be tailor-made for each individual patient.

Dose-fractionation

Conventionally fractionated radiotherapy involves the administration of 1.8 or 2 Gy per fraction, 5 fractions per week, for 7 weeks to a total dose of 70 Gy in treating NPC.[33] Accelerated hyperfractionated radiotherapy (i.e. the same total dose given in a greater number of fractions over a shorter time) has been compared in a retrospective study with conventionally fractionated radiotherapy and has been shown to yield superior local tumour control and survival. However, no prospective studies have confirmed such findings. Wang (1989) reported a 5 year-local control rate for T1–T2 NPC of 89% using hyperfractionated radiotherapy (the "BID program") and 55% using conventionally fractionated radiotherapy.[33] However his 5 year local control for T1–T2 NPC was inferior to that reported in some more modern series.[14,26,28,34] Moreover, the percentage of cases examined by CT scan/MRI before radiotherapy was not reported and it is possible in the conventional radiotherapy group treated between 1975–1979 that many cases with extra-nasopharyngeal involvement could have been understaged as T1–T2[33] tumours, thus accounting for the inferior rate of local tumour control.

In Ang's series the local control was reported to be better after concomitant boost hyperfractionated radiotherapy than after conventional radiotherapy. However as the series contained only 15 patients with NPC or pharyngeal wall cancers[35] in addition to patients with oropharyngeal cancers, the patient number for NPC alone was too small to allow for separate comparison. From 1992 to 1995, we randomized NPC patients to either conventionally fractionated radiotherapy or hyperfractionated radiotherapy[36] (*Table 1*). Interim analysis failed to show a significant difference in local control between the two kinds of radiotherapy. The trial was stopped prematurely in 1995 after the discovery of two symptomatic cases of radiation temporal encephalopathy and one radiation myelopathy in the hyperfractionated radiotherapy group despite the routine practice of separating the two daily fractions by at least 6-hours and limiting the total biological equivalent dose (BED), using an a/ß ratio of two, to a comparable level to that of conventionally fractionated radiotherapy to the cervical spinal cord and the temporal lobes[36] (*Table 2*).

Table 1. Pre-randomization investigations and trial entry criteria.

Hyperfractionated radiotherapy in NPC

Pre-randomization investigations

1. Fibreoptic nasopharyngoscopy and biopsy
2. CT scan of nasopharynx and skull base (axial and coronal)
3. MRI of nasopharynx and skull base (optional to supplement CT scan)
4. Radioisotope bone scan (for advanced T-stage[a] and/or N2/N3 lesions)
5. USG abdomen (for advanced T-stage[a] and/or N2/N3 lesions)
6. Complete blood count and bone/liver profiles
7. IgA and IgG titres versus Epstein-Barr virus antigens

↓

Trial entry criteria

1. Histologically proven NPC
2. No distant metastasis (Mo)
3. Either without cervical nodal metastasis (No), or, small upper cervical metastasis less than or equal to 4 cm (Ho's N1[b] ≤ 4 cm)
4. All T-stages eligible
5. No history of a second malignancy or severe medical illness such as stroke or myocardial infarction or connective tissue diseases
6. No history of previous radiotherapy to the head and neck region
7. Patient's informed consent obtained

↓

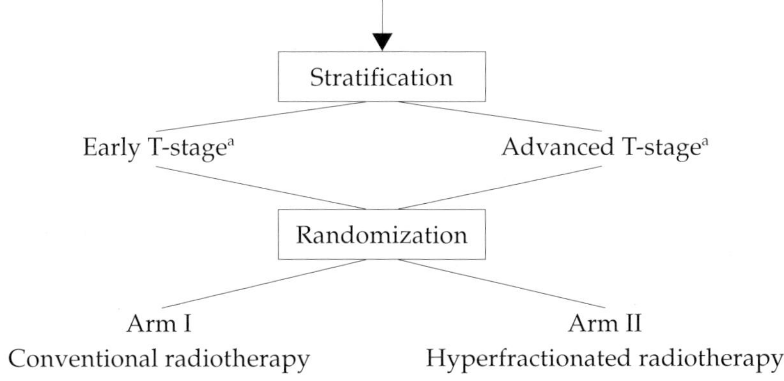

[a] Early T-stage = T1 + T2; advanced T-stage = T3 + tumour with parapharyngeal involvement.
[b] Ho's classiciation 1978.[6,7]

Previous experience in Hong Kong has shown that after conventionally fractionated radiotherapy, symptomatic temporal lobe encephalopathy is rare, while radiation myelopathy is almost unknown.[14] Thus, although not statistically significant, the increase in neurological complications after hyperfractionated radiotherapy in the randomized study,[36] suggested that this method coupled to Ho's radiotherapy technique[6,7] may do more harm than good unless the target volume can be reduced (e.g. by conformal

Table 2. Biological effective dose (BED) for various organs and tissues.

Tissue	Biological effective dose (BED)* without parapharyngeal boost Arm I	Arm II
Tumour		
Nasopharyngeal	75.0	84.4
Cervical nodal metastasis	73.1	77.2
Mucosa		
Nasopharyngeal	75.0	84.4
Oropharyngeal	75.0	84.4
Hypopharyngeal	46.9	51.0
Soft tissue		
Upper neck	117.0	118.3
Supraclavicular fossa	96.3	96.3
Central nervous system		
Temporal lobe	160.0	159.1
Upper cervical spinal chord (1st–3rd cervical vertebrae)	100.0	99.6

* BED calculated by linear-quadratic equation.
10 Gy for acute-reacting tissues including tumour tissue and mucosa; 3 Gy for soft tissue; 1.5 Gy for central nervous tissue.

radiation methods) without causing "geographical misses". To further study this important issue, we intend to initiate a new prospective randomized study which incorporates conformal radiotherapy techniques and compares conventional radiotherapy with hyperfractionated radiotherapy using concomitant boost (*Table* 3).

Dose Tumour Response

There has been a lack of consensus on the optimal time-dose-fractionation. Most series have recommended the use of a total conventional (2 Gy/fraction, 5 fractions/week) radiation dose in the order of 60–70 Gy,[1–32] below which a dose-tumour-control relationship has been demonstrated.[43] Hitherto, there has been much controversy concerning the existence of a different radiosensitivity between the various histological subtypes (WHO Type I versus II and III).[8,18,19,22,30,32,37–42] Though unproven, there is a possibility that higher total radiation dose is required for the keratinizing well-differentiated squamous cell carcinoma (WHO Type I).[42]

In T1 tumours, it has been suggested[1,44] that 60 Gy may be adequate but others[16,18,30] have demonstrated that better control can be achieved with higher doses. It was found that the total dose was the most important factor in determining local tumour control using 45.6 to 60 Gy with a fractional dose ranging from 2.5 to 4.2 Gy and a median

Table 3. Flow chart for trial HRT.

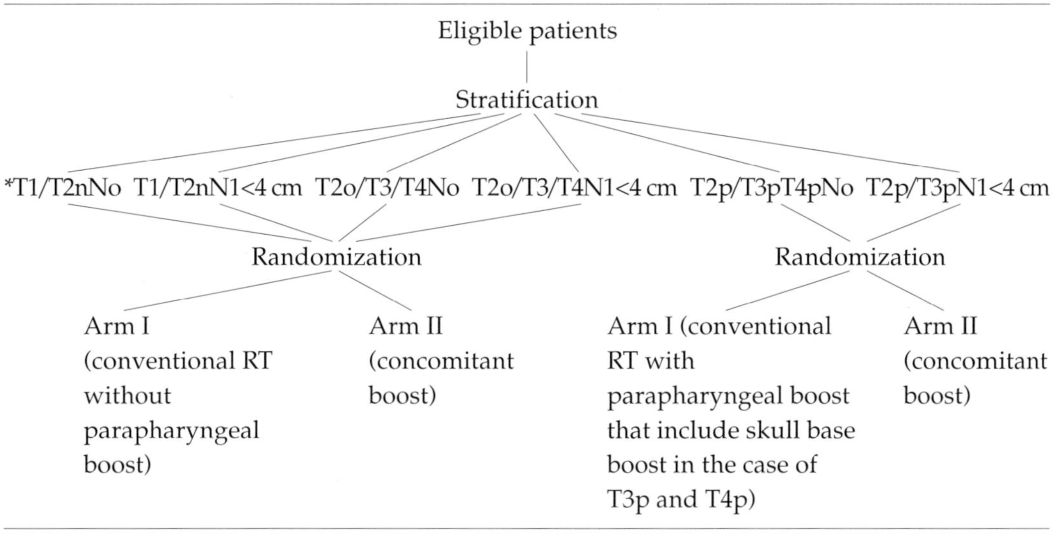

- * T1 confined to the nasopharynx.
- T2n with nasal cavity involvement only.
- T2o with oropharyngeal involvement with/without nasal cavity involvement.
- T2p with parapharyngeal involvement with/without oropharyngeal/nasal cavity involvement.
- T3 involving the skull base without T4-features and without parapharyngeal involvement.
- T3p involving the skull base and parapharynx but without T4-features.
- T4 with cranial nerve(s) palsy, intracranial extension, infratemporal fossa, laryngopharyngeal or orbital infiltration. No parapharyngeal involvement.
- T4p same as T4 except with parapharyngeal involvement.

overall time of 39 days.[43] The hazard of local failure decreased by 9% per additional Gy ($p < 0.01$).Our own experience in the Prince of Wales Hospital in Hong Kong has favoured the existence of a dose-tumour response/control relationship for NPC above the conventional tumoricidal dose of 60–70 Gy. This hypothesis is supported by the following:-

(i) The administration of booster radiotherapy for bulky parapharyngeal tumour extending to 4 cm or more lateral to the midline resulted in superior local tumour control than that of non-bulky parapharyngeal tumours without boost.[27] Retrospective study of the radiation plan for each case revealed that "geographical misses" accounted for less than 2% of the local recurrences in the non-bulky parapharyngeal tumours. Therefore, the increased number of local recurrences in the non-bulky parapharyngeal tumours was probably attributable to the omission of booster radiotherapy and the delivery of a lower total tumour dose.[27] In view of this, since 1987 all NPC's with parapharyngeal involvement were given booster radiotherapy (20 Gy) in addition to the conventional dose of radiotherapy (62.5 Gy), irrespective of the bulk of the parapharyngeal disease.

In a recent analysis of 903 patients,[34] parapharyngeal tumour involvement was significant in governing the distant metastasis rate of Ho's T2 tumours. In T2 tumours (i.e. NPC with extranasopharyngeal soft tissue infiltration only) we found that parapharyngeal tumour involvement significantly worsened the survival and increased the distant metastasis rate (*Figure 1*). The local control was adversely affected by oropharyngeal infiltration (*Figure 2*). Those patients with parapharyngeal tumour involvement who received booster radiotherapy (PPB) after conventional radiotherapy showed a trend towards improvement in local tumour control, short of statistical significance ($p = 0.06$). However, the trend towards improved local tumour control after boost existed only in Ho's T2 (*Figure 3*), and not in T3 cases. It is likely that our routine administration of booster radiotherapy (20 Gy) to all NPC cases with parapharyngeal involvement since 1987 has improved local control.[34] It is also likely that parapharyngeal tumours which were associated with skull base erosion and/or cranial nerve(s) palsy (i.e. Ho's T3) are inadequately covered by the treatment volume of the booster radiation thus rendering the boost ineffective in enhancing local control. Nonetheless, the efficacy of the boost in enhancing local control in NPC with parapharyngeal involvement but without skull base or cranial nerve infiltration,[6,7] serves as a prima facie case that a dose-tumour-response relationship exists beyond the conventional tumoricidal dose level for the tumour.

(ii) "Local persistence" diagnosed at 4–5 weeks after completion of external beam radiotherapy (ERT) has been shown to be a risk factor in predicting local failures in NPC.[45] By treating such local persistence with intracavitary brachytherapy (ICT) the local failure rate was significantly reduced where the primary tumour was confined to the nasopharynx or with extension only to the nasal cavity[45] (*Figure 4*). If this tendency to local failure in those early T-stage tumours that persist soon after ERT can effectively be reduced by ICT, it would be logical to assume that a dose-tumour-response/control relationship exists beyond the conventional ERT dose.

Based on the above and additional supporting evidence,[46,47] we can conclude, with some degree of confidence, that a dose-tumour control relationship exists beyond the conventional tumoricidal dose levels for certain NPCs. However, since the rate and severity of complications also increase with dose (see Chapter 14), the total tumour radiation dose cannot be increased indefinitely without prohibitive radiation morbidity. It is thus important to define the optimal dose level for the maximal therapeutic ratio in the modern era of 3D-conformal radiotherapy by which radiation dose to critical normal organs can be minimized.

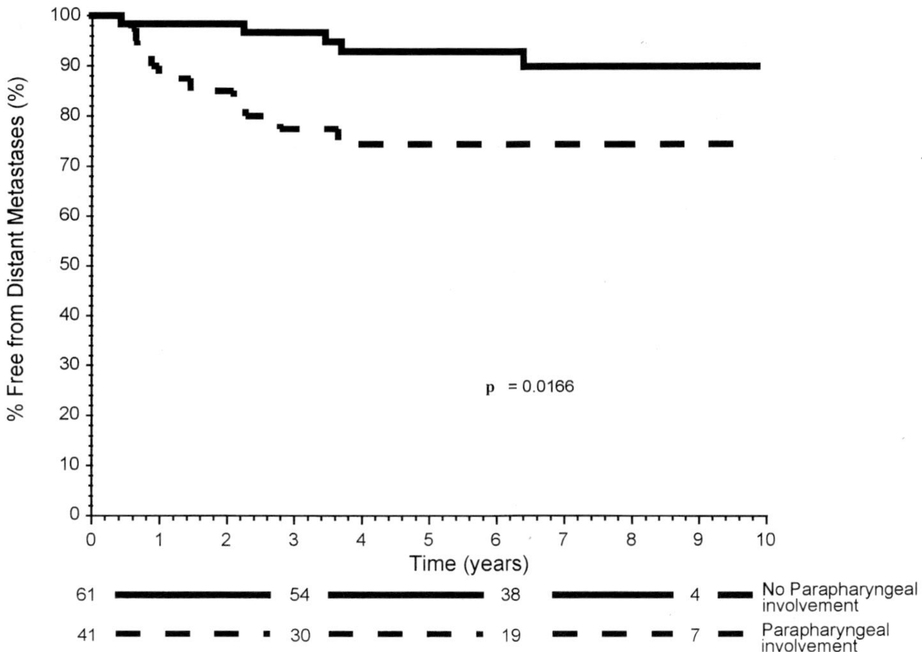

Figure 1. Comparison of the free from distant metastasis rate between T2N0 tumours with and without parapharyngeal involvement.

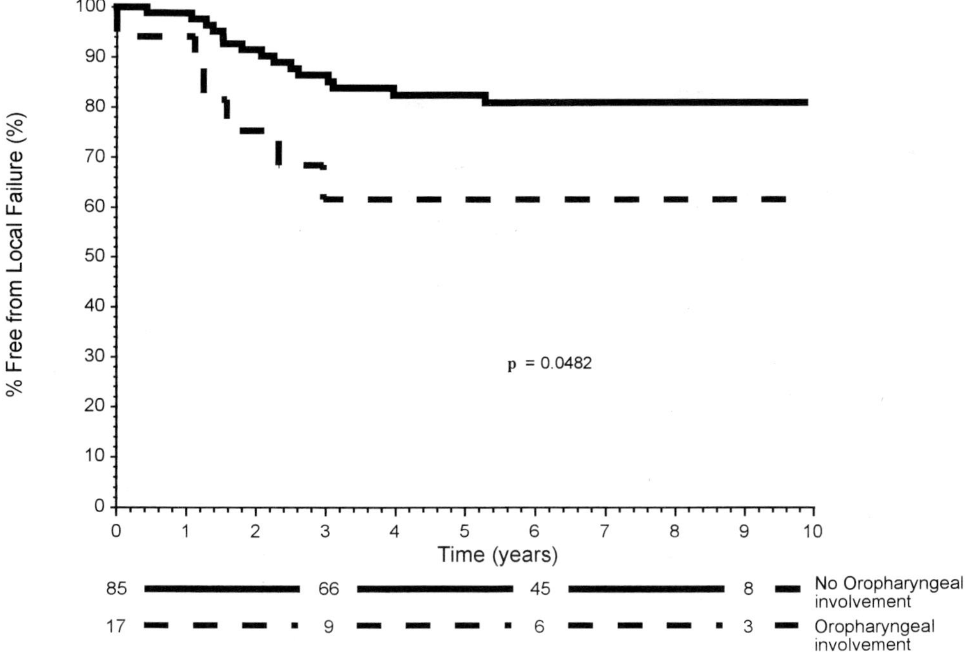

Figure 2. Comparison of the free from local failure rate between T2-tumours with and without oropharyngeal involvement.

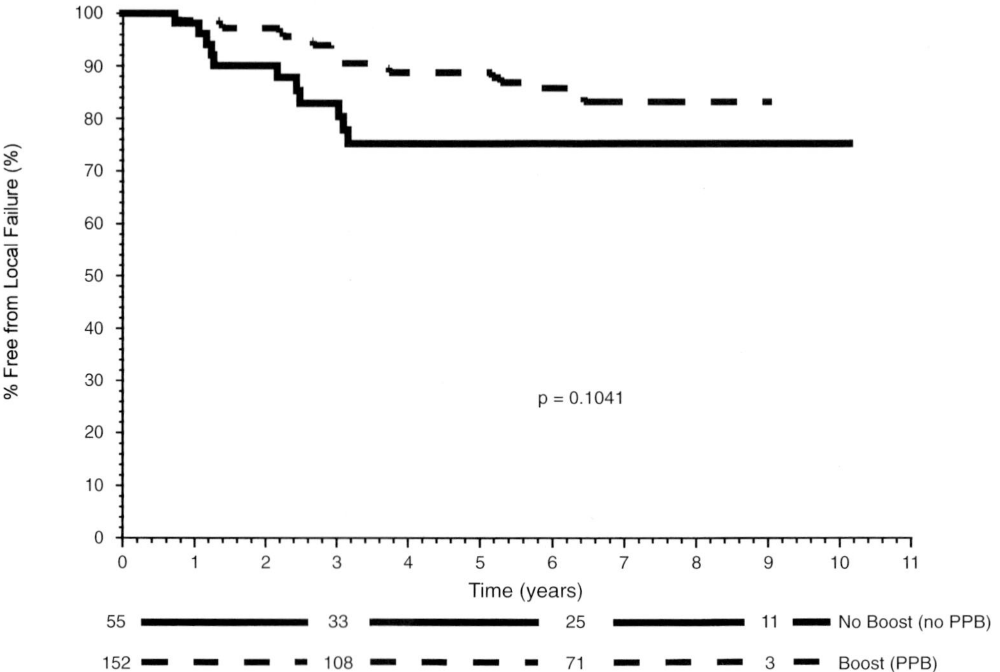

Figure 3. Comparison of the free from local failure rate between the T2 parapharyngeal tumours given booster radiotherapy with external beam (PPB) and those not given PPB.

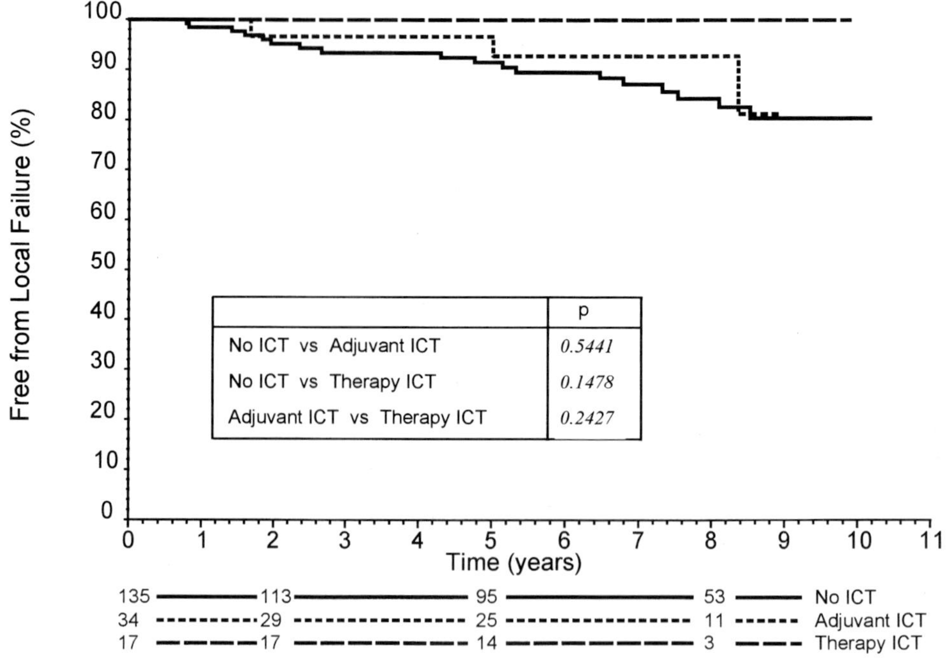

	p
No ICT vs Adjuvant ICT	*0.5441*
No ICT vs Therapy ICT	*0.1478*
Adjuvant ICT vs Therapy ICT	*0.2427*

Figure 4. Comparison of the free from local failure rate between patients given therapeutic ICT (for local persistence), patients given adjuvant ICT and patients who were not subjected to ICT.

Brachytherapy in the Primary Radical Treatment of NPC

The role of brachytherapy in the primary radical treatment for NPC can be classified according to its indication:-

1) local persistence (residual tumour within 4-months after primary radical radiotherapy; (*Table 4*),
2) adjuvant (supplementary to the primary external beam radiotherapy in the complete responders), *Table 5*, and
3) regional persistence in which brachytherapy is used in conjunction with radical neck dissection.

Local Persistence

The definition of local persistence varies between reports and the time interval between completion of primary radiotherapy and additional radiation varies from weeks to months (*Table 3*). A randomized study[46] has shown that histologically proven local persistence after primary radiotherapy runs a significantly higher risk of local failure than the histologically proven complete responders and those with local persistence given additional radiation. With the introduction of the CT scan and improved accuracy of radiotherapy, local persistence rates of 71/826 (8.6%) at 4–6 weeks and 344/4128 (8.3%) at 8–12 weeks after primary ERT were reported by Teo *et al.*[48] and Lee *et al.*[13] respectively. Therefore, the persistence within 3 months after ERT lies between 8–13%. Although spontaneous complete regression of the local persistences occurred in a half to two-thirds of the cases,[46,47] the rate of conversion to histological complete remission was significantly increased to above 90% after boost. Since achievement of the complete remission (CR) status is the first, and probably the most important, step towards final local tumour control, booster radiotherapy by increasing the CR rate of the local persistence should enhance ultimate local tumour control.

Not only will at least one third of the residual tumours diagnosed at various intervals within 3–4 months after primary ERT persist indefinitely,[13,46–48] they will also carry a higher risk of local recurrence compared to the complete responders in the T3–4 cases.[45] While intracavitary brachytherapy delivering 24 Gy/3 fractions/15 days to 1 cm perpendicularly dorsal to the midpoint of the plane of sources improved the local control for the persistent T1, it did not rectify the situation for the persistent T3+4.[45] Innovative radiation methods that can cater for a larger target volume than that possible by means of brachytherapy are required to treat the local T3 and T4 persistence adequately.[49] Stereotactic radiosurgery (SRS) or stereotactic radiotherapy (SRT) are possible options in these cases.

Adjuvant to Primary ERT

The modern standards set for the primary ERT are essentially based on the results of the series of Lee *et al.*[14,50] and Teo *et al.*[28] Lee *et al.* reported a cumulative local failure rate

Table 4. Brachytherapy for local persistence.

Author/year	Brachytherapy dose/technique	1 ERT	Interval between 1 ERT & brachytherapy or additional ERT	No. of patients	New UICC/AJC T-stage percentage T1	T2	T3	T4	% complete response	5 year local control	5 year survival
Choy 1993[58]	60 Gy 0.5 cm from implant Au-198 (4–14 grains) (mean 7 grains)	62.5 Gy	8–16 weeks	10	75		25	0	—	80%	83%
Zhang 1989[60]	a) 20 Gy at 0.25 cm submucosa in 1 fraction by ICT(HDR, Co-60)	70 Gy	1–2 weeks	14	87.5		10.9	1.7	—	95%	—
	b) 45–50Gy at 0.25 cm in 3–4 weekly fraction by ICT.	70 Gy	12 weeks	2							
Yan 1989[47]	Additional ERT, without brachytherapy, 20–50Gy; 3–4Gy/fractions; 2fractions/week)	70 Gy	0–2 weeks (additional ERT)	92	52		48		—	T1 83.3% T2–4 48%	54%
		70 Gy	— (No additional ERT)	90	36.7		63.3		21%	T1 54.5% T2–4 33%	21%

Lee 1993[13]	20Gy LDR-Co-60 ICT to 1cm submucosa	62.5 Gy (55–70 Gy)	8–12 weeks	47 (ICT alone)	32	21	47	89%	76% (10 year local control 67%)	
	(7 patients: additional ERT 20–30 Gy + 20 Gy ICT 113 patients: additional ERT 11Gy)	62.5 Gy (55–70 Gy)	8–12 weeks	120 (additional ERT ± ICT)						>60%
Teo 1994[48]	24Gy/3 fractions/15 days to 1cm from midpoint of plane of sources ICT (HDR, Ir-192)	62.5 Gy	4–6 weeks	71	59		41	74.1%	—	71% (5 year DFS 62.4%)
Yin 1995[64]	16-24 Gy/2–3 fractions/8–15 days to 1–1.2 cm from applicators	60–70 Gy	1–3 weeks	33	—		—		2 year local control 100%	—
Lin 1995[59]	5–27 Gy/1–3 weekly fractions to 1 cm from axis of the source by HDR-ICT	50–80 Gy	?	30				80%	—	—

Table 5. Brachytherapy as adjuvant boost to primary external radiotherapy.

Author/year	Brachytherapy	1 ERT	Interval after 1 ERT	No. of patients	New UICC/AJC T-stage (percentage/number) T1	T2	T3	T4	5 year local control	5 year survival
Yamashita 1986[65]	8Gy/2 fractions/8 days to 0.5cm submucosa ICT (LDR, Co-60)	66–70Gy	2 weeks	12	25 (3)	16.7 (2)	58.3 (7)		2 year 92% (only 1/12 local recurrence after mean follow-up of 21.8 months)	—
Amornmarn 1983[53]	10 Gy (? reference point) by ICT (LDR, Ra)	60 Gy	? (soon)	12	0 (0)		100 (12)		92%	5 year DFS 75%
Zhang 1989[60]	10 Gy (? reference point) by ICT (HDR Co-60)	60–66Gy	? (soon)	19	77 (?)	20 (?)	3 (?)		91.4% (with maximum follow-up of only 4-years	—
Vikram 1994[66]	160 Gy in 1 year to the max. isodose rate surface encompassing I-125 seeds (median 11 seeds)	60 Gy (50–70 Gy)	2–10 weeks (median 4 weeks)	20	35 (7)	30 (6)	35 (7)		2 year = 100% (median follow-up = 2 years; range 1–5 years)	2 year ASR 85%
Wang 1989[33]	7Gy at 0.5 cm submucosa in one fraction by ICT (LDR, Cs-137)	bid program 64 Gy q.d. program 66 Gy	2 weeks	75 (bid 38 + (q.d. 37)	100 (75)	—	—	—	T1 bid-5 year local control 89% T1 qd-5 year local control 55%	T1–T4 bid-program 5 year ASR 85%
Chang 1995[52]	5–16.5Gy/1–3 fractions to 2 cm from central axis of sources of ICT (LDR)	64.8–68.4Gy	? (soon)	129 (72.5Gy) 54 (<72.5Gy)	100 (183)	—	—	—	T1 (72.5Gy) 93%; all patients 83%	5 year ASR 85.8% (but 9% severe complication)
Levendag 1992[67]	12–18 Gy/4–6 fractions/2–3 days ICT-HDR at 0.75 cm from source axis	60–70 Gy	? (soon)	24	?	?	?	?	1 year local control 96%	—

of 24% and 5-year and 10-year local control rates of 72% and 67% respectively in 4128 patients.[50] Teo *et al.* reported a cumulative local failure rate of 20.8% and a 5-year local control of 78.8%. In both series, 2-year and 3-year local control rates of 85–90% and 80–85% respectively were achieved without routine application of adjuvant brachytherapy and despite a high proportion of T3–4 tumours (40–50%). In the absence of documentation of the local tumour status at the completion of primary ERT, it is often not possible to differentiate between reports on brachytherapy used as adjuvant treatment and to treat local persistence. Nonetheless, as only a minority of tumours persist locally after primary ERT (8–13%), the series employing brachytherapy to supplement ERT should essentially be regarded as relevant to the adjuvant use of brachytherapy (*Table 5*).

More convincing data of 5-year local control have been reported employing adjuvant brachytherapy with longer follow-up durations and larger patient numbers.[51–53] However the results of these series showed no clear superiority over those of Lee and Teo. Our own results showed no improvement in local tumour control by adjuvant intracavitary brachytherapy when comparing 52 patients (T1+T2) given adjuvant ICT (18 Gy/3 fractions/15 days) with 425 patients (T1+T2) given primary ERT.[45] Therefore the benefit of adjuvant brachytherapy in the complete responders to primary ERT has remained unproven.

Thus we may conclude that local persistence occurs in 8–13% of NPC after primary external radiotherapy. One half to two-thirds of the local persistence diagnosed within 4-months after ERT can regress completely spontaneously; the rest will persist indefinitely and result in genuine local failure. The diagnosis of local persistence at 4–6 weeks after ERT has been associated with a significantly higher rate of ultimate local failure in the T3–4 tumours. Brachytherapy has substantially increased the rate of conversion to histological complete remission of the local persistence diagnosed within 4-months after ERT. In the locally persisting early T-stage tumour, brachytherapy can improve the local control, but for the T3–4 that persists, it is ineffective. Although the morbidity of the adjuvant brachytherapy has been acceptable in all reports, its present use cannot be recommended outside the context of a clinical trial setting. Indeed at the author's institution a prospective randomized study is already planned.

Radiotherapy for Recurrent Tumour

Local Recurrence

Re-irradiation has been the most commonly employed method to treat local recurrences, although other methods such as nasopharyngectomy and photodynamic treatment are possible alternatives in selected cases. To date there have been no prospective randomized studies to compare the efficacy of the different methods for the salvage of local recurrences in NPC. Choice is based on the extent of the recurrent tumour (e.g. resectable vs non-resectable), the experience and preference of the local practice, and the cost of the treatments. Re-irradiation for local recurrences can be given by external beam, brachytherapy, or both. In either case, a tumoricidal dose of no less than 60 Gy has to be given before a significant chance of local control and survival can be realized.[50,54,55] Both advanced rT-stage and short disease-free interval predict poor survival after re-irradiation. Taking all recurrent T-stages together, the overall outcome of re-irradiation is poor, with 5- and 10-year actuarial cancer-specific survival rates of only 14% and 9%.[50] Moreover, irradiation is associated with significant acute and late complications including, trismus, temporal lobe encephalopathy,[56] cranial neuropathy, endocrine dysfunction, impairment of hearing, persistent otitis and eyeball damage.[50] With improvement in primary radiotherapy after routine use of CT-scan for tumour extent evaluation, the local failure rate has decreased[57] but any local failures seem to be more radioresistent. In addition, with escalation of the primary radiation dose, the administration of tumoricidal re-irradiation (>60 Gy) threatens increased complications.[57] We do not therefore currently recommend the routine use of external beam re-irradiation for the salvage of NPC local failures.

The option of using brachytherapy, with or without external radiotherapy, in the less advanced recurrences should always be considered. In theory at least, brachytherapy can deliver a very high and localized dose to the recurrence with relative sparing of the normal organs. The limitation of brachytherapy is that it cannot adequately irradiate any bulky tumour that erodes the skull base or infiltrates the parapharynx.[57] Nonetheless, very good local control and survival rates have been achieved in well selected patients,[51,54,58–60] (*Table 6*).

In conclusion, an overall 50–60% 5-year local tumour control can be expected from re-irradiation with brachytherapy alone for NPC local recurrence. Better local control and survival can be achieved after the exclusion of rT3 and rT4 cases with CT-scan and MRI. For early local recurrences (rT1+2), local control by brachytherapy alone seems superior to that by combined ERT+BT or a second course of ERT alone (5-year local control 50–60% versus ~30%). However, this could be due to case selection leading to brachytherapy being selected for the more favourable tumours.[49] If the rate of late complications is really not affected by the method of re-irradiation,[50] brachytherapy alone should have a higher therapeutic ratio than ERT+BT or ERT alone, at least for the smaller lesions. However, a prospective randomized study is required to prove this point. In suitably chosen cases (<5 cm tumours confined to the nasopharynx, sparing nasal septum and not particularly necrotic and friable), 5-year local control of 80% is achievable with interstitial implants which deliver a higher local dose than both intracavitary intubation and mould treatment.

With the advent of 3D-conformal external radiotherapy and stereotactic radiotherapy with relocatable frames, new horizons now open for the treatment of locally recurrent NPC. With these methods, the treatment volume conforms better to the planning target volume and the surrounding normal structures can be spared the high radiation dose to a greater degree. Therefore, the formidable task of re-irradiation can be achieved with greater precision and improved therapeutic ratio compared to

Table 6. Brachytherapy for local recurrence.

Author/year	Brachytherapy description	1 ERT	2 ERT (if any)	No. of patients	New UICC/AJC T-stage percentage (number) rT1	rT2	rT3–4	5 year local control	5 year ASR	
Choy 1993[58]	60 Gy 0.5 cm from Au-198 implant (4–14 grains) (mean 7 grains)	62.5 Gy	Nil	28	35 (10)	40 (14)	29 (9)	61%	40%	Headache Palate fistula NP necrosis
Zhang 1989[60]	15–50 Gy at 0.25 cm submucosa by HDR Co-60 ICT	60–70 Gy	45–66 Gy	29	87 (25)	11 (3)	3 (1)	? 22/29 (75.9%) crude survival with maxium 4 year follow-up with only 1/29 (4.7%) further local failure	?	—
Wang 1987[55]	20 Gy/2 fractions/8 days to 0.5 cm submucosa by LDR-ICT	a) bid-64 Gy/5½ wk b) qd-66 Gy/6½ wk	40 Gy	32	100 (32)	—	—	38%	50%	Sphenid floor necosis Cranial nerve palsy Trismus NP necrosis
Fu 1975[54]	35–55 Gy to 1.5 cm from source centre ICT (750–1200 mgh × 2)	60 Gy	30–40 Gy	42	?	?	?	53.6% (7/10 of ICT >45 Gy locally controlled i.e. 62.5%)	41%	—
Lee 1993[50]	a) 40 Gy/4 fractions/2 weeks to 1 cm from midpoint of the plane of sources ICT (LDR Co-60)	62.5 Gy	Nil	38	92 (35)		7.9 (3)	23% No difference between the different methods for local control for the rT1+rT2 100% local failure in rT3+4 by BT	14%	2 epistaxis No difference in late complicatiion rates between the different methods
	b) 20 Gy/2 fractions/1 week	62.5 Gy	40 Gy	82	91 (75)		9 (7)			
Lin 1995[59]	5–27 Gy to 1cm from axis of source in 1–3 weekly fractions	50–80 Gy	—	10	?	?	?	60% (6/10) crude local control with <2 year follow-up	Nil	Xerostonia Nasal congestion
Gerbaulet 1994[51]	60 Gy to 85% basal dose rate (Paris System) of mould-applicator ICT	?	—	14	?	?	?	50%	17%	—

conventional 2-D radiotherapy. However, until these new radiotherapy techniques are applied widely to a large number of patients and followed up for a significant period, the reduction of radiation complications or the enhancement of tumour control cannot be demonstrated.

Regional Recurrence

Isolated regional recurrences in NPC are uncommon after routine elective neck irradiation for the node-negative patients. Previously, the omission of this treatment, as practised by Lee *et al.* 1989,[61] was associated with a substantial rate of isolated regional recurrences. Not all such recurrences could be salvaged. For the radiotherapy-naive neck, regional disease can be controlled with the same degree of success in the recurrent setting, as for the primary disease. However, in the uncommon situation in which regional recurrence occurs in a previously irradiated neck, radical neck dissection is the preferred form of salvage treatment, since re-irradiation is seldom successful and is associated with a high rate of skin and soft tissue complications.

The role of radiotherapy is limited to the use of brachytherapy for the surgical bed and post-operative external radiation (with small fields and limiting the dose to 45–50 Gy). These two methods of radiotherapy are usually used mutually exclusively to eradicate tumours not completely resected by the surgeon. While Ngan *et al.* 1996[62] used low-dose rate (LDR) Ir-192 wires to afterload the applicators placed in the tumour bed, we have been employing a high dose rate (HDR) remote afterloading method with a similar degree of success. In our own experience, a single plane of applicators, 4–7 in number, spaced at 1.0–1.5 cm apart, provides effective brachytherapy to 40–42 Gy/9–10 fractions/5 days without fear of soft tissue and skin necrosis or carotid artery thrombosis or rupture. Taking into consideration the likelihood of rapid residual tumour regrowth after incomplete surgical resection and the close proximity of the after-loading applicators to the residual tumour, brachytherapy with either LDR or HDR is preferred to external radiotherapy as an adjunctive treatment to radical neck dissection.

In contrast to cases where regional recurrence occurs as an isolated event without local recurrence, simultaneous recurrence at both sites or in sequence is much more common.[14,63] There are two main treatment options. Firstly nasopharyngectomy for the primary disease and radical neck dissection for the regional recurrence and secondly radical re-irradiation for the primary disease and radical neck dissection for the regional recurrence. Although we have no proof of its superiority, our prefence is for the former method. Postoperatively, any residual tumour in the neck can be treated by HDR afterloading brachytherapy as mentioned.

Current Radiotherapy Techniques, Dosage and Treatment Results

Ho's technique has a number of drawbacks. It is a 2-D rather than a 3-D system and the field arrangements are "standard" rather than tailor-made according to the CT/MR-target volumes (planning target volume). The shielding and field borders are also "standard" and positioned at pre-determined distances from various bony landmarks in the plain-radiograph of the skull, rather than being positioned with respect to the boundary of the tumour target. This means that the field coverage is not adjusted according to the extent of the individual tumour. Recently, we have compared Ho's radiation technique and the radiation plans generated by 3-D conformal methods (3DCRT) for the dose-volume-histograms (DVH) of the planning target volume (PTV) and the DVHs of the normal critical organs. Our results show that CRT is significantly better than Ho's technique in encompassing the PTV in the prescription-isodose volume and in the dose-fall-off beyond the PTV. The addition of a vertex-field to six co-axial fields (in the axial plane) provides better isodose coverage of the PTV at the para-pharyngeal regions, which may each extend posteriorly sparing the spinal cord sandwiched between the fields at C1/C2.

If the full tumoricidal dose (66–70 Gy/33–35 fractions/61/2–7 weeks) is delivered via 3DCRT, the dose delivered to the brainstem and the spinal cord is usually less than that via the Ho technique. During the initial phase of Ho's technique, the upper cervical spinal cord is irradiated en bloc with the target volume to 40 Gy/20 fractions/4 weeks. During the latter phase, using 3-fields to treat the primary lesion and a separate anterior cervical field to treat the cervical lymphatics, the brainstem receives 20–30% of the prescribed dose via irradiation from the anterior facial field. Thus the total dose to the spinal cord at C1/C2 level exceeds 40 Gy after primary radiotherapy by the Ho technique. This presents a technical difficulty for radical re-irradiation if such is indicated for the salvage of inoperable local recurrence. Because of the dosimetric advantage of 3DCRT over the Ho technique, the latter should be systematically replaced by the former in the course of time, provided that the logistical constraints of 3DCRT can be overcome and that increased clinical experience in its application substantiates its theoretical superiority.

At present, there is no consensus as to the optimal radiation dose. However, when using the "conventional" fractionation with 2 Gy per daily fraction (10 Gy/5 fractions/week), there is strong evidence to suggest the presence of a dose-tumour-control relationship above 66 Gy–70 Gy, at least for those tumours which fail to regress completely shortly after 66 Gy–70 Gy. In such cases, dose-escalation may enhance eventual local control. On the other hand, dose-escalation to the tumour (PTV) will inevitably risk over-dosing normal critical organs. The importance of meticulous use of 3DCRT and/or stereotactic radiotherapy cannot, therefore, be overemphasized. Prospective randomized trials comparing "conventional" daily fractionation with the altered fractionation are urgently required. By employing radical radiotherapy using the Ho technique we expect to achieve a 10-year local control rate of over 70% for patients with non-disseminated NPC. This rate falls to 44% when the skull base is eroded (without cranial nerve palsy) and 31% when there is infiltration of the cranial nerves. Advances in radiation methods (including 3DCRT/dose-escalation or altered fractionation) may lead to improvement in local control.

References

1. Bedwinek, J.M., Perez, C.A., Keys, D.J. 1980. Analysis of failures after definitive irradiation for epidermoid carcinoma of the nasopharynx. *Cancer*; 45:2725–2729.
2. Bohorquez, J. 1976. Factors that modify the radio-response of cancer of the nasopharynx. *Am. J. Roentgenol.*; 126:863–876.
3. Cellai, E., Chiavacci, A., Okmi, P., Carcangiu, M.L. 1982. Carcinoma of the nasopharynx: results of radiation therapy. *Acta Radiol. Oncol.*; 21:87–95.
4. Chen, K.Y., Fletcher, G.H. 1971. Malignant tumours of the nasopharynx. *Radiology*; 99:166–171.
5. Chen, W.Z., Zhou, D.L., Luo, K.S. 1989. Long-term observation after radiotherapy for nasopharyngeal (NPC). *Int. J. Radiat. Oncol. Biol. Phys.*; 16(2):311–314.
6. Ho, J.H.C. 1978. An epidemiologic and clinical study of nasopharyngeal carcinoma. *Int. J. Radiat. Oncol. Biol. Phys.*; 4:183–198.
7. Ho, J.H.C. 1982. Nasopharynx. In: *Treatment of Cancer*, eds. Halnan, K.E., Boak, J.L., Crowther, D., von Essen, C.F., Orr, J.S., Peckham, M.J. Chapman and Hall, 249–267.
8. Hoppe, R.T., Goffinet, D.R., Bagshaw, M.A. 1976. Carcinoma of the nasopharynx. Eighteen year's experience with megavoltage radiation therapy. *Cancer*; 37:2605–2612.
9. Huang, S.C. 1980. Nasopharyngeal cacner: a review of 1605 patients treated radically with cobalt 60. *Int. J. Radiat. Oncol. Biol. Phys.*; 6:401–407.
10. Itami, J., Mikata, A., Arimizu, N., Ogata, H., Miura, K., Hayasaki, K., Kaneko, T. 1988. Radiation therapy of the nasopharyngeal cancer and its prognostic factors. *Strahlenther Onkol*; 164:446–450.
11. Larson, L.G., Seelig, I. 1976. Malignant nasopharyngeal tumours: result of radiation therapy. *Acta Radiol. Ther. Phys. Biol.*; 15:209–218.
12. Lederman, M. 1961. *Cancer of the Nasopharynx: Its Natural History and Treatment.* Illinois: Springfield.
13. Lee, A.W.M., Law, S.C.K., Foo, W., Poon, Y.F., Chan, D.K.K., O, S.K., Tung, S.Y., Cheung, F.K., Thaw, M., Ho, J.H.C. 1993. Nasopharyngeal carcinoma: local control by megavoltage irradiation. *Brit. J. Radiol.*; 66:528–536.
14. Lee, A.W.M., Poon, Y.F., Foo, W., *et al.* 1992. Retrospective analysis of 5037 patients with nasopharyngeal carcinoma treated during 1976–1985: overall survival and patterns of failure. *Int. J. Radiat. Oncol. Biol. Phys.*; 23:261–270.
15. Lin, T.M., Chen, K.P., Lin, C.C., Hsu, M.M., Tu, S.M., Chiang, T.C., Jung, P.F., Hirayama, T. 1973. Retrospective study on nasopharyngeal carcinoma. *J. Natl. Cancer Inst.*; 51:1403–1408.
16. Mesic, J.B., Fletcher, G.H., Goepfert, H. 1981. Megavoltage irradiation of epithelial tumours of the nasopharynx. *Int. J. Radiat. Oncol. Biol. Phys.*; 7:447–453.
17. Meyer, J.E., Wang, C.C. 1971. Carcinoma of the nasopharynx: factors influencing results of therapy. *Radiology*; 100:385–388.
18. Moench, H.C., Philips, T.L. 1972. Carcinoma of the nasopharynx: review of 146 patients with emphasis on radiation dose and time factors. *Am. J. Surg.*; 124:515–518.
19. Neel, H.B. 1985. Nasopharyngeal carcinoma: clinical presentation, diagnosis, treatment and prognosis. *Otolaryngol. Clin. North Am.*; 28:479–490.
20. O'Sullivan, B., Strong, E., Ho, J., Teo, P., Lee, A., Chua, J., Cai, W. 1996. The AJC/UICC nasopharyngeal carcinoma staging classification for the 5th revision of the TNM. *Abstract of 4th International Head and Neck Cancer Conference in Toronto, 1996.*
21. Payne, D.G. 1983. Carcinoma of the nasopharynx. *J. Otolaryngol.*; 12:197–202.
22. Perez, C.A., Ackerman, L.V., Mill, W.B., *et al.* 1969. Cancer of the nasopharynx: factors influencing prognosis. *Cancer*; 24:1–17.
23. Qin, D., Hu, Y., Yan, J., Xu, G., Cai, W., Wu, X., Cao, D., Gu, X. 1988. Analysis of 1379 patients with nasopharyngeal carcinoma treated by radiation. *Cancer*; 61:1117–1124.

24. Rahima, M., Rakowsky, E., Barzilay, J., Sidi, J. 1986. Carcinoma of the nasopharynx: an analysis of 91 cases and a comparison of differing treatment approaches. *Cancer*; 58:843–849.
25. Scalon, P.W., Rhodes, R.E., Woolner, L.B., Devine, K.D., McBean, J.B. 1967. Cancer of the nasopharynx: 142 patients treated in the 11 year period 1950–1960. *Am. J. Roentgenol.*; 99:313–325.
26. Sham, J.S.T., Choy, D. 1990. Prognostic factors of nasopharyngeal carcinoma: a review of 759 patients. *Brit. J. Radiol.*; 63:51–58.
27. Teo, P., Tsao, S.Y., Shiu, W., Leung, W.T., Tsang, V., Yu, P., Lui, C. 1989. A clinical study of 407 cases of nasopharyngeal carcinoma in Hong Kong. *Int. J. Radiat. Oncol. Biol. Phys.*; 17:515–530.
28. Teo, P., Yu, P., Lee, W.Y., Leung, S.F., Kwan, W.H., Yu, K.H., Choi, P., Johnson, P.J. 1996. Significant prognosticators after primary radiotherapy in 903 non-disseminated nasopharyngeal carcinoma evaluated by computer tomography. *Int. J. Radiat. Oncol. Biol. Phys.*; 36(2):291–304.
29. Thompson, R.W., Doggett, R.L.S., Bagshaw, M.A. 1970. Ten year experience with linear accelerator irradiation of cancer of the nasopharynx. *Radiology*; 97:149–155.
30. Vikram, B., Mishra, U.B., Strong, E.W., Manolatos, S. 1985. Patterns of failure in carcinoma of the nasopharynx I. failure at primary site. *Int. J. Radiat. Oncol. Biol. Phys.*; 11:1455–1459.
31. Wang, C.C. 1980. Treatment of malignant tumours of the nasopharynx. *Otolaryngol. Clin. North Am.*; 13:477–481.
32. Zhang, E.P., Lian, P.G., Cai, K.L., Chen, Y.F., Cai, M.D., Zheng, X.F., Guang, X.X. 1989. Radiation therapy of nasopharyngeal carcinoma: prognostic factors based on a 10-year follow-up of 1302 patients. *Int. J. Radiat. Oncol. Biol. Phys.*; 16:301–305.
33. Wang, C.C. 1989. Accelerated hyperfractionation radiation therapy for carcinoma of the nasopharynx techniques and results. *Cancer*; 63:2461–2467.
34. Teo, P., Lee, W.Y., Yu, P. 1996. The prognostic significance of parapharyngeal tumour involvement in nasopharyngeal carcinoma. *Radiother. Oncol.*; 39:209–221.
35. Ang, K.K., Peters, L.J., Weber, R.S., *et al.* 1991. Concomitant boost radiotherapy schedules in the treatment of carcinoma of the oropharynx and nasopharynx. *Int. J. Radiat. Oncol. Biol. Phys.*; 19:1339–1345.
36. Teo, P., K., W.H., Leung, S.F., Leung, W.T., Chan, A., Choi, P., Yu, P., Lee, W.Y., Johnson, P.J. 1996. Early tumour response and treatment toxicity after hyperfractionated radiotherapy in nasopharyngeal carcinoma. *Brit. J. Radiol.*; 69:241–248.
37. Bloom, S.M. 1961. Cancer of nasopharynx with spinal reference to the significance of histopathology. *Laryngoscope*; 71:1207–1260.
38. Chen, J.Y., Chen, C.J., Liu, M.Y., *et al.* 1989. Antibodies to Epstein-Barr virus-specific DNase as a marker for field survey of patients with nasopharyngeal carcinoma in Tai-wan. *J. Med. Virol.*; 27:269–273.
39. Fu, K.K. 1980. Prognostic factors of carcinoma of the nasopharynx. *Int. J. Radiat. Oncol. Biol. Phys.*; 6:523–526.
40. Hoppe, R.T., Williams, J., Warnke, R., Goffinet, D.R., Bagshaw, M.A. 1978. Carcinoma of the nasopharynx: the significance of histology. *Int. J. Radiat. Oncol. Biol. Phys.*; 4:199–205.
41. Saw, D., Ho, J.H.C., Fong, M., Chan, C.L., Tse, C.H., Lau, W.H. 1985. Prognosis and histology in stage I nasopharyngeal carcinoma (NPC). *Int. J. Radiat. Oncol. Biol. Phys.*; 11:893–898.
42. Shanmugaratnam, K. 1978. Histological typing of nasopharyngeal carcinoma. In: *Nasopharyngeal Carcinoma: Etiology and Control*, eds. de Thé, G., Ito, Y. Scientific Publications No. 20. Lyon: International Agency for Research on Cancer, 3–12.
43. Lee, A.W.M, Chan, D.K.K., Fowler, J.F., Poon, Y.F., Foo, W., Law, S.C.K., O, S.K., Tung, S.Y., Chappell, R. 1995. Effect of time, dose and fractionation on local control of nasopharyngeal carcinoma. *Radiother. Oncol.*; 36:24–31.
44. Chang, C., Liu, T., Chang, Y., Cao, S. 1980. Radiation therapy of nasopharyngeal carcinoma. *Acta Radiol. Oncol.*; 19 (Fasc 6):433–438.
45. Teo, P., Kwan, W.H., Yu, P., Lee, W.Y., Leung, S.F., Choi, P. 1996. A retrospective study of the role of intracavitary brachytherapy and the prognosticators determining local tumour control after primary radical radiotherapy in 903 non-disseminated nasopharyngeal carcinoma. *Clin. Oncol.*; 8:160–166.

46. Yan, J.H., Xu, G.Z., Hu, Y.H., Li, S.Y., Lie, Y.Z., Qin, D.X., Wu, X.L., Gu, X.Z. 1990. Management of local residual primary lesion of nasopharyngeal carcinoma: IL results of prospective randomized trial on booster dose. *Int. J. Radiat. Oncol. Biol. Phys.*; 18:295–298.
47. Yan, J.H., Qin, D.X., Hu, Y.H., Cai, W.M., Xu, G.Z., Wu, X.L., Li, S.Y., Gu, X.Z. 1989. Management of local residual primary lesion of nasopharyngeal carcinoma (NPC): are higher doses beneficial? *Int. J. Radiat. Oncol. Biol. Phys.*; 16:1466–1469.
48. Teo, P., Leung, S.F., Choi, P., Lee, W.Y., Johnson, P.J. 1994. Afterloading radiotherapy for local persistence of nasopharyngeal carcinoma. *Brit. J. Radiol.*; 67:181–185.
49. Teo, P. 1996. The role of brachytherapy in nasopharyngeal carcinoma. In: *Proceedings of the 4th International Conference on Head and Neck Cancer, Toronto, July 28–August 1, 1996*, 597–610.
50. Lee, A.W.M., Law, S.C.K., Foo, W., Poon, Y.F., Cheung, F.K., Chan, D.K.K., O, S.K., Tung, S.Y., Thaw, M., Ho, J.H.C. 1993. Retrospective analysis of patients with nasopharyngeal carcinoma treated during 1976–1985: survival after local recurrence. *Int. J. Radiat. Oncol. Biol. Phys.*; 26:773–782.
51. Gerbaulet, A., Haie-Meder, C., Marsiglia, H., Kumar, U., Lusinchi, A., Habrand, J.L., Mamelle, G., Flamant, F., Chassagne, D. 1994. Role of brachytherapy in treatment of head and neck cancers: institut gustave-roussy experience with 1140 patients. In: *Brachytherapy from Radium to Optimization*, eds. Mould, R.F., Battermann, J.J., Martinez, A.A., Spelser, B.L., Chap. 12. Veenendaal: Nucletron.
52. Chang, J.T.C., See, L.C., Hong, J.H., Chen, L.H., Tang, S.G. 1995. Intracavitary brachytherapy for early stage nasopharyngeal carcinoma. In: *International Brachytherapy, Program and Abstract of the 8th International Brachytherapy Conference, Nice, France, 25–28 Nov. 1995*, Chap. 36.
53. Amornmarn, R., Prempree, T., Sewchand, W., Jaiwatana, J. 1983. Radiation management of advanced nasopharyngeal cancer. *Cancer*; 52:802–807.
54. Fu, K.K., Newman, H., Theodore, P.L. 1975. Treatment of locally recurrent carcinoma of the nasopharynx. *Radiology*; 117:425–431.
55. Wang, C.C. 1987. Re-irradiation of recurrent nasopharyngeal carcinoma treatment techniques and results. *Int. J. Radiat. Oncol. Biol. Phys.*; 13:953–956.
56. Leung, S.F., Kreel, L., Tsao, S.Y. 1992. Asymptomatic temporal lobe injury after radiotherapy for nasopharyngeal carcinoma: incidence and determinants. *Brit. J. Radiol.*; 66:710–714.
57. Teo, P., Kwan, W.H., Chan, A.T.C., Lee, W.Y., King, W., Mok, C.O. 1998. How successful is high-dose (≥60 Gy) reirradiation using mainly external beams in salvaging local failures of nasopharyngeal carcinoma? *Int. J. Radiat. Oncol. Biol. Phys.*; 40(4):897–913.
58. Choy, D., Sham, J.S.T., Wei, W.I., Ho, C.M., Wu, P.M. 1993. Transpalatal insertion of radioactive gold grain for the treatment of persistent and recurrent nasopharyngeal carcinoma. *Int. J. Radiat. Oncol. Biol. Phys.*; 25:505–512.
59. Lin, Z.X., Li, D.R. 1995. Preliminary experience of HDR brachytherapy for nasopharyngeal carcinoma. In: *International Brachytherapy, Program and Abstract of the 8th International Brachytherapy Conference, Nice, France, 25–28 Nov. 1995*, Chap. 81.
60. Zhang, Y.W., Liu, T.F., Fi, C.X. 1989. Intracavitary radiation treatment of nasopharyngeal carcinoma by the high dose rate afterloading technique. *Int. J. Radiat. Oncol. Biol. Phys.*; 16:315–318.
61. Lee, A.W.M., Sham, J.S.T., Poon, Y.F., Ho, J.H.C. 1989. Treatment of stage I nasopharyngeal carcinoma: analysis of the patterns of relapse and the results of withholding elective neck irradiation. *Int. J. Radiat. Oncol. Biol. Phys.*; 17:1183–1190.
62. Ngan, K.C., Yu, H.C., Ng, M.F. Tang, S.K., Lau, W.H. 1996. Salvage treatment for recurrent advanced neck node metastases of head and neck cancer — a combined approach. *Abstract of Final Program and Abstract Book in the 4th International Conference on Head and Neck Cancer, Toronto, July 28–August 1, 1996*, No. 375.
63. Yu, K.H., Teo, P., Lee, W.Y., Leung, S.F., Choi, P., Johnson, P.J. 1994. Patterns of early treatment failure in non-metastatic NPC: a study based on CT scanning. *Clin. Oncol. R. Coll. Radiol.*; 6(3):167–171.

64. Yin, W.B., Gao, L., Xu, G.Z. 1995. Brachytherapy of nasopharyngeal carcinoma. In: *International Brachytherapy, Program and Abstracts of the 8th International Brachytherapy Conference, Nice, France, 25–28 Nov., 1995*, Chap. 106.
65. Yamashita, S., Kondo, M., Inuyama, Y., Hashimoto, S. 1986. Improved survival of patients with nasopharyngeal squamous cell carcinoma. *Int. J. Radiat. Oncol. Biol. Phys.*; 12:307–312.
66. Vikram, B., Mishra, S. 1994. Permanent Iodine-125 (I-125) boost implants after external radiation therapy in nasopharyngeal cancer. *Int. J. Radiat. Oncol. Biol. Phys.*; 28(3):699–701.
67. Levendag, P., Visser, A. 1992. Microselectron-HDR Brachytherapy for head and neck cancer with special reference to the nasopharynx and oropharynx. In: *International Brachytherapy, Program and Abstract of the 7th International Brachytherapy Working Conference, Baltimore, Washington, USA, 6–8 Sept. 1992*, Chap. 14.

CHAPTER 13

Chemotherapy

Thomas W.T. Leung and *Anthony T.C. Chan*

Nasopharyngeal carcinoma (NPC) is a chemosensitive tumour and chemotherapy has a defined role in the palliative treatment of metastastic disease and an increasing role in the primary treatment of locoregionally advanced disease. However, chemotherapy is associated with toxicities and it is therefore important to select the most active chemotherapy regimens with the most favourable toxicity profile. Hence, before describing the current status of chemotherapy in the treatment of NPC, the most commonly used cytotoxic agents and their associated toxicities are highlighted.

Cytotoxic Therapy

Drugs that are active and commonly used in NPC patients include cisplatin, carboplatin and 5-fluourouracil (5FU).[1] More recently paclitaxel has also been shown to be active.[2] The majority of patients can receive their drugs in an out-patient setting if the doctor is able to prescribe an adequate anti-emetic regimen and takes into account the side-effects from previous drug treatment. Patients undergoing chemotherapy should be aware of the nature of the treatment and its possible hazards. These include the aims of the treatment and which side effects should lead him/her to contact the hospital. The patient's age, general condition, and pre-existing medical conditions should be taken into account prior to receiving chemotherapy. The following is a brief summary of the most frequently encountered side effects of cisplatin, carboplatin, 5FU and paclitaxel.

Cisplatin

This drug is highly nephrotoxic and during administration a high urine flow is essential with intravenous fluids given before and after delivery. The nephrotoxicity is dose-dependent and the 24 hour creatinine clearance should be checked before each cycle. Mannitol is given to ensure a high urine flow. Hypokalaemia and hypomagnesaemia are common side effects. Nausea and vomiting are severe but can be controlled with the use of a prophylactic combination of 5-HT3-antagonist and dexamethasone. Other common side effects include ototoxicity and peripheral neuropathy. Myelosuppression is mild.

Carboplatin

This analogue of cisplatin has a different toxicity spectrum but is active in the same tumours. It should be given using the area under the concentration versus time curve (AUC) formula of (Glomerular Filtration Rate (ml/min) +25) × n where n is the desired multiple. It is less nephrotoxic and neurotoxic than cisplatin. Pre-hydration and post-hydration are not necessary. Myelosuppression is the principal toxicity which may be severe and typically occurs at 14–21 days. It is a more convenient drug than cisplatin to give in the outpatient setting.

5-fluorouracil

5FU has been used extensively in the treatment of head and neck cancers and has been found to have synergistic interactions with cisplatin. The toxicity is less and the activity is increased when this drug is given by continuous infusion as compared with bolus injection. This drug is generally well tolerated but toxic effects include nausea, diarrhoea, stomatitis, myelosuppression, cardiac disturbance and a cerebellar syndrome.

Paclitaxel (Taxol)

This new drug is increasingly used in the treatment of a variety of solid tumours. The dose-limiting toxicities are neutropaenia and neurotoxicity, and other side effects include myalgia and hypersensitivity, the latter being common, and therefore standard premedication using dexamethasone and anti-histamine is given prior to infusion.

Chemotherapy in Metastatic/Locally Recurrent Disease

Historically, the role of cytotoxic chemotherapy in the management of NPC has been confined to metastatic or locally recurrent disease with a palliative intent.[1] Combination chemotherapy regimens have shown higher response rates than single agent chemotherapy and therefore most recent trials have focused on the use of multi-drug regimens. Non-platinum containing regimens have not been as effective as those containing cisplatin which have achieved encouraging response rates of between 40–91% in phase II trials (*Table 1*).[3–13]

At the Institute Gustav Russy in Paris, France,[3,6,8] and at the Princess Margaret Hospital in Toronto, Canada,[5,10] response rates were clearly improved with more intensive chemotherapy but were associated with increased toxicities. The question of whether the gain in response rates is sufficient to justify the added toxicities remains to be answered. "Quality of life" measures are, to date, conspicuous by their absence in the treatment of metastatic NPC. However, in the West, randomized studies in metastatic NPC will be difficult because of the low incidence of the disease, and further phase II studies will not be able to address this issue.

At the Prince of Wales Hospital, Hong Kong, from 1984–1993, combination

Table 1. Combination chemotherapy for metastatic/recurrent NPC.

Authors (reference)	Patients	Chemotherapy	Overall response to chemotherapy (%)	Complete response to chemotherapy (%)
Boussen *et al.*[3]	41	cisplatin, bleomycin, 5FU	75	22
Chi *et al.*[4]	35	cisplatin 5FU, leucovorin	91	14
Choo *et al.*[5]	22	cisplatin-based	63	18
	28	non-cisplatin based	39	11
Cvitkovic *et al.*[6]	46	5FU, epirubicin, cisplatin, mitomycin C	61	9
Decker *et al.*[7]	17	cisplatin and non-cisplatin based	53	18
Mahjoubi *et al.*[8]	44	bleomycin, epirubicin, cisplatin	50	20
Su *et al.*[9]	25	cisplatin 5FU, bleomycin	40	4
Tannock *et al.*[10]	41	cyclophosphamide doxorubicin, cisplatin, methotrexate, bleomycin	66	12
Yeo *et al.*[11]	42	carboplatin, 5FU	38	17
Yeo *et al.*[12]	27	carboplatin, paclitaxel	59	11
Tan *et al.*[13]	31	carboplatin, paclitaxel	72	3

chemotherapy with cisplatin or carboplatin plus continuous infusion of 5FU had been the standard regimen for patients with distant metastases with or without locoregional disease. From 1987 to 1993 forty-two consecutive patients were entered into a standardized protocol using carboplatin 300 mg/m^2 on day 1 and 5FU 1 gm/m^2/day as 24 hour infusion days 1 to 3.[11] Carboplatin was used as a substitute for cisplatin to minimize nephrotoxicity and neurotoxicity. The toxicity was, indeed, minimal and the treatment was well tolerated by all the patients. However, the overall response rate was lower than in previously reported cisplatin-containing regimens at only 38% (17% CR, 21% PR). The low overall response rate may have been due to sub-optimal dosage of 5FU and carboplatin. At the time of the study, the dose of carboplatin had been calculated according to total body surface area of the patients concerned. More recent studies by Calvert and colleagues[14] have demonstrated that when the dosage of carboplatin is adjusted according to a targeted area under the concentration versus time curve (AUC), the response rates to carboplatin can be increased without excessive toxicities. Hence, the use of 5FU at 1 g/m^2/day as 24 hour infusion days 1 to 3 and carboplatin at AUC 6 mg/ml/min may constitute a more optimal regimen for patients with NPC.

We recently reported the use of combination paclitaxel at 135 mg/m^2 and carboplatin at an AUC of 6 mg/ml/min in 27 patients with locally recurrent or metastatic NPC.[12] The doses used gave an overall response rate of 59% with acceptable toxicity. A more aggressive approach with dose escalation may further improve the efficacy of this combination. This is supported by a preliminary report which recorded a response rate of 71% when paclitaxel 175 mg/m^2 was combined with carboplatin at an AUC of 6 mg/ml/min.[13] Hence this dose schedule may be the optimal outpatient regimen in patients with NPC. A multi-centre prospective randomized phase III study has been planned in which combination therapy using 5FU and carboplatin will be compared with paclitaxel and carboplatin in terms of response rates, tumour control, toxicities and quality of life measures.

Can metastatic NPC be cured?

Distant metastases in patients with NPC have, conventionally, been regarded as incurable and the aim from any form of treatment has been palliative, a view founded on observations in other head and neck cancers. However, a review of more recent experience from three centres with substantial numbers of NPC patients having undergone combination chemotherapy and achieved complete remission, suggests that metastatic NPC may indeed be curable in a small sub-group of patients. In the Institute Gustav Russy series, 9.9% of such patients remained alive and disease free at 2 years.[15] 3.2% of patients in the Princess Margaret Hospital series remained alive and disease free at 3.5 years.[10]

In a retrospective analysis of 247 NPC patients with distant metastases at the Prince of Wales Hospital, 17 of 247 (6.88%) survived 2 years or more after distant metastasis had been diagnosed.[16] Furthermore, 4 patients (1.62%) were rendered long term disease free at 5 years or more after complete response (CR) to aggressive multimodal treatments. It is clear that further studies are required to define the optimal treatment for patients with metastatic NPC.

Neoadjuvant Chemotherapy Pre-radiotherapy

Over the last two decades several phase II studies using two or three cycles of neoadjuvant cisplatin-containing regimens given 3-weekly prior to radical external radiotherapy have demonstrated highly encouraging response rates (53–98%), good tolerability and possible survival benefit when compared with historical controls (*Table* 2).[17–22] The incidence of long term side effects was not increased.

Geara *et al.*[23] from the M.D. Anderson Cancer Center reported on a matched cohort study of induction chemotherapy using cisplatin and 5FU followed by radiotherapy versus radiotherapy alone in locoregionally advanced NPC (UICC stages III and IV). The patients treated with induction chemotherapy were shown to have a significant reduction in distant failure translating into significant improvement in the 5 year disease free survival (DFS) and overall survival (OS) compared to the matched cohort. The major weakness of this study was the lack of information regarding selection for induction chemotherapy during the period of the study.

A retrospective review of 122 patients with NPC also treated at the M.D. Anderson Cancer Center was separately reported by Garden *et al.*[24] In this review the outcomes of patients treated with conventional RT or concomitant boost schedule were compared with those patients treated with or without induction chemotherapy of cisplatin-5FU. There was considerable overlap of the four different treatment strategies in the 122 patients. The results demonstrated significant improvement in OS and DFS using induction chemotherapy in stage IV patients. On the other hand, there were no significant differences in the local control rates, DFS or OS in the patients who received concomitant boost radiotherapy. This retrospective review is also limited in its value by the lack of detail as to how the patients were selected into the different treatment strategies and hence no firm conclusions can be drawn.

The International Nasopharyngeal Cancer Study Group has reported the preliminary results of a randomized trial comparing 3 cycles of neoadjuvant chemotherapy using cisplatin, epirubicin and bleomycin (BEC) plus radiotherapy versus radiotherapy alone in AJCC Stage IV (≥N2, M0) undifferentiated nasopharyngeal carcinoma.[25] The treatment toxicities of the chemotherapy arm were severe in this trial. Fourteen (8.2%) of the chemotherapy patients died from treatment-related events including acute renal failure, bleomycin-related respiratory failure, post-radiotherapy complications, anaphylactic shock and unknown causes. At a median follow up of 49 months, there was a significant difference in disease free survival favouring the chemotherapy arm ($p < 0.01$). However, bearing in mind the significant treatment-related toxicities and mortalities using this aggressive chemotherapy-radiotherapy regimen

Table 2. Neoadjuvant chemotherapy in NPC.

Authors (reference)	Patients	Chemotherapy	Overall response to chemotherapy (%)	Complete response to chemotherapy (%)	Complete response to chemo-RT (%)	Survival
Atichartakarn *et al.*[17]	28	cisplatin 5FU	NR	NR	82	64% OS
Bachouchi *et al.*[18]	39	bleomycin epirubicin cisplatin	98	66	100	NR
Clark *et al.*[19]	24	cisplatin-based	75	29	77	57% 2 year DFS
Dimery *et al.*[20]	43	cisplatin 5FU	NR	NR	86	80% 2 year OS
Galligioni *et al.*[21]	12	adriamycin bleomycin vinblastine dacarbazine	81	33	100	NR
Tannock *et al.*[22]	49	cisplatin-based	75	22	82	34% 3year OS

OS = overall survival
DFS = disease free survival
NR = not recorded

and the relatively poor figures of the radiotherapy group, the use of induction BEC cannot be recommended in locoregionally advanced NPC unless the completed trial demonstrates a statistically significant OS benefit.

Adjuvant Chemotherapy Post-radiotherapy

The use of adjuvant chemotherapy has been studied in large prospective randomized trials in other head and neck cancers, demonstrating no overall survival benefit, but a reduction in the incidence of distant relapse has been consistently shown.[26,27] However in NPC, the use of adjuvant chemotherapy has never been proven to be of benefit. The only large randomized trial with 229 patients treated in the Institute Nazionale Tumouri in Milan[28] failed to demonstrate any survival benefit in patients receiving 6 cycles of vincristine, cyclophosphamide and adriamycin compared with those receiving no adjuvant chemotherapy. However, the major criticism of this trial was the omission of cisplatin from the chemotherapy regimen. Other studies that implied survival benefit were either non-randomized or involved only small numbers of patients.[29–32] It is therefore important that an adjuvant cisplatin-containing regimen is tested in a prospective randomized trial.

Neoadjuvant and Adjuvant Chemotherapy

At the Prince of Wales Hospital in Hong Kong, between 1988 and 1991 a randomized study was completed comparing radical radiotherapy with chemoradiotherapy which comprised two cycles of neoadjuvant chemotherapy giving cisplatin and 5FU before radiotherapy and four similar cycles of adjuvant chemotherapy after radiotherapy.[33] Eighty-two patients with either Ho's N3 or any N stage with a maximal cervical node diameter of ≥4 cm were randomized, five patients being unevaluable. Thirty seven patients were subjected to chemoradiotherapy and 40 patients received radiotherapy alone. The patient characteristics including staging were comparable in both arms. Toxicities in the chemoradiotherapy arm included myelosuppression, nephrotoxicity, nausea and vomiting. The degree of mucositis was not significantly different in the two arms. There was no treatment related death. At a median follow up of 28 months, there were no differences in the OS or DFS. The main weaknesses of this study were the small number of patients randomized and the relatively short median follow up.

In a recent update analysis of 618 node-positive patients treated at the Prince of Wales Hospital between 1984 and 1989,[34] with a median follow-up of 5.5 years, patients treated with neoadjuvant, with or without adjuvant chemotherapy, using cisplatin and 5FU had significantly less local failures overall than patients treated with RT alone. This improvement in local control was especially significant for patients with Ho's T3 stage disease, and there were very few late local relapses in patients given chemotherapy. The enhancement in local control of the locally advanced NPC might be explained by the significant shrinkage of the primary tumour by the neoadjuvant chemotherapy, leading to an increased safety margin between the tumour volume and the radiation volume in the subsequent radiotherapy course.

Concurrent Chemo-radiotherapy

In head and neck cancers in general the early results using concurrent chemo-radiotherapy have been encouraging. Cisplatin is an agent with both anti-tumour activity and radiation sensitization. The major toxicities of cisplatin do not overlap with those of radiation. Myelosuppression is not commonly seen and therefore optimal doses can be delivered. The most encouraging results were reported from a randomized trial using post-operative cisplatin and radiotherapy in patients with high risk disease.[35] There was no significant increase in late radiation complications in the combined modality group.

In NPC, Al-Sarraf *et al.*[36] reported a phase II study of 27 patients with locoregionally advanced disease treated with concurrent chemo-radiotherapy using cisplatin 100 mg/m^2 every 3 weeks for 3 courses. The side effects were tolerable with no interruption of radiotherapy. When historical controls were used for comparison, the DFS, OS and incidence of distant metastasis were improved.

Hence a Head and Neck Intergroup study for AJCC Stages III and IV NPC randomized patients to receive radiotherapy alone, or concurrent chemotherapy during radiotherapy followed by further chemotherapy after completion of radiotherapy (*Figure 1*).[37] Both the 3 year progression free survival rates and the 3 year OS rates were statistically significantly improved in the combined concurrent with adjuvant chemo-radiotherapy arm. This important study has wide implications for the management of locoregionally advanced NPC. However, several important points need to be addressed before recommending the universal application of this treatment strategy to all ethnic and histological groups. In the Intergroup study, the 3 year OS for AJCC stages III and IV patients was only 47% on the radiotherapy arm and 78% on the concurrent arm. These rates of OS are poor when compared with other published series of WHO III Chinese populations where the 3 year OS is 86% for AJCC stage III and 70% for stage IV. The 3 year DFS is 72% for AJCC stage III and 60% for stage IV. These results are comparable with those of the concurrent chemo-radiotherapy arm in the Head and Neck Intergroup study and considerably better than the radiotherapy alone arm. These discrepancies may be explained by the different histological mix of the Head and Neck Intergroup patients (41% WHO III) compared to the Chinese patients (>95% WHO III), but the aggressive radiotherapy regimen used to treat the Chinese patients may also be an important factor.[38,39] Whether this aggressive radiotherapy regimen with substantially better survival figures can be improved further by the addition of concurrent chemotherapy could only be answered by a prospective randomized trial using this aggressive radiotherapy regimen as the control group.

At the Prince of Wales Hospital in Hong Kong, a prospective randomized study for patients with locoregionally advanced disease was begun in 1994. Patients are

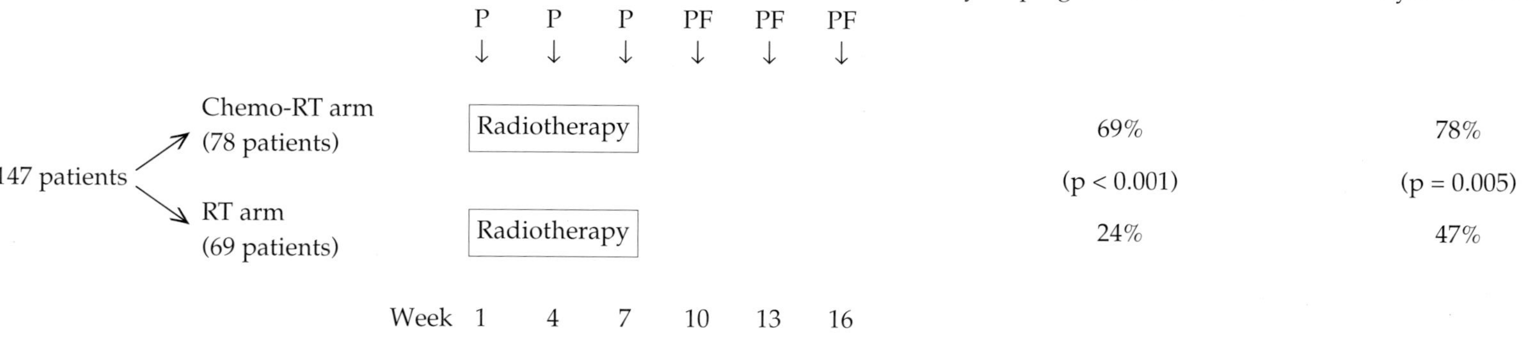

Figure 1. Head and Neck Intergroup study for locoregionally advanced NPC[33]

P = cisplatin 100 mg/m^2 D1
PF = cisplatin 80 mg/m^2 D1
5FU 1 g/m^2 D1–4

randomized to radiotherapy alone versus radiotherapy with concurrent cisplatin 40 mg/m^2 weekly given as outpatient therapy. A standard protocol of 6 weeks of chemotherapy is given concurrently with external radiotherapy (62.5 Gy). To date there have been no treatment-related mortalities and the toxicities have been tolerable. Accrual into this trial is expected to be completed by the end of 1998 and conclusive results are expected by the year 2001. Until this or similar studies mature and confirm that concurrent chemo-radiotherapy is statistically superior in terms of OS and DFS than radiotherapy alone, it is premature to recommend this strategy as standard treatment in all ethnic and histological subgroups.[1]

Concluding Remarks

Nasopharyngeal carcinoma is both radiosensitive and chemosensitive. Radiotherapy remains the gold standard of treatment and a radiotherapy arm using an optimal technique should still be used as the control for comparison with combined modality treatment. The use of neoadjuvant and adjuvant chemotherapy have yielded high response rates and although no randomized trial has demonstrated overall survival benefit, the local control rates are enhanced in locally advanced disease. The positive early results for concurrent chemo-radiotherapy together with adjuvant chemotherapy are highly encouraging, but the wider application to all ethnic and histological groups remains to be confirmed by a further prospective randomized trial done in endemic areas where NPC prevails. In the setting of metastatic disease, combination chemotherapy is recommended as a standard palliative measure.

References

1. Chan, A.T.C., Teo, P.M.L., Leung, W.T., Johnson, P.J. 1998. The role of chemotherapy in the management of nasopharyngeal carcinoma. *Cancer*; 82:1003–1012.
2. Au, E., Ang, P.T., Chuen, E.J. 1996. Paclitaxel in metastatic nasopharyngeal cancer (abstr.). *Proc. A.S.C.O.*; 15:919.
3. Boussen, H., Cvitkovic, E., Wendling, J.L., Bachouchi, M., Mahjoubi, R., Kalifa, C. 1991. Chemotherapy of metastatic and/or recurrent undifferentiated nasopharyngeal carcinoma with cisplatin, bleomycin and fluorouracil. *J. Clin. Oncol.*; 9:1675–1681.
4. Chi, K.H., Chan, W.K., Cooper, D.L., Yen, S.H., Lin, C.Z., Chen, K.Y. 1994. A phase II study of outpatient chemotherapy with cisplatin, 5-fluorouracil,and leucovorin in nasopharyngeal carcinoma. *Cancer*; 73:2:247–252.
5. Choo, R., Tannock, I. 1991. Chemotherapy for recurrent or metastatic carcinoma of the nasopharynx. A review of the Princess Margaret Hospital experience. *Cancer*; 68:2120–2124.
6. Cvitkovic, E., Mahjoubi, R., Lianes, P., Armand, J.P., Azli, N., Wibault, P. 1991. 5-fluorouracil (FU), mitomycin (M), epirubicin (E), cisplatin (P) in recurrent and/or metastatic undifferentiated nasopharyngeal carcinoma (UCNT) (abstr.). *Proc. A.S.C.O.*; 10:664.
7. Decker, D.A., Drelichman, A., Al-Sarraf, M. 1983. Chemotherapy for nasopharyngeal carcinoma: a ten-year experience. *Cancer*; 52:602–605.
8. Mahjoubi, R., Azli, N., Bachouchi, M., Soulie, P., Wibault, P. 1992. Metastatic undifferentiated carcinoma of nasopharyngeal type treated with bleomycin (B), epirubicin (E) and cisplatin (C): final report (abstr.). *Proc. A.S.C.O.*; 11:772.

9. Su, W.C., Chen, T.Y., Kao, R.H., Tsao, C.J. 1993. Chemotherapy with cisplatin and continuous infusion of 5-fluorouracil and bleomycin for recurrent and metastatic nasopharyngeal carcinoma in Taiwan. *Oncology*; 50:205–208.
10. Tannock, I.F. 1996. Chemotherapy for nasopharyngeal cancer: the CAPABLE regimen (cyclophosphamide, doxorubicin, cisplatin, methotrexate and bleomycin) (abstr.) *Proc. A.S.C.O.*; 15:916.
11. Yeo, W., Leung, T.W.T., Leung, S.F., Teo, P.M.L., Chan, A.T.C., Lee, W.Y., Johnson, P.J. 1996. Phase II study of the combination of carboplatin and 5-fluorouracil in metastatic nasopharyngeal carcinoma. *Cancer Chemother. Pharmacol.*; 38:466–470.
12. Yeo, W., Leung, T.W.T., Chan, A.T.C., Chiu, S.K.W., Mok, T.S.K., Johnson, P.J. Phase II study of combination paclitaxel and carboplatin in advanced nasopharyngeal carcinoma. *Eur. J. Cancer* (in press).
13. Tan, E.H., Khoo, K.S., Au, E. 1998. Phase II trial of paclitaxel and carboplatin in patients with metastatic undifferentiated nasopharyngeal carcinoma (abstr.). *Proc. A.S.C.O.*; 17:1477.
14. Calvert, A.H., Newell, D.R., Gumbrell, R.A., *et al.* 1989. Carboplatin dosage: prospective evaluation of a simple formula based on renal function. *J. Clin. Oncol.*; 7:1748–1756.
15. Altun, M., Fandi, A., Dupos, O., Cvitkovic, E., Krajina, Z., Eschuege, F. 1995. Undifferentiated nasopharyngeal cancer (UCNT): current diagnostic and therapeutic aspects. *Int. J. Radiat. Oncol. Biol. Phys.*; 32:859–877.
16. Teo, P.M.L., Kwan, W.H., Lee, W.Y., Leung, S.F., Johnson, P.J. 1996. Prognosticators determining survival subsequent to distant metastasis from nasopharyngeal carcinoma. *Cancer*; 77:242–231.
17. Atichartakarn, V., Kraiphibul, P., Clongsusuek, P., Pochanugool, L., Kulapaditharom, B., Ratanatharathorn, V. 1988. Nasopharyngeal carcinoma: result of treatment with cis-diaminedichloroplatinum II, 5-fluorouracil, and radiation therapy. *Int. J. Radiat. Oncol. Biol. Phys.*; 14:461–469.
18. Bachouchi, M., Cvitkovic, E., Azli, N., Gasmi, J., Cortes-Funes, H., Houssen, H. 1990. High complete response in advanced nasopharyngeal carcinoma with bleomycin, epirubicin, and cisplatin before radiotherapy. *J. Natl. Cancer Inst.*; 82:616–620.
19. Clark, J.R., Norris, C.M., Dreyfuss, A.I., Fallon, B.G., Balogh, K., Anderson, R.F. 1987. Nasopharyngeal carcinoma: the Dana-Farber Cancer Institute experience with 24 patients treated with induction chemotherapy and radiotherapy. *Ann. Otol. Rhinol. Laryngol.*; 96:608–614.
20. Dimery, I.W., Peters, L.J., Goepfert, H., Morrisone, W.H., Byers, R.M., Guillory, C. 1993. Effectiveness of combined induction chemotherapy and radiotherapy in advanced nasopharyngeal carcinoma. *J. Clin. Oncol.*; 11:1919–1928.
21. Galligioni, E., Carbone, A., Tirelli, U., Veronesi, A., Trovo, M.G., Magri, M.D. 1982. Combined chemotherapy with doxorubicin, bleomycin, vinblastine, dacarbazine, and radiotherapy for advanced lymphoepithelioma. *Cancer Treat. Rep.*; 66:1207–1210.
22. Tannock, I., Payne, D., Cummings, B., Hewitt, K., Panzarella, T. 1987. Sequential chemotherapy and radiation for nasopharyngeal cancer: absence of long-term benefit despite a high rate of tumour response to chemotherapy. *J. Clin. Oncol.*; 5:629–634.
23. Geara, F.B., Glisson, B.S., Sanguineti, G., *et al.* 1997. Induction chemotherapy followed by radiotherapy versus radiotherapy alone in patients with advanced nasopharyngeal carcinoma. *Cancer*; 79:7:1279–1286.
24. Garden, A.S., Lippman, S.M., Morrison, W.H., *et al.* 1996. Does induction chemotherapy have a role in the management of nasopharyngeal carcinoma? Results of treatment in the era of computerized tomography. *Int. J. Radiat. Oncol. Biol. Phys.*; 36:5:1005–1012.
25. International Nasopharyngeal Cancer Study Group. 1996. Preliminary results of a randomized trial comparing neoadjuvant chemotherapy (cisplatin, epirubicin, bleomycin) plus radiotherapy vs radiotherapy alone in stage IV (≥N2, M0) undifferentiated nasopharyngeal carcinoma: a positive effect on progression-free survival. *Int. J. Radiat. Oncol. Biol. Phys.*; 35(3):463–469.
26. Ervin, T.J., Clark, J.R., Weichselbaum, R.R., *et al.* 1987. An analysis of induction and adjuvant chemotherapy in the multidisciplinary treatment of squamous-cell carcinoma of the head and neck. *J. Clin. Oncol.*; 5:10–20.

27. Head and Neck Contracts Program. 1987. Adjuvant chemotherapy for advanced head and neck squamous carcinoma. *Cancer*; 60:301–311.
28. Rossi, A., Molinari, R., Boracchi, P., Vecchio, M.D., Marubini, E., Nava, M. 1988. Adjuvant chemotherapy with vincristine, cyclophosphamide, and doxorubicin after radiotherapy in local-regional nasopharyngeal cancer: results of a 4-year multicenter randomized study. *J. Clin. Oncol.*; 6:1401–1410.
29. Khoury, G.G., Paterson, I.C.M. 1987. Nasopharyngeal carcinoma: a review of cases treated by radiotherapy and chemotherapy. *Clin Radiology*; 38:17–20.
30. Rahima, M., Rakowsky, E., Barzilay, J., Sidi, J. 1986. Carcinoma of the nasopharynx: an analysis of 91 cases and a comparison of differing treatment approaches. *Cancer*; 58:843–849.
31. Tsujii, H., Kamada, T., Tsuji, H., Takamura, A., Matsuoka, Y., Usubuchi, H. 1989. Improved results in the treatment of nasopharyngeal carcinoma using combined radiotherapy and chemotherapy. *Cancer*; 63:1668–1672.
32. Dimery, I.W., Legha, S.S., Peters, L.J., Goepfert, H., Oswald, M.J. 1987. Adjuvant chemotherapy for advanced nasopharyngeal carcinoma. *Cancer*; 60:943–949.
33. Chan, A.T.C., Teo, P.M.L., Leung, T.W.T., *et al.* 1995. A prospective randomized study of chemotherapy adjunctive to definitive radiotherapy in advanced nasopharyngeal carcinoma. *Int. J. Radiat. Oncol. Biol. Phys.*; 33(3):569–577.
34. Teo, P.M.L., Chan, A.T.C., Lee, W.Y., Leung, W.T., Johnson, P.J. Significant enhancement in local control of node-positive nasopharyngeal carcinoma by adjunctive chemotherapy. *Int. J. Radiat. Oncol. Biol. Phys.* (in press).
35. Bachaud, J.-M., Cohen-Jonathan, E., Alzieu, C., David, J.-M., Serrano, E., Daly-Schveitzer, N. 1996. Combined postoperative radiotherapy and weekly cisplatin infusion for locally advanced head and neck carcinoma: final report of a randomized trial. *Int. J. Radiat. Oncol. Biol. Phys.*; 36(5):999–1004.
36. Al-Sarraf, M., Pajak, T.F., Cooper, J.S., Mohiuddin, M., Herskovic, A., Ager, P.J. 1990. Chemo-radiotherapy in patients with locally advanced nasopharyngeal carcinoma: a radiation therapy oncology group study. *J. Clin. Oncol.*; 8:1342–1351.
37. Al-Sarraf, M., LeBlanc, M., Giri, P.G.S., *et al.* 1998. Chemo-radiotherapy versus radiotherapy in patients with advanced nasopharyngeal cancer: Phase III randomized intergroup study 0099. *J. Clin. Oncol.*; 16:1310–17.
38. Teo, P., Yu, P., Lee, W.Y., *et al.* 1996. Significant prognosticators after primary radiotherapy in 903 nondisseminated nasopharyngeal carcinomas evaluated by computer tomography. *Int. J. Radiat. Oncol. Biol. Phys.*; 36(2):291–304.
39. Al-Sarraf, M., McLaughlin, P.W. 1995. Nasopharynx carcinoma: choice of treatment. *Int. J. Radiat. Oncol. Biol. Phys.*; 33(3):761–763.

CHAPTER 14

Complications of Radiation Therapy

Ann W.M. Lee

Nasopharyngeal carcinoma (NPC) with its characteristic propensity for extensive infiltration and anatomical proximity to critical structures, remains one of the most difficult cancers to treat. Surgical resection with acceptable margins is difficult, and there is little dispute that radiation therapy (RT) is the main modality for primary control. To achieve the maximum chance of cure demands accurate delivery of the highest tolerable dose to all sites of tumour infiltration within the shortest possible time. Hence, the risks of radiation-induced complications, both acute and late, are substantial. Walking the tight-rope between the risk of fatal tumour recurrence and lethal treatment complication is always a great challenge.

The target area is a complex region composed of several dissimilar structures, each having a unique response to irradiation: skin, mucosa, subcutaneous connective tissue, muscles, bones, teeth, salivary glands, ears, eyes, endocrine axis, nerves, spinal cord and brain. The clinical syndromes, pathophysiology, tolerance doses and management of the different potential injuries vary widely and multiple specialties become involved.

Diagnosis of irradiation injury can be difficult, and a high degree of awareness is demanded. Temporal lobe necrosis and endocrine dysfunction, in particular, are easily overlooked by the unwary because the majority of these patients have minimal symptoms and signs. As a substantial proportion of late damage is only observed among the long term survivors,[1] series with only 5-year results grossly under-estimate the gravity of the problem. On the other hand, before attributing abnormalities to irradiation damage, every effort must be made to exclude other possible causes. Correctly distinguishing from tumour effect is particularly critical and long periods of observation may be needed for confirmation.

Besides a balanced and comprehensive picture of all the potential risks, it is important that the differential impact of different radiation factors be thoroughly understood so that the best possible therapeutic ratio can be achieved. Unfortunately, it is not easy to learn from the literature. Only a few of the reported series have long-term results and the majority do not give detailed information on the complications observed. The reported incidence of complications varies widely and cross-study comparison is difficult (or even impossible) because of marked variations in the recording systems, statistical methods, lengths of observation, proportions of patients on regular follow-up, percentages of long-term survivors, diligence of detection and changing sensitivity of investigation methods.

In this chapter, we will try to summarize the current knowledge on the complex problems of radiation induced complications and the possible ways of minimizing the morbidity.

Overall Incidence of Complications

It is common experience that all patients develop acute reactions involving rapidly proliferating tissues within the treatment fields. While patients vary in sensitivity and pace of recovery, almost all have grade 2, or above, acute reactions based on the toxicity criteria of the Radiation Therapy Oncology Group (RTOG) and the European Organization for Research and Treatment of Cancer (EORTC).[2]

In the past, it was thought that acute reactions were only transient, and the dose-limiting factor is late damage (especially in those with serious debility). However, with experience gained from accelerated hyperfractionation, it is increasingly apparent that severe acute reactions are not only distressful to the extent of causing undesirable treatment interruption, but can also lead to late damage.[3]

The latent interval for late complications can vary from several months to years after irradiation. The majority are progressive and irreversible, but the impact on the quality of life varies. The median overall incidence of late complications is 37%,[4] and Table I summarizes the cumulative incidences of complications at different sites reported in the English literature. The serious morbidity rate was 7%,[1] and treatment mortality rate 3%.[5] The great majority of serious morbidities were due to neurological damage, especially that involving the temporal lobes and the brainstem.[1] Necrosis of soft tissue and bone only amounted to a median incidence of 3%.[6] In our review of 4527 patients treated in Hong Kong during the period 1976–1985, 1395 (31%) of patients developed one or more complications; neurological damage was detected in 450 (10%) patients, and yet this accounted for 59 out of 62 treatment deaths.[1]

Clinical Syndromes, Prevention and Management

Salivary Gland

Transient tenderness and occasionally marked swelling of the parotid glands can develop within a few hours following the first fraction of radiotherapy. This acute reaction usually subsides spontaneously within a few days, and its long-term significance is unknown. Patients should be forewarned to avoid unnecessary anxiety and a mild analgesic (e.g. paracetamol) can be prescribed to relieve the pain.

Salivary flow can decrease by 50% or more after the first week and decline to a barely measurable level by the end of the treatment's course.[7] This decrease in quantity is accompanied by increase in viscosity, concentration of sodium, chloride, calcium, magnesium and protein, together with a decrease in pH and concentration of bicarbonate and Ig A in the saliva.[7,8] As a result of these changes, the normal flora is altered to a more cariogenic spectrum. Hence, not only does this injury cause discomfort, but also increases the risk of developing dental caries.

The extent and speed of recovery vary, virtually all patients having some degree of persistent xerostomia. The major determinants of the chance of recovery include the volume of glands irradiated and the total dose. There is evidence of partial recovery after 30–40 Gy, but essentially no recovery will occur after 60–70 Gy if more than 75% of salivary glands are irradiated.[8–10] The most effective preventive measure is improvement of treatment technique to exclude as much salivary gland tissue from the high dose zone as is safely possible. Using computed tomographic simulation to localize the tumour target and the parotids, Nishioka *et al.* managed to shield the superficial lobes and reduce the total dose to the parotids from 65 Gy to 44 Gy (by changing from their conventional lateral opposed fields to a three-field technique). They demonstrated a significant improvement of mean secretion ratio and a reduction of moderate to severe xerostomia from 100% to 60% when compared with historic controls, without impairment of local control up to a median follow-up of 32 months.[11]

Treatment of established chronic xerostomia essentially relies on the use of saliva substitute and/or sialogogues. However, the latter require functional salivary gland parenchyma to be effective. Among the various stimulants tried, pilocarpine hydrochloride is the most promising, two prospective randomized clinical studies showing significant improvement when compared with placebo.[12–14] Oral pilocarpine at 5 mg three times daily for 12 weeks was effective in 30–50% patients, and no major drug-related side effects were observed.[13]

Mucocutaneous and Soft Tissues

After 20–30 Gy at conventional daily fraction of 1.8–2 Gy, the mucosa becomes erythematous. With an additional 10–20 Gy, patches of mucositis (pseudomembrane) tend to appear, and may coalesce to become confluent. Scrupulous hygiene is required. Two prospective randomized trials have shown that benzydamine HCl (a nonsteroidal drug with analgesic, anaesthetic, anti-inflammatory and anti-microbial effects) is associated with a significant decrease in mucositis when used on an elective basis.[15,16] Once established, stronger topical anesthetics (e.g. viscous xylocaine) and analgesics (e.g. dispersible aspirin) are generally beneficial, and systemic analgesics may be needed. The patient should be persuaded to give up smoking and drinking.

In conjunction with the damage to the taste buds, partial (hypogeusia) or complete (ageusia) inability to taste develops. However, the degree of alteration in taste for sweet, sour, bitter and salt varies from patient to patient. The taste cells are capable of re-populating within 4 months after treatment in most patients, although some degree of permanent impairment may remain. Clinically it is difficult to tell whether the complaint of hypogeusia/ageusia is attributed to direct damage of taste buds or to the secondary effects of xerostomia.

With all these problems in the oral cavity, together with varying degrees of nausea, anorexia and malaise, substantial weight loss (amounting to an average of 10% of initial body weight) is often observed. Dietary consultation regarding recipes with pleasing texture and taste are essential for improving the nutritional status, and sometimes more intensive support with tube feeding may be required. Trials with zinc (using zinc sulphate 220 mg twice daily) have shown promising improvements not only in taste perception, but occasionally also in saliva production.[17,18]

As cellular turnover is more rapid in mucosa than skin, similar changes in the skin lag by 1–2 weeks. With relative sparing by megavoltage photons, most patients only develop erythema, and patches of dry desquamation towards the end of the course. Extensive wet desquamation is rare except in patients with altered fractionation or chemoradiation.

Late effects on mucocutaneous tissues are characterized by paleness and thinning of the epithelium, with loss of pliability with or without the development of telangiectasia. While the great majority of cases are asymptomatic, repeated episodes of epistaxis from telangiectatic vessels in the nasal/nasopharyngeal mucosa can occur. The bleeding may be torrential and indeed fatal incidences of 1.2% and 1.4% have been reported by Mesic *et al.*[19] and Ballantyne,[20] respectively.

Although soft tissues appear impervious to irradiation during and just after treatment, there is experimental evidence to suggest that increases in collagen production occur early and are important in the pathogenesis of late mucocutaneous changes in addition to vascular injury.[21] Different degrees of submucosal/subcutaneous induration with loss of elasticity occur, and may even progress to constricting fibrosis.

Severe pharyngeal strictures have been reported in 0.5%[20] to 2%[4] of irradiated patients, the median incidence being 1.3%.[5] However, serious difficulties in swallowing are more often due to dysfunction of the ninth and tenth cranial nerves rather than mechanical obstruction.

While lymphoedema (particularly in the submental region) may occur during the post-treatment period, this tends to subside spontaneously over 3–8 months and rarely leads to persistent lymphoedema except in patients with superimposed tumour infiltration. Fibrosis of the soft tissues of the neck, with a median incidence of 14%,[5] is however a common phenomenon. The specially high incidence of 18% in our series[1] was attributed to the large fractional dose used (5.6 Gy weekly for 7 fractions). Fortunately only 0.3% had serious functional limitation. However, the possible association of fibrosis with palsies of the last four cranial nerves warrants deep concern. In addition, it may mask regional recurrence and limit the scope of salvage surgery should this prove necessary. Fractures of the clavicles have occurred in a few patients with marked contractures, but coexisting direct damage and weakening of bone by radiation could not be excluded.

Trismus resulting from fibrosis in the temporo-mandibular joints and adjacent muscles of mastication is another common late complication. The median reported incidence was 10%,[22] and could be as high as 17% among patients with re-irradiation by external beams.[23] In a minority of patients, the dental gap becomes so narrow (<0.5 cm) that feeding difficulties result.

The effects of fibrosis can be minimized by prophylactic exercise (stretching the irradiated areas 10–20 times in a row, several times each day). This is particularly useful for preventing trismus; but once contracture occurs, such manoeuvres are far less effective. Surgical release of scars is generally ineffective, and when surgical intervention becomes necessary, grafting of tissue is required.[24]

Chronic ulceration and necrosis with exposure of underlying bone and/or soft tissue are rare except in patients subjected to more than 70 Gy (especially boosts by brachytherapy) or re-irradiation. Pentoxifylline can theoretically influence soft tissue changes by improving perfusion of ischaemic tissues through increasing deformability of red blood cells, inhibiting platelet aggregations and stimulating fibrinolytic activity. A pilot study showed significant relief of pain and healing of ulceration in 7/8 necrotic sites without any significant side effects. However, further clinical evaluation is needed before this method can be recommended.[25]

Bone and Teeth

Dental complications in adults are essentially indirect effects produced by salivary changes, and not direct damage of pulpal tissues.[26] The cervical areas (along the gumline) are most typically affected, and the median reported incidence of dental caries is 9%.[4] Patients should be motivated to maintain good oral and periodontal hygiene indefinitely. Foods and drinks containing sucrose should be avoided. Hydrogen peroxide (3% H_2O_2 and equal parts of water) and/or antiseptic mouth rinses, if tolerated, are helpful in eliminating debris and controlling microbial flora. Daily topical applications of fluoride gel have been found to be very effective.[19,27,28] Prophylactic dental treatment to remove irreparable caries before commencement of radiotherapy is beneficial not only for dental health, but also for minimizing osteonecrosis, as the risk is significantly higher in dentulous patients, especially those requiring teeth extraction after radiotherapy.[29]

Osteonecrosis first manifests objectively as a nondescript erythematous change of the overlying mucosa, which then ulcerates to reveal the necrotic bone below. In the majority of cases, devitalized bone fragments will sequestrate and the lesions may thereafter stabilize spontaneously. However, some may progress and cause intolerable pain. Radiologically, lytic destruction and periosteal thickening are common; mottled sclerosis is also possible, and fracture may occur in severe cases. Fortunately, the incidence is low in the modern megavoltage era, and in our series, only 0.2% of patients developed this complication.[1] The mandible is more frequently affected than the maxilla.[29]

Antibiotics are indicated prophylactically if bone is exposed by accident or treatment, and therapeutically if pain, swelling or suppuration develop. Prevention and treatment by adding hyperbaric oxygen have been reported to be effective in some cases, but reproducible benefits remain unproven.[30,31] Experience at the University of California showed that the majority of patients could be treated by conservative means, 25% of them healing completely, while 63% had persistent but non-progressive bone necrosis. Patients with intractable pain may require resection of the affected area but post-surgical recurrence is not uncommon.[29]

Temporal Lobe

The incidence of temporal lobe necrosis following radiotherapy with once per day fractions varies from isolated case reports to 3%,[1] with a median incidence of 1%.[32] The most important radiation factors include fractional dose,[33] total dose and the volume of brain irradiated.[34,35] For patients irradiated with more than one fraction per day, the interfraction interval is a major determinant of risk. There is increasing evidence to suggest that the repair half-time is longer than anticipated, and even an interfraction interval of 6 hours may still be inadequate for complete repair to take place.[36,37] In two recent series of patients treated with altered fractionation using wide field technique, substantially higher incidences of necrosis were recorded when compared with conventional treatment.[35,38] Even in the series with a 6-h interfraction interval by Teo *et al.*,[38] 33% (4/12) showed necrotic changes on magnetic resonance imaging (MRI), and one of the four had become symptomatic within a short median follow-up of 16 months.

Besides improving the sensitivity of detection methods, the index of clinical alertness also affects the incidence observed as this sequel can be easily overlooked. In our collection of 138 patients, 26% had very vague symptoms (mild dizziness, impairment of memory and/or personality changes), and 12% were totally asymptomatic. Only 36% of patients presented with classical temporal lobe epilepsy (deja vu, hallucinations, and/or 'absence' attacks), while 25% had non-specific features of intracranial lesions (headache, mental confusion, and/or generalized convulsions). Neurological examination revealed no abnormalities other than papilloedema in 4% and sixth nerve palsy in 14%. The latent interval from completion of primary RT to the detection of cerebral necrosis ranged from 1.5–13 years (median = 5 years).[1]

The differential diagnosis includes intracranial tumour extension, meningeal spread, cerebral metastasis, second primary neoplasm and brain abscess. While histological examination is the most reliable way to establish an unequivocal diagnosis, exploration, solely for the purpose of diagnosis, is not indicated in the majority of cases. Confident diagnosis can be made based on the typical clinical picture, computed tomography (CT), MRI and correlation with the distribution of the radiation dose.[39–45]

The advent of CT is an important milestone in our ability to detect and understand this problem.[39] At the time of detection, 85% of our cases showed a small necrotic nidus at the most infero-medial portions of the temporal lobes with varying degrees of reactive oedema extending above, while the remaining 15% had already developed well-defined lesions with central liquefaction. The classical picture for the oedematous lesions consists of irregular "finger-like" hypodense shadows in the white matter in the temporo-parietal regions (*Figure 1a*). About half of the necrotic nidus do not show any enhancement after contrast injection. Differentiation from tumour recurrence with intracranial spread can be difficult in cases with florid enhancement, especially in those presenting with unilateral CT abnormalities. Diagnosis of the cystic lesions is less problematic. They manifest on CT as roundish hypodense shadows with no contrast enhancement and minimal oedema (*Figure 1b*). While early lesions are located within the irradiation portal, extensive expansion can occur as necrotic debris accumulates.

A study by Leung *et al.* showed that with a short follow-up of 1–3.5 years, more than half (5/9) of the patients with typical CT changes were totally asymptomatic, the earliest asymptomatic CT changes being detected 2.2 years after primary RT.[35] However,

a.

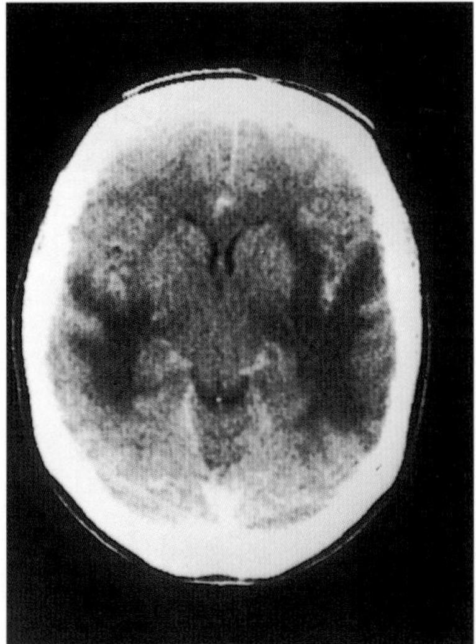

b.

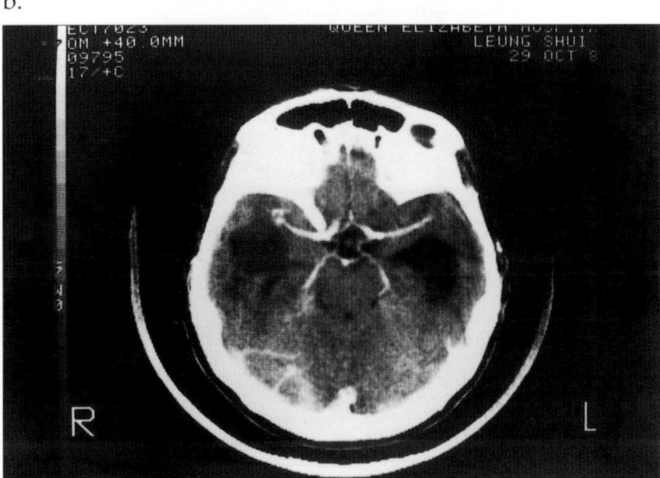

Figure 1. Computed tomographs of temporal lobe radionecrosis showing (a) irregular hypodense shadows in both temporo-parietal regions, and (b) roundish hypodense shadows with no contrast enhancement.

Table 1. Review of literature on late complications following radiation therapy for nasopharyngeal carcinoma.

Type of complication	Cumulative incidence (%) and reference Lowest	Median	Highest
Overall			
Total incidence	6 Baker (1980)[81]	37 Marks *et al.* (1982)[4]	66 Hoppe *et al.* (1976)[22]
Severe morbidity	6 Stein *et al.* (1988)[82]	7 Lee *et al.* (1992)[1]	8 Marks *et al.* (1982)[4]
Treatment death	0.7 Scanlon *et al.* (1967)[83]	3 Haghbin *et al.* (1985)[5]	6 Ballantyne (1975)[20]
Different sites			
Cerebral necrosis	0.4 Chang *et al.* (1980)[84]	1 Chatani *et al.* (1986)[32]	3 Lee *et al.* (1992)[1]
Endocrinopathies	0.7 Cellai *et al.* (1982)[51]	3 Marks *et al.* (1982)[4]	6 Mesic *et al.* (1981)[19]
Encephalomyelopathy	0.2 Huang & Chu (1981)[57]	2 Marks *et al.* (1982)[4]	18 Qin *et al.* (1988)[58]
Neuropathies	0.3 Flores *et al.* (1986)[62]	1 Mesic *et al.* (1981)[19]	6 Hoppe *et al.* (1976)[22]
Cataract	0.1 Lee *et al.* (1992)[1]	1 Chatani *et al.* (1986)[32]	3 de Schryver *et al.* (1971)[68]
Retinopathy	0.1 Lee *et al.* (1992)[1]	2 de Schryver *et al.* (1971)[68]	36 Midena *et al.* (1987)[69]
Deafness	0.7 Bohorquez (1976)[72]	7 Mesic *et al.* (1981)[19]	8 Lee *et al.* (1992)[1]
Persistent otitis	3 Lee *et al.* (1992)[1]	14 Urdaneta *et al.* (1976)[6]	44 Huang & Chu (1981)[57]
Dental caries	4 Mesic *et al.* (1981)[19]	9 Marks *et al.* (1982)[4]	17 Hoppe *et al.* (1976)[22]
Tissue necrosis*	0.8 Lee *et al.* (1992)[1]	3 Urdaneta *et al.* (1976)[6]	9 Marks *et al.* (1982)[4]
Severe epistaxis	0.6 Lee *et al.* (1992)[1]	1 Mesic *et al.* (1981)[19]	1 Ballantyne (1975)[20]
Trismus	5 Urdaneta *et al.* (1976)[6]	10 Hoppe *et al.* (1976)[22]	16 Huang & Chu (1981)[57]
Pharyngeal stricture	0.5 Ballantyne (1975)[20]	1 Haghbin *et al.* (1985)[5]	2 Marks *et al.* (1982)[4]
Neck fibrosis	2 Mesic *et al.* (1981)[19]	14 Haghbin *et al.* (1985)[5]	18 Lee *et al.* (1992)[1]
Malignancy	<0.1 Lee *et al.* (1992)[1]	1 Huang (1980)[80]	1 Ballantyne (1975)[20]

All quoted incidence rates are based on retrospective analyses using the total number of patients treated as denominator.
* Soft tissue and/or bone

the sensitivity of CT is hampered by beam-hardening artifacts from surrounding bones. Interpretation of axial cuts close to the base of skull is specially difficult. Coronal views are more useful for depicting small lesions in the most inferior parts of the temporal lobes. Even with this additional information, however, a negative CT should not be taken as conclusive evidence of exclusion.

There is little doubt that MRI is superior in sensitivity as even a minute necrotic nidus in the most inferior parts of the temporal lobes can be demonstrated.[40] The classical appearance is high signal intensity on T2-weighted spin echo sequence (*Figure 2a*), and very low intensity on T1-weighted images especially for those with liquefaction (*Figure 2b*). Another additional advantage of MRI is the ability to detect areas of liquefactive necrosis within the oedematous lesions by depicting them as roundish areas of low signal intensity on proton-density images, and this distinction is important for guiding subsequent treatment.

It is interesting to note that there is often a marked discrepancy between clinical and radiological changes. Even among those with extensive involvement of both temporal lobes, none of our patients ever showed abnormal behaviour compatible with Kluver-Bucy syndrome,[46] and many were still able to perform complex tasks with minimal difficulty. Indeed this feature was so frequently observed that this became a helpful clue to the working diagnosis.

The treatment of temporal lobe necrosis following RT for NPC is difficult. Surgical removal of the necrotic lesion is the most definitive way of achieving long-term control, but it is particularly hazardous in this situation because of bilateral involvement. While unilateral resection may result in recurrent problems on the contralateral side, bilateral temporal lobectomy is avoided as far as possible for fear of inducing Kluver-Bucy syndrome.[46] We have only treated eight patients with unilateral resection, and one (13%) of them died in the immediate post-operative period. Aspiration can only offer very short-term relief. Unilateral resection of the prominent lesion achieved good control lasting more than six months in 38% (3/8) of our patients, but all eventually relapsed.[1] One patient was so debilitated despite all conservative efforts that contralateral partial lobectomy was subsequently performed.[47] The patient showed dramatic response, regaining full mental consciousness and even resuming normal daily activities (as a housewife) with minimal neurological deficit for over six months. This is the second case of bilateral lobectomy ever reported in a human subject.[47,48] Although we cannot claim bilateral partial lobectomy to be a safe procedure based on such limited experience, it would seem reasonable to speculate that removal of cerebral tissues that have long ceased to function is unlikely to increase the risk of further deficit. This treatment is worth considering in life-threatening situations with no other effective alternative.

Conservative treatment with corticosteroids is an option for lesions in the oedematous phase. With dexamethasone 12–16 mg daily for 4–6 weeks and then gradual tapering of the dosage, we have achieved objective clinical and radiological response lasting for more than six months in 33% (27/81) of patients. Twenty per cent showed complete resolution of CT abnormalities, though minute residual areas could still be

a.

b.

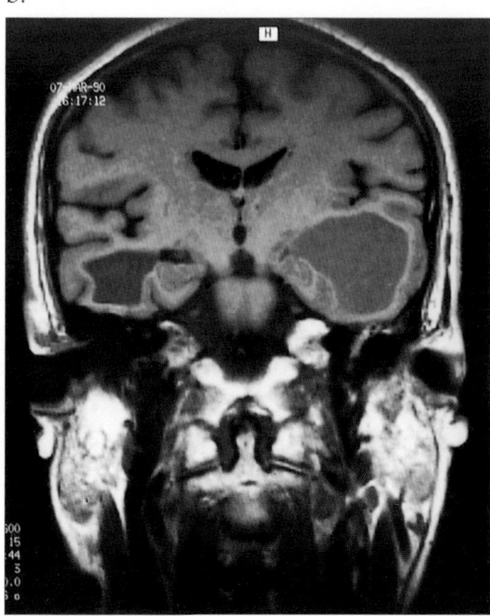

Figure 2. Magnetic resonance imaging of temporal lobe necrosis showing (a) irregular areas of high signal intensity on T2-weighted images, and (b) areas of low signal intensity on T1-weighted images suggestive of central liquefaction.

detected with MRI.[1] In addition to providing symptomatic relief, corticosteroids can have a retarding influence on the progressive pathological process during the early phase of reactive oedema.[39,41,43,49] However, once extensive liquefaction has developed, they are unlikely to offer any significant benefit, and surgical resection is the only option. Early detection and treatment of the radionecrosis are thus important. Steroid therapy however is not hazard-free. In our over-crowded environment, 14% (11/81) of patients on a prolonged course of high dose corticosteroids died of uncontrolled sepsis related to induced immunosuppression. The optimal dosage regime requires further investigation and close observation with intensive support is needed.

For patients with frequent epileptic attacks, symptomatic control with anti-convulsants (e.g. carbamazepine) is also indicated.

The natural rate of progression of the radionecrosis varies considerably not only among different patients, but between the two sides within the same patient.[39,45,50] Although the radiation doses to both sides were the same, the lesion on one side was so small that half of our patients presented with unilateral CT abnormalities, and only 10% of them subsequently became overtly bilateral. Furthermore, among the steroid responders, 12% relapsed on the side that initially appeared normal on CT.

Most patients run an indolent clinical course and even spontaneous regression has been observed. Others progress rapidly into a debilitated state attributed to intralesional hemorrhage and/or rising intracranial pressure. With a median observation period of

3 years (range = 0.5–9 years) from the detection of cerebral damage, 71% of our patients were still alive, and 62% had little functional disability; while 29% had progressed to a debilitated state and 20% died of cerebral necrosis.[1] The 5-year probability of surviving from temporal lobe necrosis or its treatment was 59% (*Figure 3a*).

Neuro-endocrinological System

Disability caused by damage to this system is generally mild, and many patients are totally asymptomatic. The reported incidence of symptomatic hormonal disturbances ranges from 0.7%[51] to 6%[19] of the exposed population, with a median at 3%.[4] Much higher incidences has been observed among survivors subjected to full endocrine scrutiny.[52,53]

The incidence of overt hypoadrenalism, hypothyroidism and/or hyperprolactineamia in our series was 4%, and the median latent interval was 5 years (range = 0.8–13 years).[1] Amenorrhoea and/or galactorrhoea resulting from hyperprolactinaemia were the commonest presenting symptoms in our female patients, but very few of our male cases complained of impotence or decreased libido. Interestingly, there was little correlation between biological evidence of hormonal disturbance and MRI features of an empty sella.

Detailed studies of the endocrine profiles in our patients by Lam *et al.* suggested that the anomalies mostly reflected secondary pituitary failure.[53–55] Biochemical disturbances could occur as early as one year after irradiation, and the initial changes included an impaired growth hormone response to insulin tolerance test, a decreased luteinizing hormone response to luteinizing hormone releasing hormone stimulation and a delayed thyroid stimulating hormone response to thyrotropin releasing hormone. The cumulative 5-year incidence of deficiencies in growth hormone amounted to 64%, gonadotrophins 31%, corticotrophin 27% and thyrotropin 15%, while hyperprolactinemia was noted in 14% of the whole series.

The overall risk of anomalies increases with increasing doses to the hypothalamic-pituitary stalk,[54] and patients subjected to neck irradiation showed a higher incidence of hypothyroidism.[53] Effective prevention of symptomatic endocrine dysfunction could be achieved by shielding the hypothalamic-pituitary axis in early cases.[34] Once developed, correction of deficiency by appropriate hormonal replacement is indicated.

Brainstem and Cervical Spinal Cord

L'hermitte's syndrome (transient tingling and paraesthesia with electric shock-like sensations on flexing the neck) occurs in a small proportion of patients several weeks after RT. Transient demyelination of sensory neurons has been suggested as the underlying pathology,[56] but all gradually recover within a few weeks.

Permanent damage to the brainstem/cervical spinal cord (encephalomyelopathy) has been reported with an incidence ranging from 0.2%[57] to 18%,[58] the median being

a.

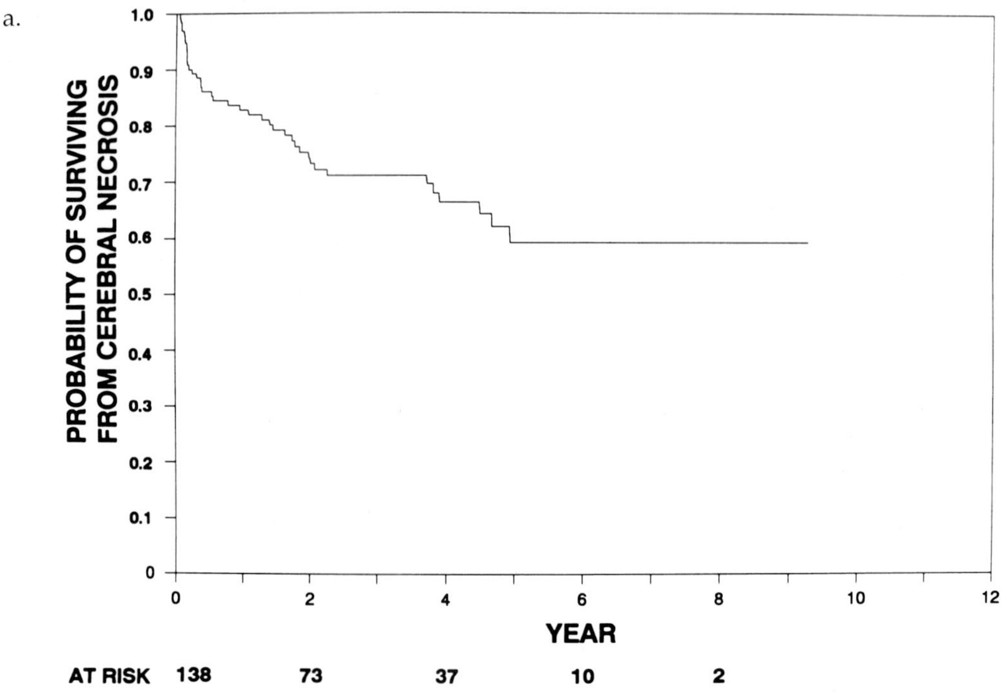

b.

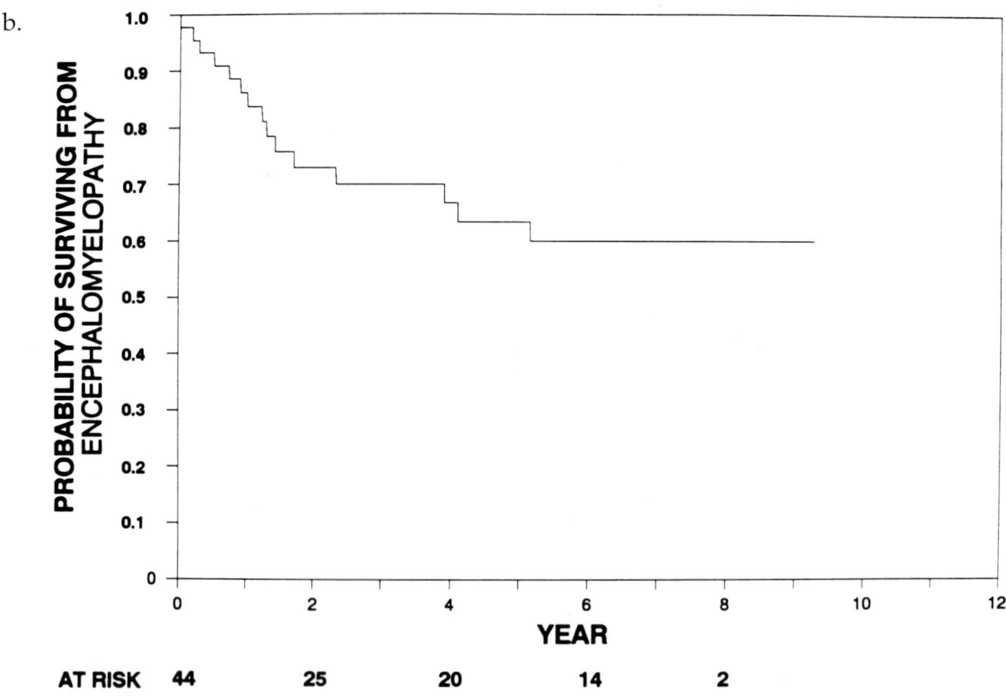

Figure 3. The probability of surviving from (a) temporal lobe necrosis or its treatment, and (b) brainstem encephalopathy/cervical cord myelopathy from the time of their detection.

2%.[4] In addition to fractional dose and total dose,[58,59] the risk depends on technique and the set-up accuracy. Of the 3% (8/251) reported by Mesic *et al.*, some could be correlated with a high dose to the spinal cord at the junction of the lateral wedge portals and the upper neck fields.[19]

A study by Tokars and Griem showed that by increasing the tumour dose from 1450 to 1750 ret (equivalent to approximately 45 to 60 Gy at conventional fractionation), a 15% gain in tumour ablation could be achieved, but the incidence of myelitis would increase from 5% to 10%.[59] Fortunately this difficult dilemma is avoided in the majority of patients as tumour erosion through the clivus is relatively rare. A greater portion of the posterior brainstem can be safely shielded in properly staged early cases, and the brainstem can be completely avoided during the final cone down. With meticulous immobilization, increased shielding and reduction of fractional dose, we have been able to reduce the incidence of brainstem damage to <0.05% without compromise of local control.[1] While the brainstem is rarely involved, postero-lateral extension into the parapharyngeal space is common, and patients with retrostyloid infiltration wrapping round the upper cervical cord pose special difficulty in RT planning.

Affected patients usually present with slowly progressing spastic paraparesis or quadriparesis, with or without multiple cranial nerve palsies. Neurological examination reveals unequivocal long tract signs, but sensory loss is mild or absent as the damage is mostly confined to the anteriorly situated corticospinal tract. The latent interval can range from 0.4 to 9 years (median = 3 years).[1] Investigations with CT, myelograms and lumbar puncture are generally non-contributory. Brainstem auditory evoked potentials help to demonstrate brainstem dysfunction,[60,61] but localization of the lesion was very difficult before the advent of MRI. The classical changes include increased intensity on T2-weighted and decreased intensity on T1-weighted scans (*Figure 4*). However, these changes are non-specific, and other aetiologies must be excluded.

Treatment is difficult as there is no effective way of reverting or arresting this pathological process. The importance of prevention cannot be over-emphasized. Physiotherapy together with symptomatic treatment using baclofen may benefit patients with spastic paresis. Nevertheless, the majority progress and develop severe motor disability. A high mortality rate of 63% (5/8) has been reported by Ballantyne.[20] In our series, 59% (26/44) of affected patients became debilitated and 34% (15/44) died, while the rest ran a slowly deteriorating course. The 5-year probability of survival from encephalomyelopathy following its detection was 63% (*Figure 3b*).

Peripheral Nerves, Eye and Ear

Although peripheral nerves are relatively resistant, radiation-induced cranial and/or cervical sympathetic nerve palsies have been reported with incidences ranging from 0.3%[62] to 6%,[22] with the median at 1%.[19] This is basically a diagnosis by exclusion, and differentiation from tumour recurrence can be difficult. There are no overt radiological signs and even MRI may only show mild non-specific thickening.

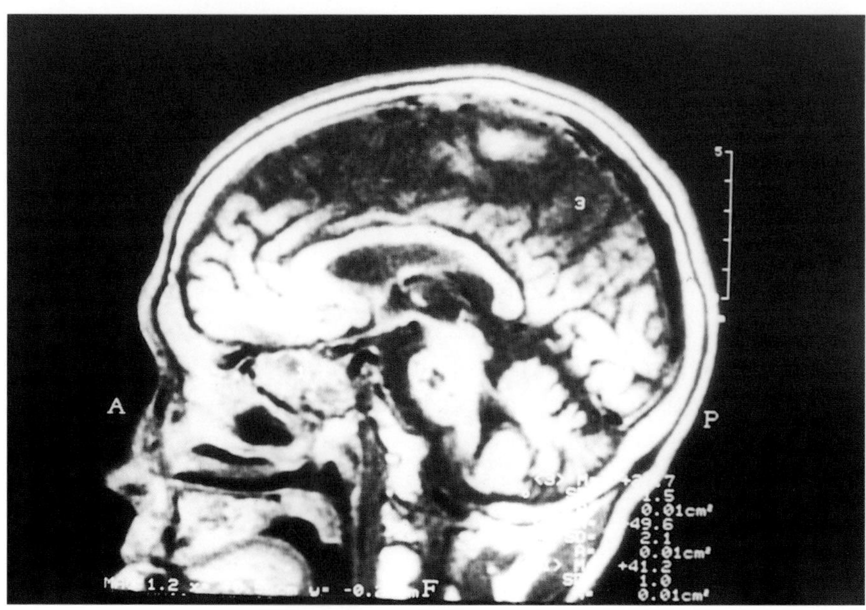

Figure 4. Magnetic resonance imaging revealing lesions in the anterior part of the brainstem.

The incidence in our series was 5% and the median latency was 5 years (range = 0.5–11 years).[1] Table II summarizes the incidence of the various nerve palsies observed. Ten per cent (23/241) of patients had additional long tract signs and were thus part of the brainstem encephalopathy syndrome. All those with fourth, fifth, and seventh nerve palsy belonged to this group. Of those who developed sixth nerve palsy, nearly half were associated with temporal lobe necrosis, and 11% (5/47) had gross papilloedema. Hence, some exhibited a false localizing sign caused by increased intracranial pressure rather than genuine nerve damage.

The last four cranial nerves (the twelfth in particular) were by far the commonest affected.[1,19,20,22,57,63] It has been suggested that perineural fibrosis in the retropharyngeal space may be a major contributing cause to the neuropathy,[22,57,63] but histological confirmation of this is not yet available. An association with marked fibrosis of soft tissues of the neck was noted in 54% (89/166) of our patients.[1] Some patients present with twitching of the respective muscles before subsequent development of paralysis and atrophy. Treatment with clonazepam might help to alleviate the irritation in patients with frequent twitching. The majority of patients present with slurring of speech, and most run a very indolent course but this complication can also be life-threatening. It should be noted that 2% (4/166) of our affected patients died of aspiration pneumonia due to severe impairment of swallowing function.

Optic nerve/chiasma damage, though non-fatal, is functionally and psychologically the most distressing complication, especially to those suffering bilateral blindness. The most important determinant is the fractional dose.[64–66] With the technique commonly adopted in Hong Kong, the optic chiasma and the proximal portion of the optic nerves

Table 2. Cumulative Incidence (%) of nerve palsy in 4527 patients with nasopharyngeal carcinoma treated by megavoltage photons in Queen Elizabeth Hospital, Hong Kong.

Nerve palsy	Total incidence	Bilateral involvement	Severe dysfunction
II	1.13	0.35	0.53
IV	0.11	0.02	
V	0.40		
VI	1.04	0.18	0.04
VII	0.11		
IX	0.33	0.11	0.07
X	0.55	0.13	0.15
XI	1.15	0.35	0.09
XII	3.25	1.39	0.51
Sympathetic	0.15	0.07	

are included at the field edge in the majority of patients. The incidence of this neurological complication in our series was 1%, with 0.4% being bilateral.[1]

With complete shielding of the eyeballs in patients without anterior tumour extension, our incidence of eyeball damage was only 0.3%, and half of those affected had an exceptionally high dose to the orbit as dictated by initial tumour infiltration.[1] Damage included corneal scarring/ulceration (0.1%), cataract (0.1%), and retinitis (0.1%).

A higher incidence of eyeball complications has been reported by other authors.[32,66–69] Accurate assessment of the true incidence is not easy, while aging and other degenerative causes must be excluded. The median reported incidences of radiation-induced cataract and retinopathy are 1%[32] and 2%,[68] respectively, of the exposed population. Ophthalmic assessment by de Schryver *et al.* showed that the corresponding incidences could be as high as 24% (19/80) and 15% (12/80) among long-term survivors.[68] Midena *et al.* even observed a 36% (4/11) retinopathy rate.[69]

Obviously, the radiation treatment technique is most important. Shielding of the eyeballs should be feasible in the majority of patients and meticulous protection (as far as possible) is warranted. Once developed, treatment is difficult; and even lens extraction may not salvage the eye-sight in those with cataract because most cases have multiple damage.[70]

Otological problems are common in patients with NPC, due to both tumour effect and radiation damage. A study by Lau *et al.* showed that 22% (11/49) of patients presented with tinnitus before treatment and 29% (24/49) complained of prolonged tinnitus 12 months after completion of RT.[71] The reported incidence of persistent otitis media and/or externa ranged widely from 3%[1] to 44%,[57] with the median at 14%.[6] Although only 3% of our patients were affected, 17% (19/111) of these had serious sepsis including meningitis.[1]

The reported incidence of hearing impairment ranged from 0.7%[72] to 8%,[1] with a median at 7%.[19] The damage may be bilateral and severe, with involvement of both conductive and sensorineural elements. Detailed otological assessment by Kwong *et al.* showed that at a median follow-up of 2.5 years, 24% of ears developed persistent sensorineural hearing loss.[73] The high frequencies are specially affected.[73,74] A higher incidence was noted in patients with post-irradiation persistent otitis media[73] and in those with higher total radiation dosage to the inner ear.[74]

Young and Hsieh recommended insertion of a ventilation tube as their study showed that the eustachian tube dysfunction was due to both organic obstruction and functional impairment.[75] A randomized comparison by Chowdhury *et al.* reported a decrease in conductive hearing loss and tinnitus in patients with prophylactic ventilation tube insertion.[76] However, the tubes are frequently associated with complications of blockage, displacement and/or infection. Both the studies by Lau *et al.*[77] and Skinner *et al.*[78] failed to show significant long-term benefits from the use of ventilation tubes.

Neuropsychological Functioning

In a small series of long-term adult survivors after treatment with large fractional doses (3.5 Gy for 17 fractions), detailed neuropsychological assessment revealed significantly poorer IQ and non-verbal memory recall, even though all patients were able to function at an acceptable level and CT did not reveal any gross anomalies.[79] The study cautions that subclinical cognitive and intellectual deficits may be more common than expected.

Radiation-induced Malignancy

Isolated cases of osteosarcoma in the irradiated parts of the maxilla,[1,20,80] squamous cell carcinoma of the palate,[20] tongue[67] and skin[19] have been reported following RT for NPC. The median incidence was 1%,[80] and the shortest latency was 10 years.[1] Treatment is difficult and the prognosis is often grave.

Concluding Remarks

With the constant fear of recurrence and late complications, it is understandable that patients with NPC face great stress. Detailed studies of their quality of life are urgently needed. While it is not advisable to compromise the chance of tumour eradication for fear of inducing morbidity, it cannot be over-emphasized that accuracy in planning and administration of treatment is vital in avoiding unnecessary damage. With increasing accuracy in delineation of tumour extent by modern investigative methods, additional shielding can be cautiously tested in properly staged early cases. Advances in technology of conformal and stereotactic radiotherapy would help to reduce the volume of normal tissues exposed to irradiation. However, new endeavours of dose escalation/acceleration, and combination with chemotherapy could lead to risks that may not yet be fully known. Cautious monitoring of the therapeutic ratio is absolutely essential, and it is hoped that the final goal of achieving the best quantity and quality of life can be effectively achieved.

References

1. Lee, A.W.M., Law, S.C.K., Ng, S.H., Chan, D.K.K., Poon, Y.F., Foo, W., O, S.K., Tung, S.Y., Cheung, F.K., Ho, J.H.C. 1992. Retrospective analysis of nasopharyngeal carcinoma treated during 1976–1985: late complications following megavoltage irradiation. *Brit. J. Radiol.*; 65:918–928.
2. Cox, J.D., Stetz, J., Pajak, T.F. 1995. Toxicity criteria of the Radiation Therapy Oncology Group (RTOG) and the European Organization for Research and Treatment of Cancer (EORTC). *Int. J. Radiat. Oncol. Biol. Phys.*; 31:1341–1346.
3. Maciejewski, B., Zajusz, A., Pilecki, B., Skiadowski, K., Dorr, W., Kummermehr, J., Trott, K.R. 1992. Escalated hyperfractionation and stimulation of acute mucosal reaction in radiotherapy for cancer of the oral cavity and oropharynx. *Semin. Radiat. Oncol.*; 2:54–57.
4. Marks, J.E., Bedwinek, J.M., Lee, F., Purdy, J.A., Perez, C.A. 1982. Dose-response analysis for nasopharyngeal carcinoma: an historical perspective. *Cancer*; 50:1042–1050.
5. Haghbin, M., Kramer, S., Patchefsky, A.S. 1985. Carcinoma of the nasopharynx: a 25-year study. *Am. J. Clin. Oncol.*; 8:384–392.
6. Urdaneta, N., Fischer, J.J., Vera, R., Gutierrez, E. 1976. Cancer of the nasopharynx: review of 43 cases treated with supervoltage radiation therapy. *Cancer*; 37:1707–1712.
7. Franzen, L., Funegard, U., Ericson, T., Henriksson, R. 1992. Parotid gland function during and following radiotherapy of malignancies in the head and neck: a consecutive study of salivary flow and patient discomfort. *Eur. J. Cancer*; 28:457–462.
8. Marks, J.E., Davis, C.C., Gottsman, V.L., Purdy, J.E., Lee, F. 1981. The effects of radiation on parotid salivary function. *Int. J. Radiat. Oncol. Biol. Phys.*; 7:1013–1019.
9. Ang, K.K., Stephens, L.C., Schultheiss, T.E. 1991. Salivary glands. In: *Radiopathology of Organs and Tissues*, eds. Scherer, E., Streffer, C., Trott, K.R. Berlin: Springer Verlag, 293–311.
10. Tsujii, H. 1985. Quantitive dose-response analysis of salivary function following radiotherapy using sequential RI-sialography. *Int. J. Radiat. Oncol. Biol. Phys.*; 11:1603–1612.
11. Nishioka, T., Shirato, H., Arimoto, T., Kaneko, M., Kitahara, T., Oomori, K., Yasuda, M., Fukuda, S., Inuyama, Y., Miyasaka, K. 1997. Reduction of radiation-induced xerostomia in nasopharyngeal carcinoma using CT simulation with laser patient marking and three-field irradiation technique. *Int. J. Radiat. Oncol. Biol. Phys.*; 38:705–712.
12. Greenspan, D., Daniels, T.E. 1987. Effectiveness of pilocarpine in postradiation xerostomia. *Cancer*; 59:1123–1125.
13. Johnson, J.T., Ferretti, G.A., Nethery, W.J., Valdez, I.H., Fox, P.C., Ng, D., Muscoplat, C.C., Gallagher, S.C. 1993. Oral pilocarpine for postradiation xerostomia in patients with head and neck cancer. *N. Engl. J. Med.*; 329:390–395.
14. Reike, J.E., Hafermann, M.D., Johnson, J.T., Leveque, F.G., Iwamoto, R., Steiger, B.W., Muscoplat, C.C., Gallagher, S.C. 1995. Oral pilocarpine for radiation-induced xerostomia: integrated efficacy and safety results from two prospective randomized clinical trials. *Int. J. Radiat. Oncol. Biol. Phys.*; 31:661–669.
15. Prada, A., Chiesa, F. 1987. Effects of benzydamine on the oral mucositis during antineoplastic radiotherapy and/or intra-arterial chemotherapy. *Int. J. Tissue React.*; 9:115–119.
16. Epstein, J.B., Stevenson-Moore, P., Jacson, S., Mohamed, J.H., Spinelli, J.J. 1989. Prevention of oral mucositis in radiation therapy: a controlled study with benzydamine hydrochloride rinse. *Int. J. Radiat. Oncol. Biol. Phys.*; 16:1571–1575.

17. Mossman, K.L., Henkin, R.I. 1978. Radiation-induced changes in taste acuity in cancer patients. *Int. J. Radiat. Oncol. Biol. Phys.*; 4:663.
18. Silverman, S. Jr., Thompson, J.S. 1984. Serum zinc and copper in oral/oropharyngeal carcinoma. *Oral Surg. Oral Med. Oral Pathol.*; 57:34.
19. Mesic, J.B., Fletcher, G.H., Goepfert, H. 1981. Megavoltage irradiation of epithelial tumours of the nasopharynx. *Int. J. Radiat. Oncol. Biol. Phys.*; 7:447–453.
20. Ballantyne, A.J. 1975. Late Sequelae of radiation therapy in cancer of the head and neck with particular reference to the nasopharynx. *Am. J. Surg.*; 130:433–436.
21. Travis, E., Mason, K.A. 1992. Late radiation damage in normal tissue. *Cancer Bull.*; 44:105–110.
22. Hoppe, R.T., Goffinet, D.R., Bagshaw, M.A. 1976. Carcinoma of the nasopharynx: eighteen years-experience with megavoltage radiation therapy. *Cancer*; 37:2605–2612.
23. Lee, A.W.M., Law, S.C.K., Foo, W., Poon, Y.F., Cheung, F.K., Chan, D.K.K., O, S.K., Tung, S.Y., Myo, Thaw, Ho, J.H.C. 1993. Retrospective analysis of patients with nasopharyngeal carcinoma treated during 1976–1985: survival after local recurrence. *Int. J. Radiat. Oncol. Biol. Phys.*; 26:773–782.
24. Larson, D.L. 1986. Management of complications of radiotherapy of the head and neck. *Head Neck Surg.*; 66:169–182.
25. Dion, M.W., Hussy, D.H., Osborn, J.W. 1989. Preliminary results of a pilot study of pentoxifylline in the treatment of late radiation soft tissue necrosis. *Int. J. Radiat. Oncol. Biol. Phys.*; 17:193–194.
26. Frank, R.M., Herdly, J., Philippe, E. 1965. Acquired dental defects and salivary gland lesions after irradiation for carcinoma. *J. Am. Dent. Assoc.*; 70:868.
27. Dreizen, S., Brown, L.R., Daly, T.E., Drane, J.B. 1977. Prevention of xerostomia-related dental caries in irradiated cancer patients. *J. Dent. Res.*; 56:99.
28. Wei, S. 1984. Clinical uses of fluoride: a state-of-the-art conference on the uses of fluorides in clinical dentistry. *J. Am. Dent. Assoc.*; 109:472.
29. Morrish, R.B., Chan, E., Silverman, S. Jr., Meyer, J., Fu, K.K., Greenspan, D. 1981. Osteonecrosis in patients irradiated for head and neck carcinoma. *Cancer*; 47:1980.
30. Fattore, L.D., Strauss, R.A. 1987. Hyperbaric oxygen in the treatment of osteoradionecrosis: a review of its use and efficacy. *Oral Surg. Oral Med. Oral Pathol.*; 63:280.
31. Katsikeris, N., Young, E.R. 1992. Postradiation dental extractions without hyperbaric oxygen. *Oral Surg. Oral Med. Oral Pathol.*; 74:155–157.
32. Chatani, M., Teshima, T., Inoue, T., *et al.* 1986. Radiation therapy for nasopharyngeal carcinoma: retrospective review of 105 patients based on a survey of Kansai Cancer Therapist Group. *Cancer*; 57:2267–2271.
33. Lee, A.W.M., Foo, W., Chappell, R., Fowler, J., Sze, W.M., Poon, Y.F., Law, S.C.K., Ng, S.H., O, S.K., Tung, S.Y., Lau, W.H., Ho, J.H.C. 1998. Effect of time, dose and fractionation on temporal lobe necrosis following radiotherapy for nasopharyngeal carcinoma. *Int. J. Radiat. Oncol. Biol. Phys.*; 40:35–42.
34. Sham, J., Choy, D., Kwong, P.W.K., Cheng, A.C.K., Kwong, D.L.W., Yau, C.C., Wan, K.Y., Au, G.K.H. 1994. Radiotherapy for nasopharyngeal carcinoma: shielding the pituitary may improve therapeutic ratio. *Int. J. Radiat. Oncol. Biol. Phys.*; 29:699–704.
35. Leung, S.F., Kreel, L., Tsao, S.Y. 1992. Asymptomatic temporal lobe injury after radiotherapy for nasopharyngeal carcinoma: incidence and determinants. *Brit. J. Radiol.*; 65:710–714.
36. Ang, K.K., Jiang, G.L., Guttenberger, R., Thames, H.D., Stephens, L.C., Smith, C.D., Feng, Y. 1992. Impact of spinal cord repair kinetics on the practice of altered fractionation schedules. *Radiother. Oncol.*; 25:287–294.
37. Bentzen, S.M., Ruifrok, A.C.C., Thames, H.D. 1996. Repair capacity and kinetics for human mucosa and epithelial tumours in the head and neck: clinical data on the effect of changing the time interval between multiple fractions per day in radiotherapy. *Radiother. Oncol.*; 38:89–101.
38. Teo, P.M.L., Kwan, W.H., Leung, S.F., Leung, W.T., Chan, A., Choi, P., Yu, P., Lee, W.Y., Johnson, P. 1996. Early tumour response and treatment toxicity after hyperfractionated radiotherapy in nasopharyngeal carcinoma. *Brit. J. Radiol.*; 69:241–248.

39. Lee, A.W.M., Ng, S.H., Ho, J.H.C., Tse, V.K.C., Poon, Y.F., Tse, C.C.H., Au, G.K.H., O, S.K., Lau, W.H., Foo, W. 1988. Clinical diagnosis of late temporal lobe necrosis following radiation therapy for nasopharyngeal carcinoma. *Cancer*; 61:1535–1542.
40. Lee, A.W.M., Cheng, L.O.C., Ng, S.H., Tse, V.K.C., O, S.K., Au, G.K.H., Poon, Y.F. 1990. Magnetic resonance imaging in the clinical diagnosis of late temporal lobe necrosis following radiotherapy for nasopharyngeal carcinoma. *Clin. Radiol.*; 41:24–41.
41. Shaw, P.J., Bates, D. 1984. Conservative treatment of delayed cerebral radiation necrosis. *J. Neurol. Neurosurg. Psychiatry*; 47:1338–1341.
42. Glass, J.P., Hwang, T.-L., Leavens, M.E., Libshitz, H.I. 1984. Cerebral radiation necrosis following treatment of extracranial malignancies. *Cancer*; 54:1966–1972.
43. Martins, A.N., Johnston, J.S., Henry, J.M., Stoffel, T.J., Di Chiro, G. 1977. Delayed radiation necrosis of the brain. *J. Neurosurg.*; 47:336–345.
44. Mikhael, M.A. 1978. Radiation necrosis of the brain: correlation between computed tomography, pathology, and dose distribution. *J. Comput. Assist. Tomogr.*; 2:71–80.
45. Chong, V.F.H., Fan, Y.F., Chan, L.L. 1997. Temporal lobe necrosis in nasopharyngeal carcinoma: pictorial essay. *Australas Radiol.*; 41:392–397.
46. Kluver, H., Bucy, P.C. 1939. Preliminary analysis of functions of the temporal lobes in monkeys. *Arch. Neurol. Psychiat.*; 42:949–1000.
47. Lee, A.W.M., Ng, S.H., Tse, V.K.C., Chiu, H.M., Myo, Thaw. 1993. Case report: bilateral temporal lobectomy for necrosis induced by radiotherapy for nasopharyngeal carcinoma. *Acta Oncol.*; 32:343–345.
48. Fontana, M., Mastrostefano, R., Bernabei, A., *et al.* 1984. Bilateral temporal lobectomy for late radionecrosis after radiotherapy for acromegaly. A case report. *J. Neurosurg. Sci.*; 28:107–112.
49. Eyster, E.F., Nielsen, S.L., Sheline, G.E., Wilosn, C.B. 1974. Cerebral radiation necrosis simulating a brain tumour: case report. *J. Neurosurg.*;39:267–271.
50. Lee, A.W.M., Yau, T.K. 1997. Complications of radiation therapy. In: *Nasopharyngeal Carcinoma*, eds. Chong, V.F.H., Tsao, S.Y. Singapore: Armour Publishing Pte. Ltd., 114–127.
51. Cellai, E., Chiavacci, P., Olmi, P., Carcangiu, M.L. 1982. Carcinoma of the nasopharynx: results of radiation therapy. *Acta Radiol. Oncol.*; 21:87–95.
52. Samaan, N.A., Vieto, R., Schulz, P.N., Maor, M., Meoz, R.T., Sampiere, V.A., Cangir, A., Ried, H.L., Jesse, R.H. Jr. 1982. Hypothalamic, pituitary and thyroid dysfunction after radiotherapy to the head and neck. *Int. J. Radiat. Oncol. Biol. Phys.*; 8:1857–1867.
53. Lam, K.S.L., Tse, V.K.C., Wang, C., Yeung, R.T.T., Ho, J.H.C. 1991. Effects of cranial irradiation on hypothalamic-pituitary function: a 5-year longitudinal study in patients with nasopharyngeal carcinoma. *Quarterly J. Med. New Series*; 78:165–176.
54. Lam, K.S.L., Tse, V.K.C., Wang, C., Yeung, R.T.T., Ma, J.T.C., Ho, J.H.C. 1987. Early effects of cranial irradiation on hypothalamic-pituitary function. *J. Clin. Endocrinol. Metab.*; 64:418–424.
55. Lam, K.S.L., Ho, J.H.C., Lee, A.W.M., Tse. V.K.C., Chan, P.K., Wang, C., Ma, J.T.C., Yeung, R.T.T. 1987. Symptomatic hypothalamic-pituitary dysfunction in nasopharyngeal carcinoma patients following radiation therapy: a retrospective study. *Int. J. Radiat. Oncol. Biol. Phys.*; 13:1343–1350.
56. Jones, A. 1964. Transient radiation myelopathy (with reference to Lhermitte's sign of electrical paresthesia). *Brit. J. Radiol.*; 37:727–744.
57. Huang, S.C., Chu, G.-L. 1981. Nasopharyngeal cancer: study II. *Int. J. Radiat. Oncol. Biol. Phys.*; 7:713–716.
58. Qin, D., Hu, Y., Yan, J., Xu, G., Cai, W., Wu, X., Cao, D., Gu, X. 1988. Analysis of 1379 patients with nasopharyngeal carcinoma treated by radiation. *Cancer*; 61:1117–1124.
59. Tokers, R.P., Griem, M.L. 1979. Carcinoma of the nasopharynx: an optimization of radiotherapeutic management for tumour control and spinal cord injury. *Int. J. Radiat. Oncol. Biol. Phys.*; 5:1741–1748.
60. Lau, S.K., Wei, W.I., Choy, D., Sham, J.S.T., Engzell, U.C. 1988. Brainstem auditory evoked potentials after irradiation of nasopharyngeal carcinoma — report on two cases with myelopathy of the brainstem. *J. Laryngol. Otol.*; 102:1142–1146.

61. Grau, C., Moller, K., Overgaard, M., Overgaard, J., Elbrond, O. 1992. Auditory brain stem responses after radiation therapy for nasopharyngeal carcinoma. *Cancer*; 70:2396–2401.
62. Flores, A.D., Dickson, R.I., Riding, K., Coy, P. 1986. Cancer of the nasopharynx in British Columbia. *Am. J. Clin. Oncol.*; 9:281–291.
63. Cheng, V.S.T., Schulz, M.D. 1975. Unilateral hypoglossal nerve atrophy as a late complication of radiation therapy of head and neck carcinoma: a report of four cases and a review of the literature on peripheral and cranial nerve damages after radiation therapy. *Cancer*; 35:1537–1544.
64. Harris, J.R., Levene, M.B. 1976. Visual complications following irradiation for pituitary adenomas and craniopharyngiomas. *Radiology*; 120:167–171.
65. Aristizabal, S., Caldwell, W.L., Avila, J. 1977. The relationship of time-dose fractionation factors to complications in the treatment of pituitary tumours by irradiation. *Int. J. Radiat. Oncol. Biol. Phys.*; 2:667–673.
66. Parsons, J.T., Fitzgerald, C.R., Hood, C.I., Ellingwood, K.E., Bova, F.J., Million, R.R. 1983. The effects of irradiation on the eye and optic nerve. *Int. J. Radiat. Oncol. Biol. Phys.*; 9:609–622.
67. John, A.C., Busby, E.R., Jones, P.H. 1980. Long-term survival in nasopharyngeal carcinoma. *J. Laryngol. Otol.*; 94:1265–1275.
68. De Schryver, A., Wachtmeister, L., Baryd, I. 1971. Ophthalmologic observations on long-term survivors after radiotherapy for nasopharyngeal tumours. *Acta Radiol. Ther. Phys. Biol.*; 10:193–209.
69. Midena, E., Segato, T., Piermarocchi, S., *et al.* 1987. Retinopathy following radiation therapy of paranasal sinus and nasopharyngeal carcinoma. *Retina*; 7:142–147.
70. Kwok, S.K., Ho, P.C., Leung, S.F., Sonal, K.F. 1994. Surgical result of radiation-induced cataract in Chinese patients with nasopharyngeal carcinoma. *Dev. Ophthalmol.*; 26:14–18.
71. Lau, S.K., Wei, W.I., Sham, J.S.T., *et al.* 1992. Early changes of auditory brain stem evoked response after radiotherapy for nasopharyngeal carcinoma: a prospective study. *J. Laryngol. Otol.*; 106:887–892.
72. Bohorquez, J. 1976. Factors that modify the radio-response of cancer of the nasopharynx. *Am. J. Roentgenol.*; 126:863–876.
73. Kwong, D.L.W., Wei, W.I., Sham, J.S.T., Ho, W.K., Yuen, P.W., Chua, D.T.T., Au, D.K K., Wu, P.M., Choy, D.T.K. 1996. Sensorineural hearing loss in patients treated for nasopharyngeal carcinoma: a prospective study of the effect of radiation and cisplatin treatment. *Int. Rad. Oncol. Biol. Phys.*; 36:281–289.
74. Grau, C., Moller, K., Overgaard, M., Overgaard, J., Elbrond, O. 1991. Sensori-neural hearing loss in patients treated with irradiation for nasopharyngeal carcinoma. *Int. J. Radiat. Oncol. Biol. Phys.*; 21:723–728.
75. Young, Y.H., Hsieh, T. 1992. Eustachian tube dysfunction in patients with nasopharyngeal carcinoma, pre- and postradiation. *Eur. Arch. Otorhinolaryngol.*; 249:206–208.
76. Chowdhury, C.R., Ho, J.H.C., Wright, A., Tsao, S.Y., Au, G.K.H., Tung, Y. 1988. Prospective study of the effects of ventilation tubes on hearing after radiotherapy for carcinoma of nasopharynx. *Ann. Otol. Rhinol. Laryngol.*; 97:142–145.
77. Lau, S.K., Wei, W.I., Sham, J.S.T., *et al.* 1992. Effects of irradiation on middle ear effusion due to nasopharyngeal carcinoma: a prospective study. *Clin. Otolaryngol.*; 17:246–250.
78. Skinner, D. W., Lesser, T. H., Richards, S. H. 1988. A 15 year follow-up of a controlled trial of the use of grommets in glue ear. *Clin. Otolaryngol.*; 13:341–346.
79. Lee, P.W.H., Hung, B.K.M., Woo, E.K.W., Tai, P.T.H., Choi, D.T.K. 1989. Effects of radiation therapy on neuropsychological functioning in patients with nasopharyngeal carcinoma. *J. Neurol. Neurosurg. Psychiatry*; 52:488–492.
80. Huang, S.C. 1980. Nasopharyngeal cancer: a review of 1605 patients treated radically with cobalt 60. *Int. J. Radiat. Oncol. Biol. Phys.*; 6:401–407.
81. Baker, S.R. 1980. Nasopharyngeal carcinoma: clinical course and results of therapy. *Head Neck Surg.*; 3:8–14.

82. Stein, M., Kuten, A., Arbel, M., Ben-Schachar, M., Epelbaum, R., Wajsbort, R., Klein, B., Cohen, Y., Robinson, E. 1988. Carcinoma of the nasopharynx in Northern Israel: epidemiology and treatment results. *J. Surg. Oncol.*; 37:84–88.
83. Scanlon, P.W., Rhodes, R.E., Woolner, L.B., Devine, K.D., McBean, J.B. 1967. Cancer of the nasopharynx: 142 patients treated in the 11 year period 1950–1960. *Am. J. Roentgenol.*; 99:313–325.
84. Chang, C., Liu, T., Chang, Y., Cao, S. 1980. Radiation therapy of nasopharyngeal carcinoma. *Acta Radiol. Oncol.*; 19:433–438.

CHAPTER 15

Role of Surgery

Kee Chee Soo

The role for surgery in the management of nasopharyngeal carcinoma is limited as the tumour is radiosensitive and radiotherapy is the mainstay of treatment. The nasopharynx is an anatomical site where access is difficult. Morever, it is close to several vital structures such as the brain, skull base, eye, and internal carotid artery. This makes oncological resection a difficult exercise. Also, the disease tends to be submucosal and it may not be possible to define margins of resection especially after radiotherapy. A sizeable proportion of the patients present late and up to 10% of all patients have systemic metastases at initial diagnosis.[1] Surgery can be hazardous because patients have invariably had prior radiation therapy and a good proportion of them may even have had a second course of radiation. Thus the role of surgery in nasopharyngeal carcinoma has to be clearly defined.

Indications

Indications for surgery include:

- (i) the diagnosis of the disease and the occasional need for examination and biopsy of the nasopharynx and/or the cervical nodes,
- (ii) the surgical treatment of residual or recurrent nodal disease,
- (iii) exposure of, and access to, the nasopharynx for local excision, implantation radiotherapy or after-loading brachytherapy,
- (iv) various surgical procedures for the management of complications of radiation therapy e.g. trismus necessitating feeding gastrostomy, otitis media requiring myringotomy or cricopharyngeal myotomy for aspiration.

Diagnosis of the Disease

The diagnosis of the disease and the occasional need for examination and biopsy of the nasopharynx or the cervical nodes under anaesthesia are outlined in Chapter 7. However it is recognized that open neck biopsies are most often unnecessary. There are only occasional instances when these may have to be performed. These include the scenario where fine needle aspiration cytology of a neck mass is equivocal in the presence of persistently negative biopsies of the nasopharynx, or for confirmation of recurrent or residual disease at the primary site or in lymph nodes. The lymph node biopsy should be carried out under general anaesthesia. It is often preceded by examination and curettage of the nasopharynx and frozen section processing of the specimens from the nasopharynx, thereby aiming to avoid a neck biopsy. The node after biopsy should be sent fresh for immunological processing to exclude lymphoma. The incision for the biopsy is placed appropriately to allow for subsequent radical neck dissection if necessary.

Residual and Recurrent Nodal Disease

Lymph node metastases in nasopharyngeal carcinoma are extremely common and have been observed in 60% to 88% of the patients.[2,3] Despite the sensitivity of the tumour to radiotherapy, there is a recurrence rate of 9% to 10% in the neck after therapeutic or prophylactic neck irradiation.[3,4] The diagnosis of recurrent or residual nodal disease can then be difficult to confirm. The irradiated neck is difficult to palpate because of soft tissue and skin induration and there is often an underestimation of positive lymph node involvement.[5] MRI and CT scans can sometimes show and confirm the presence of node enlargement. Fine needle aspiration cytology is useful but there is a false negative rate of 39%.[6] Clinically false positive findings are also not uncommon and a negative resection rate of 12% to 22% has been reported from various centres.[6,7,8] Although radiotherapy has been used as definitive treatment,[9] surgery is now the treatment of choice. Surgery gives a survival rate from 40% to 80% compared to a survival rate of only 19% to 28% with a second course of radiation therapy.[6,9,10] Though lymph node excision has been performed in the past, it is now well recognised that radical neck dissection is necessary because of inaccuracy in the preoperative assessment of lymph nodes involved and the finding of multiple levels of lymph node involvement in up to 60% of the patients.[5,10] There has also been the observation of a very high incidence of extra capsular spread of 70% or more in the lymph nodes involved in this group of patients.[5,10] Radical neck dissection should be considered in the absence of local recurrence or systemic metastasis. In our experience a significant proportion of the patients will require extensive sacrifice of overlying involved skin and regional flaps will have to be used to achieve wound cover.[10] In addition, because of extensive soft tissue involvement, we have often utilised after loading catheters for postoperative brachytherapy as adjuvant treatment. The mortality and morbidity rates with radical neck dissection are low and the 5-year actuarial survival has been reported to be as high as 80% with a 5-year disease free survival of 59%.[10] Multivariate analysis has shown that neither the pre-treatment staging nor the disease free interval appear to affect subsequent neck control and survival. The only significant prognostic variable was the number of positive lymph nodes at the time of radical neck dissection.[8,10]

Recurrent or Residual Disease in the Nasopharynx

The majority of cases have been treated with a second course of radiation either externally or by implants or by the use of stereotactic irradiation,[12,13] though there are increasing reports of surgical attempts at removal of locally recurrent or residual disease.[14,15,16,17,18] The good results obtained from the surgical treatment of nodal disease would suggest that in a highly selected group of patients, surgical resection of the nasopharynx may be appropriate.

Contraindications to surgery include the presence of systemic metastases, intracranial involvement, cranial nerve involvement, skull base erosion and carotid artery encasement. MRI assessment is particularly useful for local extension of disease especially with regard to intracranial spread and cranial nerve involvement.[11]

Surgical approaches to the nasopharynx

There have been numerous approaches described to gain access to the nasopharynx. The internal carotid artery is in close proximity to the lateral nasopharynx whatever the approach, and care must be taken to avoid inadvertent injury to the artery. Exposure with most approaches is less than satisfactory and margins are difficult to assess intraoperatively even with frozen sections. Tumours can easily extend to the parapharyngeal space or along the eustachian tube to the middle ear, frequently giving rise to failure despite an extensive operation.

The nasopharynx can be approached inferiorly (transpalatal, mandibular swing), anteriorly (Lefort I osteotomy, subtotal maxillectomy, maxillary swing), or laterally (infra-temporal approach). Recently we have described an endoscopic approach for resection of localised recurrence of nasopharyngeal carcinoma.[19]

CT or MR imaging is required to assess the extent of the disease especially as it is frequently submucosal making endoscopic assessment difficult and inaccurate. These scans are also vital as they may show up certain contraindications to nasopharygectomy i.e. intra-cranial extension, cranial nerve involvement, extensive skull base erosion or carotid artery encasement.

In all the techniques described, it is important to appreciate the close proximity of the internal carotid artery especially when the disease extends laterally. The extent of the disease will determine the optimal approach to the nasopharynx and a combined approach may often be necessary. The resection can usually be done without a tracheostomy. The handling of the tissues must be meticulous because they have been irradiated. We usually isolate the internal carotid artery in the neck and this artery is then traced into the skull base. A piece of gauze is placed around it to protect it from inadvertent injury. The external carotid is looped with a vascular sling for control of bleeding if necessary. Resection of the nasopharyngeal mucosa is carried to the bony surface of the clivus which may also require drilling. The resection margins require meticulous frozen section assessment as some of the techniques of approach are too tedious for a reoperation if the frozen section margins subsequently turn out to be falsely negative. The exposed bone at the skull base can be re-lined by the turbinate or nasal mucosa but in recent times we have used a free radial forearm flap. This provides healthy vascularised tissue for a heavily irradiated area.

Inferior Approach

Transpalatal. (*Figure* 1) Up till now this has been the simplest approach. It is used primarily for insertion of intracavitary radium or for biopsy and occasionally for resection of small tumours.[7] To enable greater access a posteriorly based mucoperiosteal flap preserving the greater palatine neurovascular bundle can be used. The hard palate and the posterior aspect of nasal septum require removal to provide better exposure (*Figure* 2). The mucoperiosteal flap can then be reapproximated and this has to be done with care as wound breakdown, which is not uncommon, results in very troublesome palatal regurgitation. This, when coupled with the other swallowing problems that such patients have, including trismus and aspiration, make management very difficult. Sometimes the soft palate has to be removed especially when there is extension of disease to the soft palate itself. In such circumstances, a dental prothesis will be necessary.

Mandibular Swing. (*Figure* 3) This is a useful technique for disease that has extended inferiorly into the oropharynx and to the parapharyngeal space. Exposure is adequate

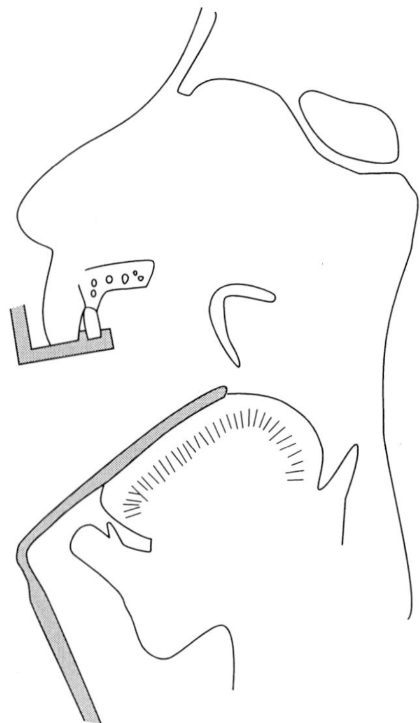

Figure 1. Transpalatal approach. Sagittal section with Dingman mouth gag in place.

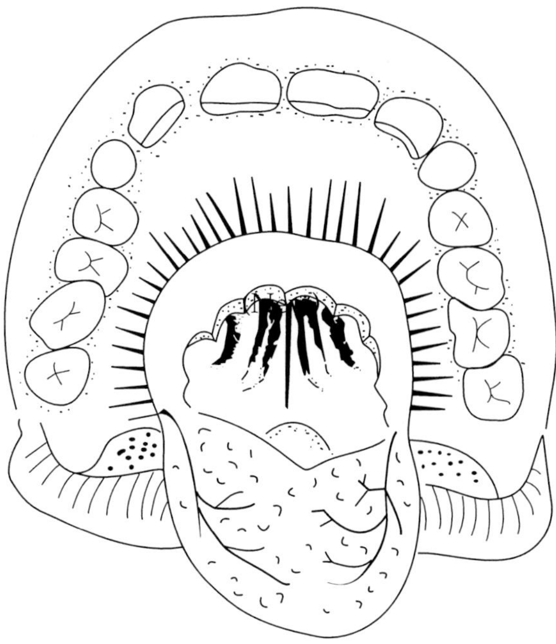

Figure 2. Transpalatal approach. Inferior view through the partially resected hard palate and posteriorly based soft palatal flap.

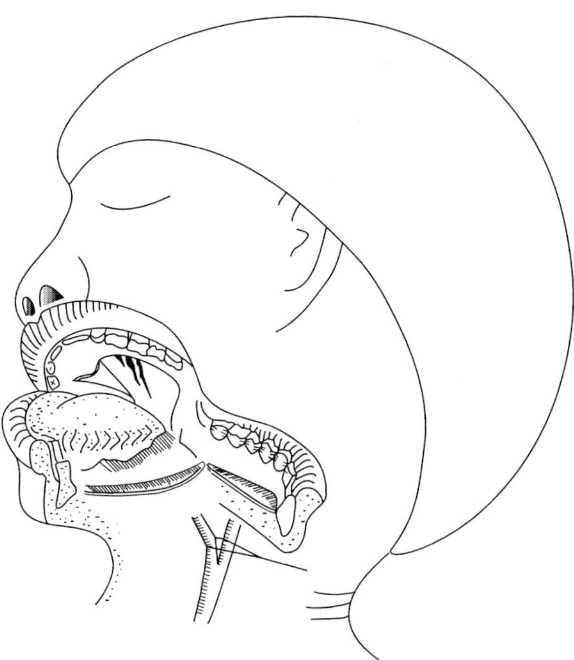

Figure 3. Mandibular Swing. Incision and retraction of soft palate to expose the nasopharynx. Internal carotid artery traced to the base of skull and protected after neck dissection.

especially if the soft palate is split. Through the neck incision, the internal and external carotids are exposed and isolated. A concomitant neck dissection can be performed and the retropharyngeal lymph nodes can also be dissected. The exposure will also facilitate the inset and microvascular anastomosis of the free radial forearm flap. Only one osteotomy is required and it is at the penumbra of the radiation field. There is also probably less problem with trismus in the postoperative period.

Lateral Approach

This approach was described by Fisch.[14] It is a useful approach for disease that has extended laterally to the parapharyngeal space. The internal carotid as it enters the skull base is safely identified and protected. The disadvantages include the need for dissection and preservation of the facial nerve, the destruction of the auditory organ and the postoperative conductive deafness that follows. There is also difficulty obtaining adequate exposure of disease extending towards the midline or to the opposite side.

Anterior Approaches

These approaches all involve resection or osteotomy of the malar bone complex in order to expose the nasopharynx.

Lefort I Osteotomy. (*Figure 4*) This involves the down fracture of the entire palate and the inferior maxilla. The nasal septum may also need to be resected. The procedure provides good exposure to the skull base including the nasopharynx.[15,16] The osteotomies are plated after the resection of the nasopharynx and as the incision is made sublabially, there are no facial scars.

Subtotal Maxillectomy. This provides exposure of the skull base if, in addition to the conventional maxillectomy, the coronoid process and posterior nasal septum are also removed. To some extent, this operation is replaced by the maxillary swing.

Maxillary Swing. (*Figure 5*) This operation was described by Wei *et al.*[18] It essentially, as the name indicates, involves swinging the maxilla laterally after multiple osteotomies (*Figure 6*). The blood supply of the maxilla is now dependent on the cheek flap and masseter muscle. With this approach there is good exposure of the nasopharynx and the parapharyngeal space. Resection can be adequately carried out and the resultant bone is covered over with a free mucosal flap held in place by packing or with a Foley's balloon catheter. This technique involves multiple osteotomies in an irradiated field with the potential of impaired bone healing and osteoradionecrosis unless plating and fixation are done with accuracy and care. Trismus can be a significant problem postoperatively, though in most instances this is transitory. There is also a palatal fistula rate of 27%.[18]

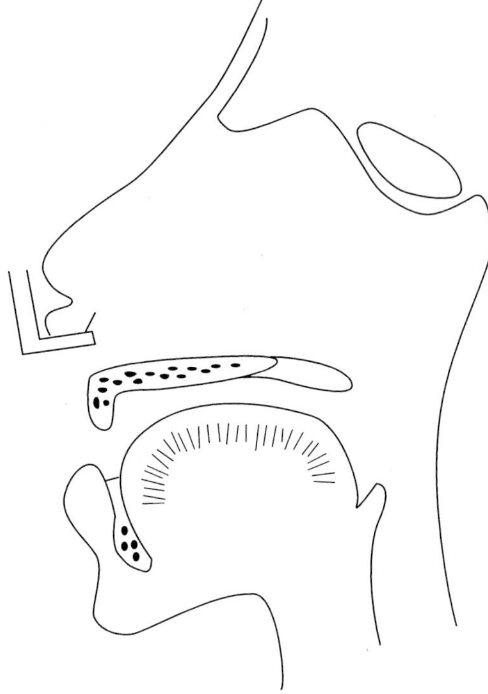

Figure 4. LeFort I Osteotomy using a sublabial incision and osteotomy of the inferior maxilla and nasal septum.

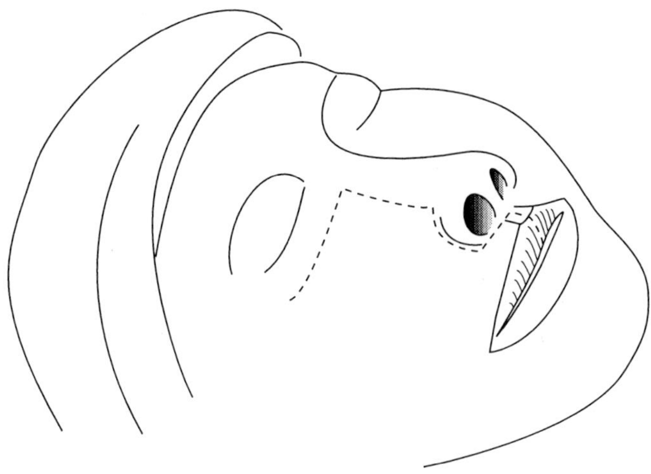

Figure 5. Maxillary Swing. The Weber-Ferguson-Longmire incision.

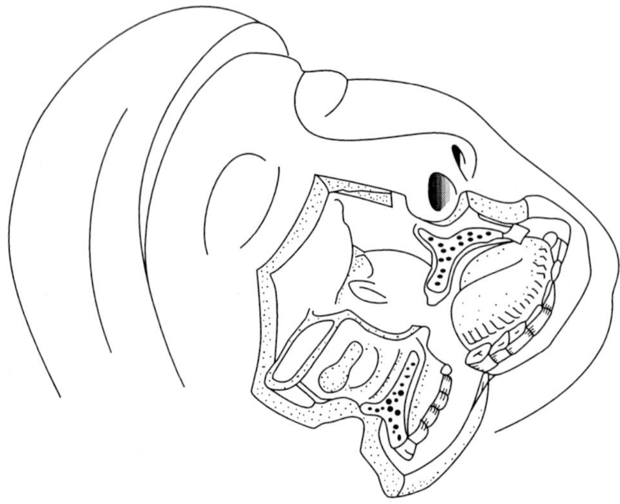

Figure 6. Maxillary Swing. Multiple maxillary osteotomies based on the myocutaneous cheek flap.

Endoscopic nasopharyngectomy

We have, recently described endoscopic resection of the nasopharynx.[19] This involves using the techniques of functional endoscopic sinus surgery for visualisation and resection of the nasopharynx. The neck is initially exposed and the internal carotid artery traced to the skull base for protection. The external carotid artery is looped in case of significant bleeding during the resection. The nasal and the nasopharyngeal mucosae are then infiltrated with epinephrine to reduce the bleeding. The posterior nasal septum is removed. Resection commences at the floor of the sphenoid adjacent to the roof of the nasopharynx using both scalpel and diathermy. The underlying bone is drilled to obtain further tumour clearance of that area. At completion of the operation the exposed area is covered with septal mucosa as a free graft. This technique is useful as visualisation is much improved with the help of the videotelescope. Also as there are no osteotomies nor extensive soft tissue dissection, the postoperative rehabilitation is rapid and trismus is much less of a problem. Its limitation is probably the inability to accomplish extensive lateral resection. This technique will require further evaluation.

Results of Nasopharyngectomy

The results of nasopharyngectomy are few. While the initial reports were dismal, subsequent reports have been quite promising, with a 5-year survival rate of 44% in one series[7] and a 3-year actuarial survival of 42.5% in another.[18] Fee[17] achieved an overall local control rate of 31%. All these series represent highly selected groups of patients. It may never be possible to know whether surgical excision of the resectable tumour is superior to a second course of irradiation unless randomised trials are done on large enough numbers of patients.

Surgical Management of Complications of Radiation Therapy

Palliation of trismus

Trismus is often a problem especially after irradiation of the nasopharynx. Jaw opening exercises can be undertaken especially after a surgical procedure, e.g. maxillary swing, as a prophylactic measure though it is debatable whether it will significantly reduce the trismus. Palliation can be achieved by feeding via a fine nasogastric tube or by a formal gastrostomy. Percutaneous endoscopic gastrostomy can be attempted but as the problem is of difficulty in opening the mouth, it may be impossible to insert the gastroscope orally. Division of both coronoid processes has been advocated to relieve the trismus but again the efficacy of such a procedure is questionable because of the extensive soft tissue fibrosis in the pterygoid and masseter muscles.

Treatment of otitis media

Occasionally myringotomy may is carried out for middle ear effusion due to dysfunction of the eustachian tube resulting from tumour spread, fibrosis or surgery. At times, there may be a need for insertion of a ventilation tube (Chapter 17).

Dysphagia and aspiration

Involvement of the 9th and 10th cranial nerves by the tumour may lead to difficulties in swallowing and aspiration of secretions. Cricopharyngeal myotomy has been carried out with success in the relief of this problem.[20]

References

1. Skinner, P.W., van Hascurt, C.A., Tsao, S.Y. 1991. Nasopharyngeal carcinoma: a study of the modes of presentation annals of otology. *Rhinol. Laryngol.*; 100:544–551.
2. Sham, J.S.T., Choy, D., Wei, W.I. 1990. Nasopharyngeal carcinoma: orderly neck node spread. *Int. J. Radiat. Oncol. Biol. Phys.*; 19(4):929–933.
3. Huang, S.C. 1980. Nasopharyngeal cancer: a review of 1605 patients treated radically with cobat 60. *Int. J. Radiat. Oncol. Biol. Phys.*; 6:401–407.
4. Yu, J.H., Hu, Y.H., Gu, X.Z. 1983. Radiation therapy of recurrent nasopharyngeal carcinoma. *Acta Radiol. Oncol.*; 22:23–28.
5. Wei, W.I., Ho, C.M., Wong, M.P., *et al.* 1992. Pathological basis for surgery in the management of post-radiotherapy cervical metastasis in nasopharyngeal carcinoma. *Arch. Otolaryngol. Head Neck Surg.*; 118:923–929.
6. Wei, W.I., Lam, K.H., Ho, C.M., *et al.* 1990. Efficiency of radical neck dissection for the control of cervical metastasis after radiotherapy for nasopharyngeal carcinoma. *Am. J. Surg.*; 160:439–442.

7. Tu, G.Y., Hu, Y.H., Xui, G.Z., Ye, M. 1988. Salvage surgery for nasopharyngeal carcinoma. *Arch. Otolarygol. Head Neck Surg.*; 114:328–329.
8. Lim, D.T.H., Khoo, M.L.C., Fong, F.W., *et al.* 1996. Prognostic variables in patients undergoing radical neck dissection for nodal metastases in nasopharyngeal carcinoma. In: *Abstract, International Head and Neck Cancer Meeting, Toronto, 1996.*
9. Sham, J.S.T., Choy, D. 1991. Nasopharyngeal carcinoma: treatment of neck node recurrence by radiology. *Australas Radiol.*; 35:370–373.
10. Soo, K.C., Lim, D.T.H., Khoo, M.L.C., *et al.* 1997. The biological basis for surgical treatment of recurrent and residual nodal disease in nasopharyngeal carcinoma. *Abstract, Royal Australasian College of Surgeons, Annual Scientific Meeting, Brisbane, 1997.*
11. Chong, V.F.H., Fan, Y.F. 1997. Pterygopalatine fossa and maxillary nerve infiltration in nasopharyngeal carcinoma. *Head Neck*; 19(2):121–125.
12. Wei, W.I., Sham, J.S.T., Choy, D., Ho, C.M., Lam, K.H. 1990. Split palate approach for gold grain implantation in nasopharyngeal carcinoma. *Head Neck Surg.*; 116:578–582.
13. Zhang, E.P., Liang, P.G., Li, Z.Q., *et al.* Ten year survival of nasopharyngeal carcinoma: a report of 1302 cases. *Chin. Med. J.*; 100:419–424.
14. Fisch, U. 1983. The infra-temporal fossa approach for nasopharyngeal tumours. *Laryngoscope*; 93:36–44.
15. Belmont, J.R. 1988. The LeFort I osteotomy approach for nasopharyngeal and nasal fossa tumours. *Arch. Otolarygol. Head Neck Surg.*; 114:751–754.
16. Uttley, D., Moore, A., Archer, D.J. 1989. Surgical management of midline skull base tissues: a new approach. *J. Neurosurg.*; 7:705–710.
17. Fee, W.E., Roberson, J.B., Goffinet, D.R. 1991. Long term survival after surgical resection for recurrent nasopharyngeal cancer after radiotherapy failure. *Arch. Otolarygol. Head Neck Surg.*; 117:1233–1236.
18. Wei, W.I., Ho, C.M., Yuen, P.W., Fung, C.F., Sham, J.S.T., Lam, K.H. 1995. Maxillary swing approach for resection of tumours in and around the nasopharynx. *Arch. Otolarygol. Head Neck Surg.*; 121:638–642.
19. Sethi, D.S., Hong, G.S., Soo, K.C. 1998. Endoscopic nasopharyngectomy. *Abstract, UICC Conference on Nasopharyngeal Carcinoma, Feb. 1998, Singapore.*
20. Mills, C.P. 1993. Dysphagia in pharyngeal paralysis treated by cricopharyngeal sphincterotomy. *Lancet*; 1993(3):455–457.

CHAPTER 16

Recent Treatment Modalities

C. Andrew van Hasselt and *Michael C.F. Tong*

Dissatisfaction with the results of conventional therapy, particularly for advanced and recurrent tumours, has prompted clinicians and research workers to study and apply technological developments and other forms of treatment which in time might supplement or even replace standard methods of treatment. Mention will therefore be made of these although in most cases their clinical value has yet to be proven.

Lasers

Laser therapy has not as yet fulfilled a definitive role in the treatment of nasopharyngeal cancer (NPC). The increasing popularity and widened acceptance of laser therapy in medicine has rendered it inevitable that its value be assessed. Recent reports in the literature have focused on three different modes of application, namely:

(i) Laser vaporization
(ii) Laser-induced thermotherapy (LITT)
(iii) Photodynamic therapy (PDT)

(i) Laser Vaporization

The carbon dioxide (CO2) laser is capable of precise tissue vaporization so that destruction of surrounding tissue is minimal and morbidity is slight. The procedure may be repeated frequently without a theoretical dose-limit. As the laser beam cannot be conveniently delivered via a fibre-optic cable, use of this method requires a direct approach to the tumour preferably via transpalatal fenestration. Alternatively, a steel reflector can be used transorally with endoscopic guidance. A self-retaining device allowing the surgeon to operate with both hands has also been used in two patients.[1] The Holmium-YAG (Ho-YAG) laser delivered through a fibre-optic system has also been used for attempted tumour ablation.[2] The effectiveness of this and other new lasers such as the surgical diode and Erbium-YAG (Er-YAG) types have not as yet been fully evaluated.

"En bloc" tissue resection is not practical with ablative laser surgery as the laser acts by vapourization. Tumour margins are therefore difficult to visualize and repeated biopsies of the margins are required in order to differentiate normal from malignant tissue. Vapourization of persistent or recurrent NPC has been suggested as an alternative approach to surgical resection for palliative purposes[3] but the technique has not gained wide acceptance.

(ii) Laser-induced Thermotherapy (LITT)

Insterstitial LITT is a recently developed technique for local tumour destruction within solid organs. An optic fibre delivering low power Nd-YAG laser light through an insulated diffusing applicator is inserted into the centre of the tumour mass. The thermal destruction is monitored instantaneously by magnetic resonance (MR) thermometry. Three patients with NPC have been relieved of pain following one session of treatment.[4]

(iii) Photodynamic Therapy (PDT)

PDT is a therapeutic concept based on the ability of a number of photosensitizing drugs (photo-sensitizers) to concentrate in tumour tissue. Light of a specific wavelength illuminating the sensitized cells can then be used to cause selective necrosis of the tumour.[5] In theory the potential advantages offered by PDT for treating NPC are appealing. The tumour is readily illuminated by fibreoptic delivery of light energy thus facilitating selective tumour destruction while sparing surrounding tissue. Squamous cell carcinomas of the head and neck have been shown to respond favourably to PDT.[6–8] The first generation photo-sensitizer, haematoporphyrin derivative (HPD) or its active puratives, Photofrin II or Photosan III, have been selectively used in the treatment of NPC.[7–14] These compounds which fix on the cellular organelles including the mitochondria and rough endoplasmic recticulum are activated by red light (630nm) produced by an argon pumped dye laser,[7–8,10–11] a helium-neon laser[9] or a gold-vapour laser .[13–14] A series of photochemical reactions follow which result in free radicals and oxygen singlet formation with subsequent cell injury or cell death.[15] Clinical observation by endoscopic assessment however suggests that a vascular event, ie. vasculitis and occlusion with subsequent avascular necrosis, could occur and reduce the selectivity of destruction but at the same time improve the overall tumoricidal effects.[14] This is further supported by the improved response rate in one Chinese study using an argon laser (514nm) which theoretically does not trigger a maximal photochemical reaction.[11]

Studies in China in over 150 subjects dating back to 1984 utilizing PDT to treat residual or recurrent NPC after radiotherapy have shown a 90%–100% overall response rate with an initial complete response rate of 40%–60%.[9–11] Long-term follow-up showed 3-year and 5-year survival rates of 45.6% and 26.2% respectively.[11] Two patients with small T1 primary tumours have also been treated with success.[10]

In the Prince of Wales Hospital in Hong Kong, the authors have undertaken a study to evaluate the response of NPC to PDT since 1992.[14] The following criteria were used to select candidates for the trial: (1) recurrent local NPC after completion of full-course radiotherapy (to 60 Gy); (2) recurrence situated in an area that could be exposed to light of 630nm wavelength via an optic fibre; (3) no potentially curative therapy available; (4) patient's age between 25 and 65 years; (5) no evidence of distant metastasis on pretreatment investigation; and (6) no evidence of porphyria or pregnancy.[14] Forty-eight hours after the injection of 5mg/kg of HPD, the patients were exposed to a total of 150–200 J/cm^2 of laser light energy under local anaesthesia. This was achieved using pure red light (wavelength 630nm) generated from a gold vapour laser unit through a 400 um optic fiber with a spherical diffuser head. The power delivered was approximately 0.5 Watt while the treatment time varied from 20 to 80 minutes. A total of 16 patients have currently been subjected to one or more PDT treatments and followed for 4 to 38 months. All patients showed macroscopic and radiological evidence of tumour regression at six months. Ten patients with tumours of approximately 1 cm or less in thickness were treated with curative intent. Two of these patients were still disease free more than 3 years post treatment. Six patients were palliated for the symptoms of nasal obstruction, epistaxis and dysphagia with varying degrees of success. One patient with metastatic neck disease was treated with dramatic response (*Figures 1a and b*). Complications including local infection were attributed mainly to previous radiotherapy treatment. Two patients developed significant skin hypersensitivity which responded to conservative measures.

Experience in Western Countries is limited but there are reports from the 1980s citing PDT treatment of 4 previously treated NPC's[7–8] with complete disappearance of the tumour in 2 and no response in one patient. A recent report from Sweden of 4 patients with nasopharyngeal squamous cell carcinoma (SCC) and 1 patient with adenocarcinoma showed encouraging long-term results. The patient with adenocarcinoma and 2 of the patients with SCC remained disease-free for more than 4 years. The treatment was well tolerated, there were minimal side effects with no immunological compromise of the patients. These results prompted the authors to suggest that PDT might be the treatment of choice for Stage I disease[10] and a better option than radiotherapy (RT) for small recurrent disease.[10–11,13–14] Furthermore, repeated treatment is possible and other treatment modalities are minimally affected.

In summary, PDT is maturing as a mode of treatment and is the most encouraging alternative form of therapy to arise in recent times. It is no longer in the experimental category. However, until it can be shown to be at least as effective as conventional forms of therapy, it should be reserved for those patients who have failed all other accepted forms of treatment. Further studies to evaluate its role as a primary treatment are awaited with interest. Studies in China using PDT as an adjuvant to radiotherapy in NPC have shown significant improvement in primary control rates.[12] The emergence of a second generation of photosensitizers such as the chlorins and phthalocyanines with improved differential uptake by tumour cells opens new frontiers for researching PDT in NPC.[15]

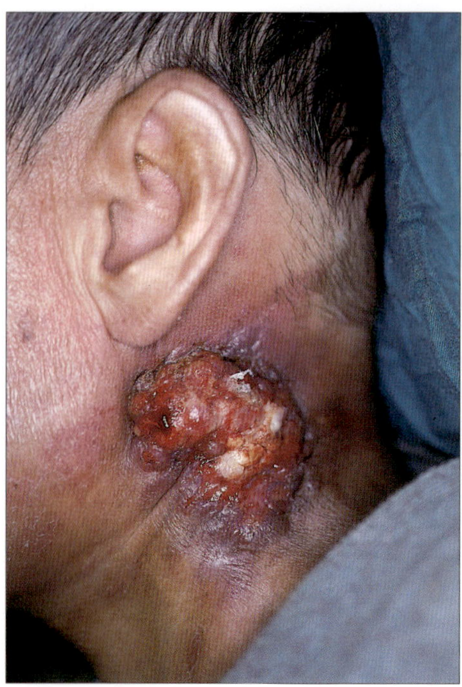

Figure 1a. An ulcerated, fungating NPC neck metastasis.

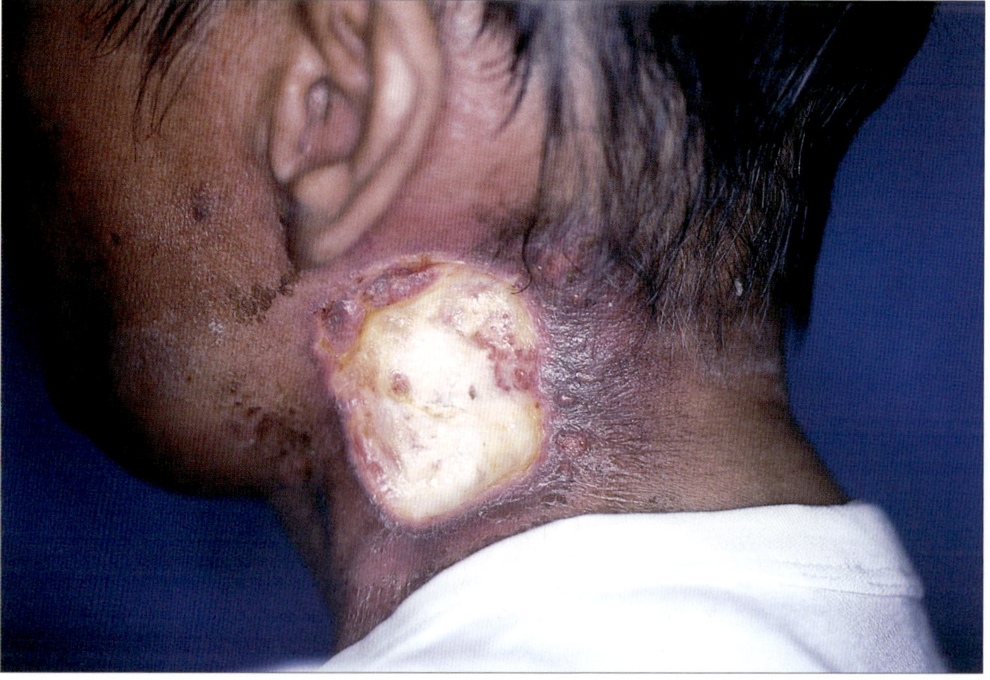

Figure 1b. The same lesion in *Figure 1* two weeks after photodynamic therapy.

Thermotherapy and Microwave Therapy

The use of hyperthermia to treat head and neck tumours has been undertaken since the mid-80s.[16–17] Both insterstitial and external hyperthermia have been applied. Interstitial hyperthermia is administered through an optic fibre from a laser source (LITT)[4] or through a catheter from a microwave generator.[16] An external microwave generator with wavelenghts of 915 MHz,[16] 410 MHz or 2450 MHz[17] is used to apply external hyperthermia in combination with chemo-radiotherapy for metastatic neck disease.

The control rates for neck disease in 60 NPC cases treated with thermo-radiotherapy showed response rates of 69%, 84% and 93% for groups treated with microwaves of 410MHz, 2450MHz and a combination of 410MHz + 2450 MHz respectively.[17] Another study in China also showed an improvement in local control rate of 10% when compared with radiotherapy alone.[18]

Radiosurgery and Other Techniques

Conventional radiotherapy techniques have been criticized for their relatively low selectivity in tumour destruction and high complication rates. In recent years, stereotactic irradiation techniques have evolved through advances in both software and hardware technology. These include the Gamma knife, Linac radiosurgery and 3-dimensional conformal radiotherapy. The techniques allow precise delivery of high doses of radiotherapy without affecting adjacent vital structures. These modalities were used initially to treat intracranial tumours but their application to NPC has been reported by few centres.

The Leksell Gamma Knife with a 201 ^{60}Co source has been used to treat 4 primary and 32 recurrent NPCs. A report from China revealed that the tumours "became smaller or even disappeared" with a high local symptom control rate.[19] Repeated nasopharyngeal biopsies in 12 patients showed no recurrence of disease. However neither the survival nor the follow-up of these cases was mentioned. In another report, using the Gamma Knife on 3 NPC patients with skull base involvement, no symptomatic relief or tumour response was encountered with this treatment.[20]

Linac radiosurgery is a single fraction form of stereotactic radiosurgery using a conventional linear accelerator as the source. From a series of 3 patients with locally recurrent NPC who were treated by this means,[21] one patient remained disease-free after 1 year. A second patient who had previously undergone treatment with both conventional radiotherapy and the Gamma Knife was further treated by linac radiosurgery for local recurrence in the nasopharyngnx eroding the clivus. Neurological deterioration including blindness and temporal lobe abnormalities occurred 6 months after radiosurgery and death followed shortly afterwards. The third patient recurred 6 months after radiosurgery and died of disease. In another series of 9 NPC patients,[22] 7 of 12 "lesions" had complete response after a median follow-up of 17 months. In the same report, radiosurgery was also used as a booster with doses ranging from 7 to 16

Gy in 11 patients with T2 to T4 lesions. With a median follow-up of 18 months, all 11 patients remained locally controlled but one patient with recurrence at the jugular foramen required salvage by a second course of radiosurgery. Complications included facial nerve palsy in one patient in the recurrent group but none in the booster group.

The technique of 3-dimensional conformal radiotherapy to complement conventional techniques is being tested in the Prince of Wales Hospital. The M.D. Anderson group are currently treating newly diagnosed nasopharyngeal tumours with this enhanced fractionated technique with encouraging initial results.[23]

Although only a few patients are being treated with these advanced techniques, questions are raised when comparisons are drawn with conventional radiotherapy techniques.[24] The newer techniques require sophisticated planning procedures involving more manpower and expense, thus limiting the number of centres capable of offering the treatment. Their use is therefore currently restricted to the management of isolated cases or case series. Perhaps the strongest indication for radiosurgery in NPC as suggested by the Stanford group is as an adjunct to conventional radiotherapy.[22] We believe however that a well-planned controlled trial is essential to further evaluate efficacy and complications associated with these techniques in comparison to conventional fractionated radiotherapy.

Immunotherapy and Gene Therapy

A deficiency in cellular immunity has been cited as one of the reasons for treatment failure in patients with NPC.[25] Attempts to enhance immuno-responsiveness have been made using OK-432 (streptococcal preparation) and lymphocyte transfer in Japan[25] and recently Interleukin 2 (IL 2) in China.[26,27]

In one study dividing 200 late stage (III and IV) NPC patients into 4 parallel groups,[27] the 6-month control rates (primary tumour 92% versus 82% and cervical nodes 88% versus 80%) were significantly higher in the lymphokine activated killer cell (LAK)/IL2 and RT treated group than in the patients treated with RT alone. The one-year survival rate in the former group of 93% compared favourably with the latter group (82%). LAK/IL2 was also used in combination with Lycium barbarum polysaccharides (LBP) which are said to enhance immuno-stimulant properties in the treatment of patients with advanced NPC.[26] Combination treatment with another immunostimulant PSK (Krestim) in 67 patients with different kinds of head and neck, breast , brain and other cancers was tried in Taiwan.[28] Analysis of the 21 NPC patients within the group showed a significantly better survival than historical controls (28% versus 17% 5-year survival rate, $p < 0.05$).[28] However in 13 patients with local recurrence or metastatic disease, gamma interferon was not found to be useful in reducing the size of the tumour either in the nasopharynx or the neck.[29]

New approaches in immunotherapy are being targeted towards the presence of EB viral genomes within the cancer cells.[30,31] A 108-fold differential has been achieved between cells containing or lacking EBNA-1 expression by a method combining an oriP/EBNA-1 dependent EBV Cp promoter with delayed assay of reporter gene. This has been suggested as a potential therapeutic strategy in treating NPC.[30] Other promising strategies include enhancement and targeting of viral antigen or enzyme expression (such as thymidine kinase) with demethylating agents or protein kinase C activators respectively, and rendering tumour cells sensitive to destruction by cytotoxic T cells or anti-viral agents.[31] Researchers have also directed their efforts towards gene therapy in head and neck cancers[32] though we do not expect this to precede the decoding of cancer and normal human genes.

Herbal and Alternative Medicine

Traditional Chinese medicine (TCM) supposes that carcinogenesis results from the accumulation of stagnant and toxic substances at various sites within the body.[33] Multi-drug therapy, under the collective name of "Destagnation" has been used in China to improve micro-circulation in order to clear stagnant substances, thus acting as an anti-cancer agent. Impressive results using collective Chinese herbal medicine, consisting of ten drugs, in combination with chemotherapy for the treatment of NPC have been reported in a prospective randomized trial.[34] The success rate, judged by freedom of local recurrence after 5 years, was 53% for the combined RT-destagnation group compared with 37% in the control (RT alone) group ($p < 0.005$). Destagnation was noted to be particularly effective for advanced lesions. No side effects or complications of this treatment were reported. Observations on the rate of tumour response to treatment between the two groups suggest that destagnation may act as a radiosensitizer.

The concept of combining Chinese herbs with radiotherapy and chemotherapy has been frequently applied in China. One study utilizing the "de-toxification" method combined with RT in 38 patients showed decreased residual disease in the neck from 79% (RT only) to 12% (combined treatment).[35] Another study showed that the use of two different Chinese herbs significantly diminished complications of radiotherapy.[36]

Contradictory results on the use of traditional Chinese medicine have been reported. Dietary and epidemiological research[37] have shown a higher risk of patients developing NPC if they consume Chinese herbal tea (Odds ratio = 4.2, $p = 0.02$). On the other hand, the use of Fuchunpian[38] as a radiosensitizer in 60 patients resulted in the treated group having a significantly higher rate of metastasis within 5 years than the control group (36.7% versus 10.0%). Random use of Chinese herbs is therefore not recommended.

Scientific studies into the anti-cancer properties of Chinese herbs have been undertaken in China and Hong Kong. In an in-vitro study using an NPC cell-line, 54 herbs were tested for their anti-growth and tumoricidal properties in an attempt to identify suitable agents for subsequent clinical trials.[39] It is believed that continuous scientific research into traditional Chinese practice may be rewarding in the future.

References

1. Heher, W. 1996. Micro-laser surgery in nasopharyngeal tumors with steel reflector, report of experiences with an improved technique. *Laryngorhinootologie*; 75(11):700–702. (in German)
2. Kautzky, M., Susani, M., Steurer, M., Hofler, H. 1993. Holmium: YAG laser surgery of nasopharyngeal cancer. *Laryngorhinootologie*; 72(4):181–186. (in German)
3. Rontal, M., Rontal, E. 1983. Treatment of recurrent carcinoma at the base of skull with carbon dioxide laser. *Laryngoscope*; 93(10):1261–1265.
4. Vogl, T.J., Mack, M.G., Muller, P., Phillip, C., Bottcher, H., Roggan, A., Juergens, M., Deimling, M., Knobber, D., Wust, P., Felix, R. 1995. Recurrent nasopharyngeal tumors: preliminary clinical results with interventional MR imaging-controlled laser-induced thermotherapy. *Radiology*; 196(3):725–733.
5. Dougherty, T.J., Kaufman, J.E., Goldfarb, A., Weishaupt, K.R., Boyle, D., Mittleman, A. 1978. Photoradiation therapy for the treatment of malignant tumours. *Cancer Res.*; 38(8):2628–2635.
6. Gluckman, J.L., Weissler, M.C. 1986. The role of photoradiation therapy in the management of early cancers of the upper aerodigestive tract. *Lasers Med. Sci.*; 3:217.
7. Wile, A.G., Coffey, J., Nahabedian, M.Y., Bagldassarian, R., Mason, G.R., Berns, M.W. 1984. Laser photoradiation therapy of cancer. *Laser Surg. Med.*; 4:5–12.
8. Edge, C.J., Carruth, J.A.S. 1988. Photodynamic therapy and the treatment of head and neck cancer. *Br. J. Oral Maxillofac. Surg.*; 26(1):1–11.
9. Zhao, S.P., Tao, Z.D., Xiao, J.Y., Peng, Y.Y., Yang, Y.H., Zeng, Q.S., Liu, Z.W. 1990. Photoradiation therapy of animal tumours and nasopharyngeal carcinoma. *Ann. Otol. Rhinol. Laryngol.*; 99(6)(Pt.1):454–460.
10. Sun, Z.Q., Lo, G.Y. 1990. Photodynamic therapy of nasopharyngeal cancer: a trial of 57 cases. *Chung Hua Chung Liu Tsa Chih (Chinese Journal of Oncology)*; 12:120–122. (in Chinese)
11. Sun, Z.Q., Lo, G.Y. 1992. Photodynamic therapy of nasopharyngeal carcinoma by argon or dye laser- an analysis of 137 cases. *Chung Hua Chung Liu Tsa Chih (Chinese Journal of Oncology)*; 14(4):290–292. (in Chinese)
12. Hu, Y.L., Shen, M.X., Cui, S.R., Guan, S.C., Liu, D.W., Wang, R.Z., Gao, Y.J., Zhao, Y.Z. 1992. Preliminary observation of combined radiotherapy and laser-HPD in the treatment of nasopharyngeal carcinoma. *Proceedings of the Sixth National Nasopharyngeal Cancer Congress, Quangzhou, May 1992*, 148. (in Chinese)
13. Lofgren, L.A., Hallgren, S., Nilsson, E., Westerborn, A., Nilsson, C., Reizenstein, J. 1995. Photodynamic therapy for recurrent nasopharyngeal cancer. *Arch. Otolaryngol. Head Neck Surg.*; 121(9):997–1002.
14. Tong, M.C., van Hasselt, C.A., Woo, J.K. 1996. Preliminary results of photodynamic therapy for recurrent nasopharyngeal carcinoma. *Eur. Arch. Otorhinolaryngol.*; 253(3):189–192.
15. Dougherty, T.J. 1993. Photodynamic therapy. *Photochem. Photobiol.*; 58(6):895–900.
16. Engin, K., Tupchong, L., Waterman, F.M., Nerlinger, R.T., Hoh, L.L., McFarlane, J.D., Leeper, D.B. 1993. Thermoradiotherapy with combined interstitial and external hyperthermia in advanced tumours in the head and neck with depth > or = 3 cm. *Int. J. Hyperthermia*; 9(5):645–654.
17. Deng, A.W., Hu, G.Q., Zhao, B.D. 1992 An analysis of 60 cases of metastatic cervical lymph node response to microwave treatment of various wavelengths. *Proceedings of the Sixth National Nasopharyngeal Cancer Congress, Quangzhou, May 1992*, 149. (In Chinese)
18. Zhang, Y.J. 1992 Report of the results of microwave hyperthermia combined with radiotherapy in 30 nasopharyngeal carcinoma cases. *Proceedings of the Sixth National Nasopharyngeal Cancer Congress, Quangzhou, May 1992*, 149. (In Chinese)
19. Dong, R.H., Gao, Z.U., Hu, Z.Q., Xu, W.M., Pan, L. 1996. Preliminary application of Gamma Knife in the treatment of nasopharyngeal carcinoma. *Stereotact. Funct. Neurosurg.*; 66(Suppl. 1):201–207.
20. Miller, R.C., Foote, R.L., Coffey, R.J., Gorman, D.A., Earle, J.D., Schomberg, P.J., Kline, R.W. 1997. The role of stereotactic radiosurgery in the treatment of malignant skull base tumors. *Int. J. Radiat. Oncol. Biol. Phys.*; 39(5):977–981.

21. Buatti, J.M., Friedman, W.A., Bova, F.J., Mendenhall, W.M. 1995. Linac radiosurgery for locally recurrent nasopharyngeal carcinoma: rationale and technique. *Head Neck*; 17(1):14–19.
22. Cmelak, A.J., Cox, R.S., Adler, J.R., Fee, W.E. Jr., Goffinet, D.R. 1997. Radiosurgery for skull base malignancies and nasopharyngeal carcinoma. *Int. J. Radiat. Oncol. Biol. Phys.*; 37(5):997–1003.
23. Harrison, L. 1998. Personal communication and Plenary Lecture. *'98 International & 5th National Head and Neck Cancer Congress, 9 June 1998, Hong Kong*.
24. Cooper, J.S. 1997. Editorial: Current and future therapy of nasophayrngeal cancer. *Int. J. of Rad. Oncol. Biol. Phys.*; 37(5):973–974.
25. Tsukuda, M., Sawaki, S. 1985. Immunological basis and immunotherapy of nasopharyngeal carcinoma. *Auris Nasus Larynx*; 12(Suppl. 2):S161–165.
26. Cao, G.W., Yang, W.G., Du, P. 1994. Observation of the effects of LAK/IL-2 therapy combining with Lycium barbarum polysaccharides in the treatment of 75 cancer patients. *Chung Hua Chung Liu Tsa Chih (Chinese Journal of Oncology)*; 16(6):428–431. (in Chinese)
27. Zhang, S.H., Cai, Y.C., Gu, Y.L. 1996. Combination treatment of late nasopharyngeal carcinoma: an analysis of short-term therapeutic results in 200 cases. *Chung Hua Chung Liu Tsa Chih (Chinese Journal of Oncology)*; 18(1):70–72. (in Chinese)
28. Chung, C.H., Go, P., Chang, K.H. 1987. PSK immunotherapy in cancer patients — a preliminary report. *Chin. J. Microbiol. Immunol.*; 20(3):210–216.
29. Mahjoubi, R., Bachouchi, M., Munck, J.N., Busson, P., Gasmi, J., Azli, N., Brandely, M., Tursz, T., Cvitkovic, E., Armand, J.P. 1993. Phase II trial of recombinant interferon gamma in refractory undifferentiated carcinoma of the nasopharynx. *Head Neck*; 15(2):115–118.
30. Evans, T.J., Brooks, L., Farrell, P.J. 1997. A strategy for specific targeting of therapeutic agents to tumour cells of virus-associated cancers. *Gene Ther.*; 4(3):264–267.
31. Ambinder, R.F., Robertson, K.D., Moore, S.M., Yang, J. 1996. Epstein-Barr virus as a therapeutic target in Hodgkin's disease and nasopharyngeal carcinoma. *Semin. Cancer Biol.*; 7(4):217–226.
32. Breau, R.L., Clayman, G.L. 1996 Gene therapy for head and neck cancer. *Curr. Opin. Oncol.*; 8(3):227–231.
33. Department of Oncology, Hospital of Traditional Chinese Medicine. 1978. *A Practice in Oncology*, Vol. 1. Beijing: The People's Medical Publishing House, 19–21. (in Chinese)
34. Xu, G.Z., Cai, W.M., Qin, D.X., Yan, J.H., Wu, L., Zhang, H.X., Hu, Y.H., Gu, X.Z. 1989. Chinese herb "destagnation" series I: Combination of radiotherapy with destagnation in the treatment of nasopharyngeal carcinoma (NPC): a prospective randomized trial on 188 cases. *Int. J. Radiat. Oncol. Biol. Phys.*; 16(2):297–300.
35. Yan, Y., Huang, Q.Z., Zhu, C.D. 1992. An analysis of early results of combined radiotherapy and yang yin de-toxification with larger metastatic cervical lymph nodes from NPC. *Proceedings of the Sixth National Nasopharyngeal Cancer Congress, Quangzhou, May 1992*, 179. (In Chinese)
36. Wang, D.J. 1992. Preliminary observation of lycopodium casuarinoides spring in the treatment of nasopharyngeal cancer. *Proceedings of the Sixth National Nasopharyngeal Cancer Congress, Quangzhou, May 1992*, 180. (In Chinese)
37. Zheng, Y.M., Tuppin, P., Hubert, A., Jeannel, D., Pan, Y.J., Zeng, Y., de Thé, G. 1994. Environmental and dietary risk factors for nasopharyngeal carcinoma: a case-control study in Zangwu County, Guangxi. China. *Brit. J. Cancer*; 69(3):508–514.
38. Han, J.Q., Chen, Y.T., Man, Y.Y. 1995. Clinical study on the effect of combined treatment of fuchunpian with radiotherapy on nasopharyngeal carcinoma. *Chung Kuo Chung Hsi I Chieh Ho Tsa Chih*; 15(12):710–712. (in Chinese)
39. Zhao, M.L., Luo, C.M., Long, F., Chen, J., Tang, L.Y. 1988. Growth capability of an epithelial cell line of human poorly differentiated nasopharyngeal carcinoma and its response to Chinese medicinal herbs and marine drugs. *Chung Hua Chung Liu Tsa Chih (Chinese Journal of Oncology)*; 10(2):98–101. (in Chinese)

CHAPTER 17

Related Ear Problems

C. Andrew van Hasselt and *Alan G. Gibb*

The close association between nasopharyngeal carcinoma (NPC) and the ear has long been recognized. In one of the earliest reviews Jackson (1901)[1] reported ear symptoms in no fewer than 43% of cases. A similar pattern emerged from a more recent study by Skinner *et al.*[2] in Hong Kong. While in most instances the ear problem is related to the presence of the tumour itself, standard radiation treatment may aggravate, or even initiate, the condition.

Symptomatology

Deafness, usually mild and unilateral and often accompanied by tinnitus is by far the commonest ear complaint in the early stages of the disease. Thus hearing loss is of great significance diagnostically. In fact, as long ago as 1911, Trotter[3] focused attention on the importance of what he termed "Eustachian tube type" deafness as the first symptom of nasopharyngeal carcinoma. We would strongly endorse Trotter's sentiment, which underlines the importance of careful examination of the nasopharynx in all cases of unexplained conductive deafness in the adult. If examination is negative, repeated follow-up visits are essential until a definitive diagnosis is established.

Interestingly however, many NPC patients with an established middle ear effusion either remain unaware of, or fail to complain of, hearing loss, as the degree of deafness is usually not severe.[4] In a study at the Prince of Wales Hospital, Hong Kong, it was found that 36% of patients with evidence of an ear effusion on routine tympanometric testing did not complain of hearing loss when attending the doctor.[2]

Other ear symptoms encountered in NPC such as otorrhoea and otalgia are diagnostically of lesser importance, being associated as a rule with advanced tumours. At the same time they may adversely affect the quality of life. These symptoms are often aggravated or caused by radiation treatment of the tumour.

Deafness of sensorineural type is mainly seen in advanced tumours of longstanding. The condition may rarely be due to tumour invasion of the cochlea or 8th cranial nerve. However, as nearly all cases have also received high doses of radiation, the deafness has frequently been attributed to the radiotherapy, albeit without scientific validation, as has the rare symptom of vertigo.

Pathogenesis

Hearing loss

Hearing loss is almost invariably conductive in nature and results from derangement of eustachian tube function by the tumour. Numerous studies have been carried out in an effort to determine the exact mechanism involved. Although the answer still remains uncertain, the evidence points to a functional rather than a mechanical obstructive problem in most cases.[5,6,7]

Research Studies

Su and Juan (1985)[8] discovered that although active opening of the eustachian tube was impaired in nearly all symptomatic cases of middle ear effusion in NPC, the passive opening pressure of the tube, as measured by an air pump, was within normal limits (< 400 mm H_2O) in 75% of cases. The results suggested that external compression of the tube or tumour growth into the lumen were not normally the cause of the problem. Attention was accordingly focused on the action of the tensor veli palatini muscle which is responsible for opening the tube. Casselbrandt *et al.*[9] in experiments in Rhesus monkeys, were able to induce serous otitis media by paralysing this muscle using botulinum toxin. However Su *et al.*[10] using CT scanning, MR imaging and electromyographic recording showed that in stage 1 and some stage 2 tumours the function of tensor veli palatini is undisturbed. Thus factors other than muscular inhibition must be operative in some cases of serous otitis media. Su *et al.*[10] proposed the theory that tubal dysfunction might be caused in some instances by altered compliance of the tubal cartilage due to tumour erosion. This view has recently been supported by Low *et al.*[11] who consider that erosion involving the outer lamina of the tubal cartilage only is sufficient to alter its compliance.

Honjo[12] in extensive research studies, supported a multifactorial pathogenesis, indicating three different mechanisms which may underlie the tubal derangement in NPC:- (a) alteration of dynamic function caused by interference with the action of the tensor veli palatini muscle, (b) reduction of ciliary clearance due to inflammatory changes in the middle ear mucosa and (c) lateral displacement of the tubal cartilage by large tumours. He confirmed that compression or invasion of the lumen of the tube are rare and encountered only in advanced tumours. We have been able in the Prince of Wales Hospital, Hong Kong to confirm both the muscular and displacement theories of Honjo by high resolution, multiplanar magnetic resonance imaging (MRI).[13] Reduced ciliary clearance could not be confirmed by imaging but we do not dispute the validity and importance of this theory.

Comment

Dynamic derangement due to muscular dysfunction appears to be the most important factor in the majority of cases. This is caused by direct invasion of the tensor veli palatini muscle or infiltration of its innervating nerve as it traverses the parapharyngeal space.[10] As invasion of these areas is extremely common in view of their immediate proximity to the fossa of Rosenmüller, the action of the tensor muscle is often already impaired by the time the patient first presents to the doctor.

Honjo[12] found a direct relationship between the effusion incidence and the size and extent of the tumour and our MRI investigations confirmed this.[13] The most dramatic rise in the incidence of effusion matches the spread of the tumour into the parapharyngeal space,[12] which in our imaging series was associated with an effusion rate of 95%.[13] In such cases tumour infiltration not only causes inactivation, or paralysis, of the tensor veli palatini muscle but also tubal displacement and cartilage invasion with altered tubal compliance.

Disordered ciliary function, especially following radiotherapy, is also a significant factor in the pathogenesis of middle ear effusions. Inflammatory changes of the mucosa within the tympanic cavity and eustachian tube associated with the presence of the tumour, especially if ulcerated, are inevitably aggravated by radiation with damage to ciliated cells and secretory glands. Thus secretions may become more viscid and difficult to evacuate due to the reduced population of functionally effective ciliated cells.

Very large tumours may infiltrate widely enough to affect both tubes causing bilateral loss of hearing.

In rare instances the cochlea and eighth nerve have been directly infiltrated by tumour resulting in profound or even total sensorineural deafness.[14] The role of radiation treatment in the aetiology of sensorineural loss will be discussed later. (*vide infra*).

Tinnitus

Tinnitus is usually accompanied by hearing loss and occurs with almost the same frequency.[2] It is unusual to encounter tinnitus as an isolated symptom in the absence of other aural complaints. It's close association with hearing loss in NPC suggests that, in the majority of cases, especially in those with early disease, the symptoms are related to eustachian tube dysfunction and middle ear effusion. In late cases in which there is a sensorineural component to the deafness, tinnitus is more likely to be due to vascular or cellular degenerative changes in the cochlea or neural pathway.

Otalgia

Jackson (1901)[1] described the otalgia encountered in NPC as either a deep dull ache, vaguely referable to the ear, or a sharp, stabbing pain arising in the ear. In some cases pain is due to an inflammatory reaction in the middle ear or temporal bone but frequently it takes the form of a neuralgia due to tumour infiltration of the glossopharyngeal nerve which carries sensory fibres to the middle ear. Invasion of this nerve occurs where it courses in close proximity to the nasopharynx between the jugular foramen and the oropharyngeal region. Otalgia is less common than one might expect in view of the frequency of erosion of the skull base and infiltration of the parapharyngeal regions.

Effects of Radiation Therapy

Due to the anatomical proximity of the ear to the nasopharynx and the importance of limiting damage to the brain stem, the ear is inevitably exposed to significant radiation energy during a standard course of radiotherapy for NPC. External radiation is most often delivered in two opposing fields. Virtually the entire ear is exposed to these effects and the vestibular and cochlear nerves also receive a variable dose at the edges of the field. The effects of radiation depend not only upon the exposure, but also upon the type of radiation, method of delivery and total dose given to the tumour, which may vary according to the extent of the disease. For example, a parapharyngeal boost of radiation may be given for parapharyngeal extension of disease, and intra-nasopharyngeal brachytherapy may be given as a boost to enhance local control. The estimated exposure to the ear in an average standard course of treatment is 55 Gy delivered in fractions of 1.8–2 Gy over a period of 6 weeks.[15] The fraction size has an important bearing on the degree of late damage to neural tissue.[16] According to Evans,[17] if fractions can be kept below 2–3.3 Gy, permanent sensorineural hearing impairment is unlikely to occur.

The precision of present day imaging in providing accurate delineation of disease, coupled with modern radiation delivery techniques permit precise and customized planning with consequent reduction of exposure to the ear. The incidence of immediate side effects is therefore likely to show a progressive decrease with ever improving techniques. However, this may be counter-balanced by longer survival times; Moretti[18] has suggested that the survival interval of patients is often less than the time required for sensorineural hearing loss to become manifest. A delay of 8 years post-radiotherapy has been reported.[19]

External ear

As in radiotherapy to other areas, skin reactions are common. Initially there is redness, swelling and "weeping" of the skin, but with time the ear canal becomes dry and scaly with diminished wax secretion due to epithelial damage and destruction of sebaceous and apocrine glands.[20] In some instances infection may supervene, resulting in active otitis externa. Destruction of the skin and osteoradionecrosis may also occur and areas of exposed bone, usually in the floor or anterior wall of the meatus, with or without sequestration, may be encountered.[21]

Tympanic membrane

Permanent changes of the tympanic membrane are rarely encountered, but a dull thickened drum has been reported several months after radiation treatment.[22]

Middle ear

The middle ear mucosa suffers direct damaging effects from radiation exposure. In the acute stage, "radiation otitis media" takes the form of mucositis, desquamation and oedema.[23] Effusion with associated conductive deafness may develop, often *de novo*, due exclusively to the radiotherapy reaction. An increase in collagenous fibrous tissue and the formation of new glands, albeit with reduced activity, have been observed in the middle ear mucosa several months after completion of radiotherapy.[22] Vascular changes, similar to radiation induced changes in other parts of the body[23] are reported to occur, including endothelial swelling, duplication of the basement membrane and fibrosis and thickening of the vessel walls, with narrowing of the lumen to the point of occlusion. If eustachian tube function remains inadequate, either from involvement by the tumour or reaction to treatment, adhesive otitis media may represent the final outcome.[24]

Although necrosis of auditory ossicles has been reported as a complication of radiation therapy, it has not to our knowledge been encountered after treatment for NPC. Late avascular necrosis of the lenticular process of the incus was reported in a patient who received 99 Gy for treatment of a brain tumour.[25] Conductive deafness due to necrosis of the long process of incus was also recorded in six cases 6–11 months following the administration of 65–85 Gy for head and neck malignancies not situated within the temporal bone.[22]

Inner ear

Cellular nuclear changes affecting the post-mitotic phase of the sensory epithelium and altered vascular physiology, interfering with the supply of oxygen and metabolites may follow radiation of the cochlea.[18]

In endemic areas, cases of NPC subjected to one or more courses of radiotherapy frequently show a slowly progressive or even sudden hearing loss of sensorineural or mixed type in advanced or long standing cases of NPC . In such circumstances, radiation therapy rightly or wrongly has invariably been incriminated as the causative factor.[26]

Research Studies

The original concept that the cochlea, lying within the dense otic capsule, might be protected from the effects of radiation[18] has been shown to be erroneous in animal research.[27,28] Radiation effects in the inner ear were first noted by Ewald in pigeons in 1905.[29] At a later date, Winther,[30] in experiments in guinea pigs found early degeneration of the outer hair cells in the basal turns of the cochlea after a single exposure to 6,000 cGy. Similar effects were not however seen with lower dosage. It has been estimated, applying Dale's equation,[31] that a single large dose of radiation multiplies the dangers to the cochlear hair cells up to 6 times compared to small dosage fractions given over a period of weeks.[17] Thus the clinical significance of Winther's experiment[30] is doubtful. While there is undoubted danger to the cochlea in radiation treatment of temporal bone malignancies, especially if the otic capsule is eroded, the potential for damage in the treatment of NPC, where the inner ear is not the main focus of radiation, is far less.

Clinical Trials

Reports in the literature of radiation reactions are conflicting, frequently retrospective and mostly relate to tumours other than NPC.

However, a prospective controlled trial was carried out by Chowdhury *et al.*[32] involving 115 irradiated NPC patients. They reported only slight deterioration in the bone conduction (BC) threshold average ($p < 0.01$). Oddly, no BC deterioration occurred in subjects using ventilation tubes, but the reason for this remained unexplained.

Choy *et al.*[33] are currently engaged in a carefully controlled prospective study of 79 patients, with no ear problems, given curative-intent radiation therapy for NPC. The exact dose of radiation delivered to the cochlea was calculated in each case; the median dose to the inner ear was 66 Gy and ranged from 33.5 to 80.4 Gy in individual patients. In a preliminary analysis a mild neurosensory deficit averaging 4.96 dB was present at the end of 18 months. However, the degree of hearing loss showed no correlation with the radiation dosage so that any inter-relationship remains speculative. Later results are not yet available.

Evans *et al.*,[17] in a study in parotid tumours in which the ipsilateral temporal bone was fully exposed to irradiation of 5500–6000 cGy in 200–220 cGy fractions daily for 6 weeks found no significant deafness in 20 cases after a mean follow-up of 8 years. They stressed the importance of fraction size in avoiding damage to neural structures.

Histological Evidence

Histological confirmation of cochlear damage after NPC therapy in humans is lacking. The authors were able to trace only one necropsy report in the literature.[34] The light microscope findings in this case were unhelpful, being distorted by severe chronic middle ear suppuration with probable labyrinthitis so that the cochlear destruction was almost certainly of inflammatory origin rather than radiation damage. Against this background, the findings of a recent case collected by one of the authors, in which histological studies were carried out at the Harvard Laboratory in Boston, U.S.A., acquire added significance.

A 42 year old Chinese female resident in Singapore, was seen initially in 1986 suffering from undifferentiated NPC with a staging of $T_4 N_0 M_0$. She received two radiation courses by external beam therapy using a Cobalt-60 machine for both treatments with additional therapy by linear accelerator in the latter course. The total radiation dose was 11,000 cGy. She died 8 years later from advanced local spread of tumour with a marked symmetrical mixed hearing loss. Despite her high radiation dosage, the histological report from Harvard showed that "the organ of Corti and other sensory cells were well preserved". The deafness in this case was probably the result of severe degeneration of the cochlear nerves. The histopathologist's comment, "it is remarkable that hair cells are present in nearly normal numbers, given the extremely high radiation dose", serves to underline the relative immunity of the cochlea from high doses of irradiation. Furthermore, it should be recognized that in the absence of histological studies, the clinical diagnosis of radiation damage to the organ of Corti would have remained unchallenged.

The above case supports the conclusion of Dias[35] that irradiation in the head and neck area, even in high doses, when judiciously applied, does not appear to cause serious hearing impairment and post-radiation disturbances are related mainly to eustachian tube function. In conclusion, a diagnosis of radiation-induced sensorineural deafness should be made with caution in the absence of histological confirmation.

Temporal bone

Two patterns of osteoradionecrosis of the temporal bone may occur at variable time intervals after radiotherapy.[19,21] The less serious, localized necrosis of the tympanic ring is observed in patients who have been irradiated for lesions adjacent to the ear, such as NPC. This condition usually presents with mild otalgia and a picture similar to chronic otitis externa. An area of exposed dead bone, usually in the floor of the external meatus, may become evident. A sequestrum forms and separates gradually, leaving a defect which heals with the disappearance of symptoms. The entire process may take years to resolve. Localized osteoradionecrosis has been reported 6–12 years after treatment with radiation doses ranging between 30 and 90 Gy delivered to the nasopharynx.[21] Wang has suggested that no area of the temporal bone should receive more than 72 Gy if osteoradionecrosis is to be avoided.[36]

The more severe effect of radiotherapy is diffuse osteonecrosis,[19] but this is rare following radiation for NPC and usually follows treatment of temporal bone tumours. It is manifested clinically by severe pain with evidence of chronic otitis media, mastoiditis and a foul discharge due to the presence of bony sequestra. In addition, sensorineural deafness, vertigo, ataxia and occasional attacks of nausea may result from fistulization of the labyrinth, which in turn may lead to meningitis, brain abscess and death.[19]

Effects of Chemotherapy

The more commonly used cytotoxic agents, are known to be ototoxic. These include the most effective tumoricidal agent, cisplatin, currently employed in the treatment of NPC. Sensorineural deafness and tinnitus may be encountered following drug administration, especially if concomitant nephrotoxicity impairs renal excretion. The effects may be temporary or permanent, depending on the length and severity of the toxicity.

Investigations

The diagnosis and monitoring of ear disease involves the employment of standard tests. The use of tympanometry in eustachian tube related problems merits special mention. These tests are indispensable in the investigation of serous otitis media and mild tubal dysfunction, especially if the tympanic membrane appears normal. Serial tympanometric and audiometric tests are also invaluable for monitoring progress and response to treatment.

Other standard otological investigations may be indicated, imaging being of special value in cases of bone erosion or radionecrosis.

Management

Otitis externa

The treatment of otitis externa follows routine principles. Avoidance of water, regular cleaning and the application of appropriate local medications are generally adequate in controlling the condition. Areas of exposed bone or sequestra may interfere with healing, but these are not necessarily associated with discharge or other symptoms if the ear is kept free from infection.

Middle ear problems

Otologists undertaking treatment of NPC patients should be aware that standard procedures successful in other conditions, will not necessarily yield similar results in NPC cases. For this there are two main reasons. Firstly, the primary tumour in the nasopharynx, which is the cause of the ear problem may persist or recur despite treatment. Either treatment may fail or the tumour may be so extensive that palliation is the only option. Secondly, radiotherapy, the standard treatment, not only causes an inflammatory reaction in the middle ear but also impairs healing. Thus radiation therapy may actually cause the ear problem or, if already present, may interfere with resolution.

Serous Otitis Media

Cases of middle ear effusion due to NPC require careful consideration before treatment is undertaken and the problem should be thoroughly explained and discussed with the patient. If hearing loss is the only complaint, the clinician may be tempted to proceed with conventional treatment, namely myringotomy and insertion of a ventilation tube, as this will invariably relieve the symptom and provide at least temporary patient satisfaction.[4] However, various studies suggest that caution should be exercised, since a substantial proportion of patients ranging from 38%[4] to 64%[37] subsequently develop otorrhoea. Furthermore, the otorrhoea showed resistance to treatment in 92% of cases in the latter series[37], presumably due to impaired healing following radiation therapy. If, on the other hand, the serous otitis media is left untreated and a course of radiation is administered to the tumour, more than half the pre-treatment effusions resolve spontaneously[38]; cases failing to clear up receiving higher radiation doses. Furthermore 16% of unaffected ears develop an effusion after radiotherapy.[38]

Our current regime is therefore to withhold ventilation treatment in serous otitis media in view of its liability to initiate otorrhoea and, in some instances pain, which may add to the patient's misery and reduce the quality of life.

One other scenario merits consideration. This concerns the adult who attends the doctor for hearing loss with an obvious serous otitis media but with no visible nasopharyngeal tumour. In this circumstance treatment of the effusion should be delayed until a full diagnostic regime has been carried out to exclude NPC (Chapter 7).

In summary, great caution and careful judgement should always be exercised before resorting to the insertion of ventilation tubes. A hearing aid may well constitute a more acceptable alternative.

Otorrhoea

The management of chronic suppurative otitis media in cases of NPC presents the otologist with a difficult problem, especially if radiotherapy has been given. Persistent disease in the nasopharynx or eustachian tube in the form of tumour or infection, often combined with an impaired healing response following radiotherapy, compound the difficulties facing the otologist. Under these circumstances ambitious procedures are ill-advised. Conservative treatment, including frequent thorough aural toilet, plays the main role in controlling the problem and keeping the patient comfortable. Surgical reconstructive measures are, in our view, contra-indicated and the benefits of salvage procedures such as radical mastoidectomy are also dubious[26] in view of the impaired healing response of irradiated tissues. If an open cavity mastoid operation is unavoidable, we consider it desirable to line the cavity with vascularised tissue to assist healing. The Hong Kong Flap[39] has proved effective for this purpose in our hands.

Sensorineural hearing loss

Sensorineural deafness occurring in NPC patients does not dictate any particular form of management. Routine evaluation including careful inspection of the external canal and hearing aid fitting is advised, as for other forms of sensorineural hearing loss. In patients with bilateral profound hearing loss and satisfactory tumour control, we have found cochlear implantation, although expensive, to be a positively rewarding procedure towards improving the quality of life.

Tinnitus

Tinnitus is occasionally troublesome, but is generally overshadowed by more serious or debilitating symptoms. The management follows standard principles. If the tinnitus is caused by eustachian tube dysfunction, improvement frequently follows middle ear ventilation.[32]

Osteoradionecrosis

Spontaneous sequestration and eventual healing occurs in the localized type of osteoradionecrosis. Although the process is slow and may take several years to run its course, a conservative approach to management is advised. Diffuse necrosis on the other hand, which fortunately is very rare in NPC, carries a high risk of involvement of adjacent structures.[21] The condition is frequently associated with considerable pain and symptomatic control enhances the quality of life. The necrotic bone is highly susceptible to infection and the ear should be kept as clean as possible by regular aural toilet. Any loose sequestra should be removed. In view of the dangers of spread to other structures, a case may be made for early radical exploration of the mastoid in an attempt to remove as much necrotic bone as possible. In spite of extensive debridement and removal of sequestra, meningitis is a frequent complication to which most patients eventually succumb.[19]

Concluding Remarks

Loss of hearing, usually in one ear, if conductive in type, is an important early sign of NPC. A tumour of the nasopharynx must be carefully excluded in all adults exhibiting this presentation. The hearing loss usually results from eustachian tube dysfunction leading to middle ear effusion. Radiotherapy treatment tends in many cases to aggravate the ear problems and interferes with healing. In such cases surgical procedures such as ventilation of the middle ear, mastoidectomy and reconstructive operations require very careful consideration as in some instances they may be detrimental rather than beneficial to the patient's comfort and well being.

Longer survival times resulting from improvements in tumour management may uncover more cases of delayed deafness. On the other hand advances in imaging techniques and increasing precision in radiation delivery should help to reduce otological problems and provide hope for the future.

References

1. Jackson, C. 1901. Primary carcinoma of the nasopharynx: a table of cases. *J.A.M.A.*; 37:371–377.
2. Skinner, D.W., van Hasselt, C.A., Tsao S.Y. 1991. Nasopharyngeal carcinoma: a study of the modes of presentation. *Ann. Otol. Rhinol. Laryngol.*; 100:544–551.
3. Trotter, W. 1911. On certain clinically obscure malignant tumours of the nasopharyngeal wall. *Brit. Med. J.*; 2:1057–1059.
4. Wei, W.I., Engzell, U.C.G., Lam, K.H., Lau, S.K. 1987. The efficacy of myringotomy and ventilation tube insertion in middle-ear effusions in patients with nasopharyngeal carcinoma. *Laryngoscope*; 97:1295–1298.
5. Neel, H.B. III. 1986. Malignant neoplasms of the nasopharynx. In: *Otolaryngology — Head and Neck Surgery*, Vol. 2, eds. Cummings, C.W., Schuller, D.E. St. Louis: C.V. Mosby Co., 1399–1409.
6. Bluestone, C.D. 1983. Eustachian tube function: physiology, pathophysiology, and role of allergy in pathogenesis of otitis media. *J. Allergy Clin. Immunol.*; 72:242–251.

7. Choa, G. 1981. Nasopharyngeal carcinoma. In: *Otolaryngology*, Vol. 5, ed. English, G.M. Philadelphia: Harper & Row, 1–35.
8. Su, T.Y., Juan, K.H. 1985. Eustachian tube function in patients with nasopharyngeal carcinoma. *Kaohsiung J. Med. Sci.*; 1:53–62.
9. Casselbrandt, M.L., Cantekin, E.I., Dirkmaat, D.C., Doyle, W.C., Bluestone, C.D. 1988. Experimental paralysis of tensor veli palatini muscle. *Acta Otolaryngol.* (Stockh.); 106:178–185.
10. Su, C.Y., Hsu, S.P., Lui, C.C. 1993. Computed tomography, magnetic resonance imaging, and electromyographic studies of tensor veli palatini muscles in patients with hasopharyngeal carcinoma. *Laryngoscope*; 103:673–678.
11. Low, W.K., Lim, T.A., Balakrishnan, A. 1997. Pathogenesis of middle-ear effusion in nasopharyngeal carcinoma: a new perspective. *J. Laryngol. Otol.*; 111:431–434.
12. Honjo, I. 1988. *Eustachian Tube and Middle Ear Diseases*. Tokyo: Springer-Verlag.
13. King, A.D., Kew, J., Tong, M., Leung, S.F., Lam, W.W.M., Metreweli, C., van Hasselt, C.A. Magnetic resonance imaging of the eustachian tube in nasopharyngeal carcinoma: correlation of patterns of spread with middle ear effusion. (in press)
14. Ho, J.H.C. 1970. The natural history and treatment of nasopharyngeal carcinoma (NPC). In: *Proceedings of the 10th International Cancer Congress,* Vol. 4, *Oncology,* eds. Lee-Clark R., Cumley, R.W., McCay, J.E., Copeland, M. Chicago: Year Book Medical Publishers, 1–14.
15. Leung, S.F. 1991. Institutional data, Prince of Wales Hospital.
16. Wara, W.M., Phillips, T.L., Sheline, H.E., Schwayde, J.G. 1975. Radiation tolerance of the spinal cord. *Cancer*; 35:1558–1562.
17. Evans, R.A., Liu, K.C., Azhar, T., Symonds, R.P. 1988. Assessment of permanent hearing impairment following radical megavoltage radiotherapy. *J. Laryngol. Otol.*; 102:588–589.
18. Moretti, J.A. 1976. Sensorineural hearing loss following radiotherapy to the nasopharynx. *Laryngoscope*; 86:598–602.
19. Schuknecht, H., Karmodey, C.S. 1966. Radionecrosis of the temporal bone. *Laryngoscope*; 76:1416–1428.
20. Lederman, M. 1985. Malignant tumours of the ear. *J. Laryngol. Otol.*; 79:85–119.
21. Ramsden, R.T., Bulman, C.H., Lorigan, B.P. 1975. Osteoradionecrosis of the temporal bone. *J. Laryngol. Otol.*; 89:941–955.
22. Elwany, S. 1985. Delayed ultrastructural radiation induced changes in the human mesotympanic middle ear mucosa. *J. Laryngol. Otol.*; 99:343–353.
23. Mass, W.T. 1959. *Therapeutic Radiology*. St. Louis: C.V. Mosby, 104.
24. Gibb, A.G. 1979. Non-suppurative otitis media. In: *Diseases of the Ear, Nose and Throat*, Vol. 2, 4th edn., ed. Scott-Brown's. London: Butterworths, 217.
25. Gyorkey, J., Pollock, F.J. 1960. Radiation necrosis of ossicles. *Arch. Otolaryngol.*; 20:263–290.
26. Choa, G. 1991 Personal communication.
27. Kelemen, G. 1955 Experimental defects in the ear and the upper airways induced by radiation. *Arch. Otolaryngol.*; 61:405–418.
28. Bohne, B.A., Marks, J.E., Glasgow, G.P. 1985. Delayed effects of ionizing radiation on the ear. *Laryngoscope*; 95:818–828.
29. Ewald, J.R. 1906. Radiation effects on the inner ear. *Die Wirkung des Radiums und das Labyrint. Zentralblatt fur Physiologie*; 19:297–298.
30. Winther, F.O. 1969. X-ray irradiation of the inner ear of the guinea pig. Early degenerative changes in the cochlea. *Acta Otolaryngol.*; 68:98–117.
31. Dale, R.G. 1985. The application of the linear quadratic dose-effect equation to fractioned and protracted radiotherapy. *Brit. J. Radiol.*; 59:515–528.
32. Chowdhury, C.R., Ho J.H.C., Wright, A., Tsao, S.Y., Au, G.K.H., Tung, Y. 1988. Prospective study of the effects of ventilation tubes on hearing after radiotherapy for carcinoma of the nasopharynx. *Ann. Otol. Rhinol. Laryngol.*; 97(1):142–145.

33. Choy, A.T.K., Leung, S.F., Woo, J.K.S., van Hasselt, C.A. Sensorineural hearing loss following radiation therapy for patients with nasopharyngeal carcinoma. (in press).
34. Schuknecht, H.E., Karmody, C.S. 1966. Radionecrosis of the temporal bone. *Laryngoscope*; 76:1416–1428.
35. Dias, A. 1966. Effects on hearing of patients treated with irradiation in the head and neck area. *J. Laryngol. Otol.*; 80:276–287.
36. Wang, C., Doppke, K. 1976. Osteoradionecrosis of the temporal bone — consideration of nominal standard dose. *Am. J. Rad. Oncol. Biol. Phys.*; 1:881–883.
37. Skinner, D.W., van Hasselt, C.A. 1991. A study of complications of grommet insertion for secretory otitis media in the presence of nasopharyngeal carcinoma. *Clin. Otolaryngol.*; 16:480–482.
38. John, D.G., Woo, J.K.S., van Hasselt, C.A., Leung, S.F. 1996. Middle ear effusion in patients with nasopharyngeal carcinoma: occurrence, progression and the effect of radiotherapy. *Abstracts of the 7th Asean ORL — Head and Neck Congress, Kuala Lumpur, Malaysia, December 1996*, 142.
39. van Hasselt, C.A. 1994. Mastoid surgery and the Hong Kong flap. Toynbee Memorial Lecture. *J. Laryngol. Otol.*; 108:825–833.

CHAPTER 18

Disease in Non-endemic Areas

Alan G. Gibb and *Philip W. Allen*

The main endemic areas for nasopharyngeal carcinoma (NPC) are Southern China, Alaska and Greenland. The average incidence in Southern China is approximately 20 cases per 100,000 population per year, rising as high as 50 per 100,000 in some areas, while in Alaskan and Greenland Eskimos, the incidence is from 15 to 20 per 100,000.[1] An intermediate incidence is encountered in Peninsular Malaysia, Borneo, North Africa, Southern Italy, Greece, Turkey and other countries around the Mediterranean basin together with Jamaica, Central Africa and the Philippines.[1] In other parts of the world, the disease is non-endemic in the native populations with an incidence of less than 1 per 100,000 per year.

Since much of the information incorporated elsewhere in this volume is related to a southern Chinese population, highly susceptible to NPC, where the incidence is the highest in the world, a clinician practising in a non-endemic area may doubt the relevance of the information to his own particular situation. We will therefore address this question and outline some of the problems he is liable to encounter.

Problems Influencing Diagnostic Accuracy

Population factors

In a non-endemic area, the likelihood of the clinician encountering a case of NPC is fairly remote, at least as far as the indigenous population is concerned. As a consequence his sense of awareness may be less acute, especially when dealing with younger or middle aged patients in which cancer in general is unusual, yet NPC is not uncommon.

However, there are few places in the present day world where a society remains exclusively indigenous and for this reason the overall incidence of NPC is progressively increasing. This relates particularly to the Cantonese, who integrate easily, being adventurous, hard working and ambitious. Significant population movements have occurred in the USA,[2] Canada[3] and Australia,[4] while many of the world's largest cities have acquired their own "Chinatowns".

Apart from migratory movements, short-term travel for business or recreational purposes may also be responsible for a rise in incidence especially in cities or holiday areas favoured by Asian communities.

Cantonese immigrants retain the propensity to develop nasopharyngeal carcinoma for more than one generation although the susceptibility becomes progressively reduced.[5–8] Accordingly countries affected by migration are already experiencing a rising incidence of NPC and further increases can be expected over the next twenty or thirty years. Interestingly, evidence suggests that populations migrating from non-endemic to endemic locations also exhibit a rise in incidence of NPC. Jeannel and associates[9] found that the incidence of nasopharyngeal carcinoma amongst males of French origin who had lived in North Africa for more than 15 years, or were born there, was 5.7 times higher than in males of French origin born in France.

Clinical expertise

In non-endemic areas, local clinicians- general practitioners or specialists-, may "miss" the primary lesion due to lack of familiarity with the disease. However, even in a non-endemic area, all clinicians should be constantly alert to the importance of examining the nasopharynx in all patients presenting with a "silent" node in the neck. In reports from the United Kingdom and Canada, the nasopharynx proved to be by far the commonest site of the "unknown primary".[10,11] In addition, clinicians should realize that serous otitis media occurring in an adult also mandates careful examination of the nasopharynx.

Specialists practising in non-endemic areas suffer from disadvantages compared to their counterparts in endemic regions as they are less experienced in examining the nasopharynx, and even if they possess a modern endoscope they are likely to be less familiar with the varied appearances and characteristics of the tumour. Furthermore, they may not appreciate the importance of obtaining an adequate and representative sample of tissue by a deep biopsy taken under clear vision.

Investigations

Specialists unfamiliar with NPC may not fully realise the value of organ imaging and may order inappropriate investigations, such as plain X-rays or fail to interpret or appreciate the significance of the findings on imaging by CT or MR.

Pathologists with limited experience of NPC may overlook small clusters of malignant cells or wrongly report the tumour as a squamous cell carcinoma.[12] This may have far reaching implications affecting prognosis and treatment. According to most reports, well differentiated tumours of squamous type, which comprise only 3% of nasopharyngeal cancers in endemic areas, account for a considerably higher percentage of tumours in non-endemic areas.[6,13] Indeed, in one small European series, squamous tumours were actually in the majority.[14]

Relevant serological investigations may or may not be available, even in teaching hospitals, as they are seldom required or requested. However, as these tests depend on the development of antibodies to the Epstein-Barr virus (EBV) in contrast to well differentiated tumours of squamous cell type which are not EBV-related, the value of testing in non-endemic areas, where the incidence of the latter is substantial, could be questioned. The relevance of these tests in the Western world was studied by Pearson *et al.*[15] In a co-operative multi-centre investigation in the USA, specimens of sera were collected from a mixed population with diverse racial and ethnic backgrounds. Most of the patients were Caucasian, but American Chinese, Alaskan Eskimos and American Indians were also included. The sera from patients with tumours reported as undifferentiated carcinomas showed positive antibodies to IgA anti-viral capsid antigen in over 80% of cases, while less than 20% of sera from patients with well-differentiated tumours gave positive results. It was concluded that in the USA serological testing is useful for the detection of poorly differentiated and undifferentiated NPC but has no value in the detection of well differentiated cancers.

The above results lead us to the conclusion that serological investigations have a worthwhile place in sporadic as well as endemic areas in detecting EBV-related undifferentiated NPC, in view of the fact that this is the commonest type of tumour in virtually all areas.[13]

The antibody titres against EBV-specific antigens in NPC in diverse communities throughout the world are summarized in Chapter 9 (*Table 2*). Elevated antibody levels were found in all the countries and groups investigated.

Treatment Deficiencies

The success of treatment , as judged by the recurrence and survival rates, is likely to be affected by the experience and expertise of local physicians and the way they are co-ordinated into an experienced team. In non-endemic areas, even though few NPC tumours are encountered, lack of experience may be counter-balanced in centres of excellence by expertise in dealing with other malignancies. The availability of the best and most appropriate radiotherapy equipment with supporting technologists backed up by experienced radiotherapists, oncologists, surgeons, radiologists and pathologists, maximises the cure rate and minimises complications. Clinicians in non-endemic areas should consult with centres of expertise if they wish their patients to have the best chance of survival. With modern methods, the five year survival for patients with the endemic or EBV-related tumour should be at least 50%, a considerably better figure than for squamous cell carcinoma of the nasopharynx. This latter type of cancer, being less responsive to radiotherapy,[13] normally requires a special treatment regime involving higher radiation dosage: even then, the local recurrence rate is higher than in undifferentiated carcinoma. Furthermore, in the squamous cell variety, metastatic neck nodes may be better treated by surgery than by radiation.

Research Benefits

The changing incidence and occasional unexplained "pockets" of disease in non-endemic areas provide opportunities for research into the aetiology, pathogenesis and possible inherited characteristics of nasopharyngeal carcinoma. For example, the death rate from nasopharyngeal carcinoma observed in the North of China around Xiangyuan and Lucheng Counties, Shanxi Province from 1973 to 1975 approached that in Southern China, but rates in adjacent regions were equal to, or less than, the national average.[16] This epidemiological enigma does not appear to have been investigated or explained and could prove a fruitful field for study.

Concluding Remarks

Although nasopharyngeal carcinoma varies greatly in both its racial and geographical incidences, it varies little in its behaviour or management worldwide. Even in non-endemic areas, poorly- or un-differentiated carcinoma (EBV-related) is by far the commonest nasopharyngeal cancer. Although the clinician in a non-endemic area seldom encounters the tumour, its incidence is increasing in many regions and he must remain ever alert to its unexpected appearance and harness all available facilities in establishing a diagnosis in a suspicious case. If the diagnostic or management team lacks experience or the necessary facilities for expert treatment, referral to, or consultation with, a centre of excellence should be undertaken in the best interests of the patient.

References

1. Fandi, A., Altun, M., Azli, N., Armand, J.P., Cvitkovic, E. 1994. Nasopharyngeal cancer: epidemiology, staging, and treatment. *Semin. Oncol.*; 21:382–389.
2. Burt, R.D., Vaughan, T.L., McKnight, B. 1992. Descriptive epidemiology and survival analysis of nasopharyngeal carcinoma in the United States. *Int. J. Cancer*; 52:549–556.
3. Dickson, R.I., Flores, A.D. 1985. Nasopharyngeal carcinoma: an evaluation of 134 patients treated between 1971–1980. *Laryngoscope*; 95:276–283.
4. Grulich, A.E., McCredie, M., Coates, M. 1995. Cancer incidence in Asian migrants to New South Wales, Australia. *Brit. J. Cancer*; 71:400–408.
5. Zippin, C., Tekawa, I. S., Bragg, K.U., Watson, D., A., Linden, G. 1962. Studies on heredity and environment in cancer of the nasopharynx. *J. Natl. Cancer Inst.*; 29:483–490.
6. Dickson, R.I. 1981. Nasopharyngeal carcinoma: an evaluation of 209 patients. *Laryngoscope*; 91(3):333–354.
7. Parkin, D.M., Iscovich, J. 1997. Risk of cancer in migrants and their descendants in Israel: II. Carcinomas and germ-cell tumours. *Int. J. Cancer*; 70:654–660.
8. King, H., Haenszel, W. 1972. Cancer mortality among foreign and native-born Chinese in the United States. *J. Chron. Dis.*; 26:623–646.
9. Jeannel, D., Ghnassia, M., Hubert, A., Sancho-Garnier, H., Eschwege, F., Crognier, E., de Thé, G. 1993. Increased risk of nasopharyngeal carcinoma among males of French origin born in Maghreb (North Africa). *Int. J. Cancer*; 54:536–539.
10. Shaw, H.J. 1970. Metastatic carcinoma in cervical lymph nodes with occult primary tumour-diagnosis and treatment. *J. Laryngol. Otol.*; 84:249–265.
11. Dickson, R.I., Vargas, D.R. 1979. Occult primary of the Head and Neck. *J. Otolaryngol*, 8(5):427–434.
12. Nageris, B., Elidan, J., Hansen, M.C., Ankhol, O., Veshler, Z. 1994. Nasopharyngeal carcinoma among the population in Jerusalem. *Am. J. Otolaryngol.*; 5:190–192.

13. Applebaum, E.L., Mantravadi, P., Haas, R. 1982. Lymphoepithelioma of the nasopharynx. *Laryngoscope*. 92(5):510–514.
14. Huygen, P.L., Fischer, A.J., van den Broek, P. 1980. Nasopharyngeal cancer: a clinical study with special reference to age and occupation. *Clin. Otolaryngol.*; 5(1):37–47.
15. Pearson, G.R., Weiland, L.H., Neel, H.B., Taylor, W., Earle, J., Mulroney, S.E., Goepfert, H., Lanier, A., Talvot, M.L., Pilch, B., Goodman, M., Huang, A., Levine, H., Hyams, V., Moran, E., Henle, G., Henle, E. 1983. Application of Epstein-Barr Virus (EBV) serology to the diagnosis of North American nasopharyngeal carcinoma. *Cancer*; 51:261–268.
16. Editorial Committee for the Atlas of Cancer Mortality in the People's Republic of China under the auspices of the Ministry of Health and Chinese Academy of Sciences. 1979. *Atlas of Cancer Mortality in the People's Republic of China*. Beijing: China Map Press, 79–86.

CHAPTER 19

Screening

C. Andrew van Hasselt and *Sing Fai Leung*

In areas of high prevalence, the question of cancer screening is justifiably raised. The prime objective is to provide the opportunity for early diagnosis and treatment that offers a real chance of cure with the ultimate aim of lowering the mortality rate of the population at large. Actuarial predictive calculations to determine a financial balance-sheet are theoretically feasible, but there remains the question of costing human suffering and life itself. Unless an absolute detection mechanism exists, or the prevalence of the cancer is so great that crisis management dictates the necessity for screening, the subject will remain controversial.

The complexity of evaluating screening programmes has delayed critical scrutiny in this area which is currently only just beginning. The United Kingdom National Screening Committee (NSC) identified almost three hundred screening programmes in that country, many at the research stage, but nearly one hundred currently in practice.[1] The NSC may have been optimistic in naming only four of these programmes that met their criteria for both quality and evidence of effectiveness. These were breast cancer and cervical cancer screening, and neonatal blood spot screening for phenylketonuria and hypothyroidism.

General Principles of Cancer Screening

The existence of evidence that screening reduces cancer mortality or morbidity from prospective randomised trials is the best justification for a cancer screening programme. However, this level of evidence is not yet available for nasophayngeal carcinoma (NPC). Nonetheless, design of investigational screening should take the following considerations into account:

i) The consequences of the cancer are costly to both the individual and the community.
ii) Detection of preclinical or early cancers offers the chance for effective or curative treatment, with a higher cure rate or reduced morbidity compared to advanced disease.

iii) Effective and safe methods of detection are utilized, cost being an important factor.
iv) The target cancer occurs with high frequency.

When evaluating the evidence for the screening programme, the inclusion of non-attendants in the intervention group and comparison with a control group is desirable as it allows a more complete assessment and accurate quantification of costs and additional benefits of the programme. The control group also reflects any change in prevalence of the disease over time which can otherwise be wrongly ascribed to the cancer screening tests.

Requirements of the Screening Tests

The tests should be easily performed with little inconvenience to the public. Markers readily obtainable from blood, urine, saliva or exfoliated cells can be used.

In choosing the best screening tests the four relevant parameters are the sensitivity, specificity, positive predictive value and negative predictive value. Sensitivity is defined as the percentage of positive tests in proven cancer cases. The positive predictive value is the percentage of proven cancer cases amongst all positively tested subjects.[2] This is an indication of the likelihood that a person labelled as positive by a screening test actually has cancer. A high sensitivity does not necessarily imply a high predictive value. Depending on their specificity, the positive predictive value of current screening tests is generally around 0.5%.[3] Ruling out cancer in more than 99.5% of those patients labelled as positive by the screening test is extremely costly, not to mention the psychological effect on the normal subjects. Identification of a high risk group is appropriate as this alone would increase the disease prevalence within the group and positive predictive value of the tests.

Consideration can be given to utilizing several screening tests in combination or in sequence[3] (see Chapter 9). In this event predictive values would rise, albeit at the expense of the combined battery of tests.

The Case for Nasopharyngeal Cancer

The high incidence of NPC in endemic areas is undisputed. In these locations the disease occurs in a significantly younger age group than other comparable malignancies.[4] Detection occurs at a relatively advanced stage of the disease in the vast majority of individuals,[5] despite wide public awareness of the prevalence of the tumour. Since early-stage disease has a better prognosis and allows the use of treatment techniques that afford a greater degree of sparing of unaffected tissues than advanced disease,[6–8] screening for this cancer is an attractive proposition. The identification of non-invasive dysplastic changes and carcinoma in situ in the nasopharynx[9–12] further indicates that there is a period of time during which the susceptible individual may be identified before the disease becomes frankly invasive.

Selection of a high risk population can be achieved by focusing on the peak incidence age group, the sex in which the tumour predominates and blood relatives of NPC patients. As the genetic pattern of this disease unfolds and typing becomes inexpensive and practical to implement, individuals detected with a genetic susceptibility to NPC (see Chapter 3) could then be closely monitored.

Methods

The most widely applied tests for NPC screening have been the EBV-related serum markers. Exfoliative cytological studies of the nasopharynx have the ability to identify tumour cells,[13–15] however the specific requirements for the collection of cells would limit this application in a mass screening programme. The detection of subclinical disease is also reported to be possible by endoscopic examination in individuals identified by positive blood tests.[16]

The EBV-related Tumour Markers

The IgA sub-class antibodies to the EBV Viral Capsid Antigen (VCA) and Early Antigen (EA) have been widely studied and used in an attempt to detect NPC. Furthermore, these antibodies are known to be present for at least one year prior to the development of clinically detectable disease.[17] The most impressive results for any reported test show that sensitivities and specificities of 95% and 97% respectively can be achieved.[3,18–22] Positive predictive values in unselected population groups are low at about 0.5% for the most specific of these tests. However, due to their labour intensive technique of assay and the fact that their subjective interpretation has delivered variable results, immunofluorescence tests for IgA anti-VCA and anti-EA have in general been difficult to apply for mass screening. Enzyme-linked immune assays (ELISA) currently under refinement and evaluation would simplify the procedure and reduce costs. These tests are likely to be of comparable efficiency to current techniques[18–19] and therefore offer promising prospects for mass screening.

There are also encouraging reports that EBV-coded proteins in recombinant expression systems with western blot analysis have a useful diagnostic capacity.[23] EBV-coded thymidine kinase and DNase potentially achieve sensitivities of 95% even for early stage disease[23–25] and promise to be useful antigens to act as markers for NPC. ELISA assays based on these proteins will make rapid and cost effective diagnostic tests feasible.

The foremost weakness of existing tests is the lack of sensitivity in detecting early disease. When quoting the efficiency of various tests in an attempt to justify screening, it must be remembered that, with few exceptions,[19,24] the results are almost exclusively based on hospital populations. These results may therefore be biased by a predominance of advanced tumours and do not necessarily represent a true reflection of the efficacy for early disease detection in the general population. It is vital to target and identify patients with early disease as it is this group that screening programmes aim to draw from the population at large. Under these circumstances performance is of prime importance in aiming to select tests to implement general population screening.

A pilot screening programme using the immunofluorescence tests for IgA anti-VCA titres testing 1330 first degree relatives of patients with NPC identified four patients all with early stage disease without regional nodal metastases.[26] One patient had a borderline IgA anti-VCA titre (1/5). The sensitivity of this test , taking a titre level of >1/5 as abnormal, was 75% but the positive predictive value at this low cut off level was only 0.4%.

A precedent for large scale screening has been set by Zeng *et al.*,[17] who were able to detect a greater proportion of early disease using the IgA anti-VCA test than surfaced spontaneously in a comparable unscreened group. Furthermore, detection of early and even subclinical disease has been achieved by Sham *et al.* by detailed examination of a "high risk" group identified by "positive" serological tests.[16]

Strategy for Mass Screening

To be cost effective, screening for NPC should be restricted to selected population groups. The incidence of NPC predominates in males by 3:1 and starts to peak at 40 years of age.[5] Based on the aggregation of familial cases[27,28] and the occurrence of NPC among twins,[29,30] the increased risk in families is well recognized. However, as the population of NPC patients with a positive family history is small, screening of family members alone will not make any impact on the population mortality rate.

The strategy, therefore, to initiate mass screening would be to subject a selected high risk group of the population to the most effective and practical test available. The formulation of the group is arbitrary, but the inclusion of all relatives and males within a ten year period and females within a five year range, on either side of the peak age incidence, would be logical. All individuals with "positive" tests would then be referred to specialists and subjected to detailed endoscopic examination of the nasopharynx and biopsy of any suspicious area.

A simultaneous Health Education programme would be vital in order to ensure that screening methods presently available were both implemented and received in a responsible way. An understanding public is of paramount importance in working towards a successful programme.

Almost all available tests will be positive in some patients with disease other than NPC. (This may, of course, be viewed as a bonus.) The benefits of using screening tests to identify a relatively broad "at risk" population group are offset by the potential psychological disturbance in a great number of normal subjects by causing them to be aware of the increased risk that they carry. This raises ethical issues for clinicians. When a health intervention is initiated by clinicians rather than the patient, the clinician is under greater obligation to ensure that the benefits outweigh the harm.[31]

With currently available tests, individuals who are clearly at risk of developing NPC, even though they may not do so, can be identified and closely followed. This group of people may provide further information, lacking at present, as to how the disease progresses through the early pre-invasive phase before spread of the tumour occurs. Only through a screening programme can sufficient information concerning the early changes be unearthed to enhance our understanding of the natural history of NPC.

Given that the detection of NPC most often occurs at an advanced stage, it is entirely feasible that the implementation of effective screening could result in earlier diagnosis and treatment of this disease with consequent reduction in morbidity and mortality rates.

Concluding Remarks

Screening programmes should be subjected to quality assurance measures, their success being judged by the number of early stage cancers detected and reduction in morbidity and mortality rates when viewed in the setting of high quality randomised controlled trials. The attempt to initiate screening programmes for NPC should thus be addressed in a responsible way with due attention to costs. The high incidence in certain population groups and potential rewards from early diagnosis provide strong motivation for effective programmes. Current work towards the development of less expensive, more sensitive and specific tests and the improvement in diagnostic techniques offer an encouraging outlook for NPC screening in the future. Identification of the best possible tumour marker by the most efficient cost effective method remains the ultimate challenge.

References

1. National Screening Committee. *Annual Report*. Milton Keynes: National Screening Committee, 1998.
2. Chamberlain, J. 1982. Screening for early detection of cancer: general principles. In: *The Prevention of Cancer*, ed. Alderson, M. London: Edward Arnold, 227–258.
3. Chan, S.H. 1989. Screening for NPC. *Ann. Acad. Med. Singapore*; 18:80–82.
4. Sham, J.S.T., Poon, Y.F., Wei, W.I., Choy, D. 1980. Nasopharyngeal carcinoma in young patients. *Cancer*; 65:2606–2610.
5. Skinner, D.W., van Hasselt, C.A., Tsao, S.Y. 1991. Nasopharyngeal carcinoma: a study of the modes of presentation. *Ann. Otol. Rhinol. Laryngol.*; 100:544–551.
6. Tsao, S.Y., Shiu, W.C.T. 1990. Radiotherapy and chemotherapy for nasopharyngeal carcinoma. *Ear Nose Throat J.*; 69:272–278.
7. Tsao, S.Y., Chua, E.T. 1991. Current problems in radiotherapy chemotherapy and staging of nasopharyngeal carcinoma (NPC). *Ann. Acad. Med. Singapore*; 20(5):649–655.
8. Sham, J., Choy, D., Kwong, P.W., Cheng, A.C., Kwong, D.L., Yua, C.C., Wan, K.Y., Au, G.K. 1994. Radiotherapy for nasopharyngeal carcinoma:shielding the pituitary may improve therapeutic ratio. *Int. J. Radiat. Oncol. Biol. Phys.*; 29(4):699–704.
9. Liang, P.C., Chen, C.C., Chu, C.C., Hu, Y.F., Chu, H.M., Tsung, Y.S. 1962. The histologic classification, biological characteristics and histogenesis of nasopharyngeal carcinomas. *Chin. Med. J.*; 81:629–658.

10. Zong, Y.S., Li, Q.X. 1986. Histopathology of paracancerous nasopharyngeal carcinoma in situ. *Chin. Med. J.*; 99:763–771.
11. Lee, J.C.K., Suen, M.W.M. 1986. Intraepithelial neoplasia in mucosa of human nasopharyngeal carcinoma. In: *Abstracts of the XVI International Congress of the International Academy of Pathology, Vienna.*
12. Cheung, F., Pang, S.W., Hioe, F., Cheung, K.N., Lee, A., Yau, T.K. 1998. Nasopharyngeal carcinoma in situ: two cases of an emerging diagnostic entity. *Cancer*; 83(6):1069–1073.
13. Dong, H., Shen, S., Huang, S., *et al.* 1983. The cytologic diagnosis of nasopharyngeal carcinoma from exfoliated cells collected by suction method. *J. Laryngol. Otol.*; 97:727–734.
14. Chan, M.K.M., Huang, D.P. 1990. The value of cytologic examination for nasopharyngeal carcinoma. *Ear Nose Throat J.*; 69:268–271.
15. Lau, S.K., Hsu, C.S., Sham, J.S., Wei, W.I. 1991. The cytological diagnosis of nasopharyngeal carcinoma using a silk swab stick. *Cytopathology*; 2(5):239–246.
16. Sham, J.S.T., Wei, W.I., Zong, Y.S., Choy, D., Guo, Y.Q., Tan, L., Lin, Z.X., Ng, M.H. 1990. Detection of subclinical nasopharyngeal carcinoma by fibreoptic endoscopy and multiple biopsy. *Lancet*; 335:371–374.
17. Zeng, Y., Zhong, J.M., Li, L.Y., *et al.* 1983. Follow-up studies on Epstein-Barr Virus IgA/VCA antibody-positive persons in Zangwu County, China. *Intervirology*; 20:190–194.
18. Ho, J.H.C., Lau, W.H., Kwan, H.C., Chan, C.L., Au, G.K.H., Saw, D. 1981. *Immunology and Diagnosis of Nasopharyngeal Carcinoma*. Excerpta Med. Int. Congr. Ser., No. 571.
19. Zeng, Y., Zhang, L.G., Li, H.Y., *et al.* 1982. Serological mass survey for early detection of nasopharyngeal carcinoma in Wuzhou City, China. *Int. J. Cancer*; 29:139–141.
20. Hsu, M.M., Chen, J.Y., Liy, M.Y., Lynn, T.C., Tu, S.M., Yang, C.S. 1984. Antibody to Epstein-Barr Virus specific DNase in sera of nasopharyngeal carcinoma and other nine most common cancer patients in Taiwan. *Chung Hua Min Kuo Wei Sheng Wu Chi Mien I Hsueh Tsa Chih*; 17(3):131–137.
21. Chow, K.C., Ma, J., Lin, L.S., Chi, K.H., Yen, S.H., Liu, S.M., Liu, W.T., Chen, W.K., Chang, T.H., Chen, K.Y. 1997. Serum responses to the combination of Epstein-Barr Virus antigens from both latent and acute phases in nasopharyngeal carcinoma: complementary test of EBNA-1 with EA-D. *Cancer Epidemiol. Biomarkers Prev.*; 6(5):363–368.
22. Liu, M.Y., Chang, Y.L., Ma, J., Yang, H.L., Hsu, M.M., Chen, C.J., Chen, J.Y., Yang, C.S. 1997. Evaluation of multiple antibodies to Epstein-Barr Virus as markers for detecting patients with nasopharyngeal carcinoma. *J. Med. Virol.*; 52(3):262–269.
23. Littler, E., Baylis, S.A., Zeng, Y., Conway, M.J., Mackett, M., John, R.A. 1991. Diagnosis of nasopharyngeal carcinoma by means of recombinant Epstein-Barr Virus proteins. *Lancet*; 337:685–689.
24. Chen, J.Y., Chen, C.U., Liu, M.Y., *et al.* 1989. Antibody to Epstein-Barr Virus-specific DNase as a marker for field survey of patients with nasopharyngeal carcinoma in Taiwan. *J. Med. Virol.*; 27:269–272.
25. Chen, H.F., Huang, D. 1989. An approach to the method for detecting the titers of antibody against Epstein-Barr Virus-specific DNase in sera from patients with nasopharyngeal carcinoma. *Chin. Biochem. J.*; 5:131–135. (in Chinese)
26. Prince of Wales Hospital data.
27. Williams, E.H., de Thé, G. 1974. Familial aggregation in nasopharyngeal carcinoma. *Lancet*; 2:295.
28. Chan, S.H., Day, N.E., Kunaratnam, N., Chia, K.B., Simons, M.J. 1983. HLA and nasopharyngeal carcinoma in Chinese — a further study. *Int. J. Cancer*; 32:171–176.
29. Nevo, S., Meyer, W., Altman, M. 1971. Carcinoma of nasopharynx in Twins. *Cancer*; 28:807–809.
30. Ho, J.H.C. 1975. Epidemiology of nasopharyngeal carcinoma. *J. R. Coll. Surg. Edinb.*; 20:223–235.
31. Sackett, D., Holland, W.W. 1975. Controversy in the detection of disease. *Lancet*; ii:357.

Cited Authors Index

Subject Index